# CYSTIC FIBROSIS: HORIZONS

# 9th INTERNATIONAL CYSTIC FIBROSIS CONGRESS

## MEDICAL/SCIENTIFIC PROGRAMME COMMITTEE

*Chairman*   David Lawson
*Members*    John Dodge
             Duncan Geddes
             Robert Johnson
             Robert D. McCreery
             Edward Tempany
             Robert Williamson

## ALLIED HEALTH PROFESSIONALS PROGRAMME ADVISERS

John Dodge
Diana Gaskell
Elizabeth Martin
Maureen Maxwell
Margaret Mearns
Ann Murdoch
Philip Pinkerton
Barbara Webber

## CONGRESS CO-ORDINATOR

Ron Tucker

## SECRETARIAT

Sandra Kennedy
Lilian Uden

# CYSTIC FIBROSIS: HORIZONS

PROCEEDINGS OF THE
9th INTERNATIONAL CYSTIC
FIBROSIS CONGRESS
BRIGHTON, ENGLAND.
JUNE 9th–15th 1984

edited by
**DAVID LAWSON, MD, FRCP**

Hosted on behalf of the
International Cystic Fibrosis (Mucoviscidosis)
Association
*by*
Cystic Fibrosis Research Trust
Alexandra House, 5 Blyth Road,
Bromley, Kent, England BR1 3RS

*A Wiley Medical Publication*

JOHN WILEY & SONS
*Chichester · New York · Brisbane · Toronto · Singapore*

*Library of Congress Cataloging in Publication Data:*

International Cystic Fibrosis Congress (9th : 1984 :
   Brighton, East Sussex)
   Cystic fibrosis.

   (A Wiley Medical publication)
   1. Cystic fibrosis: Horizons—Congresses. I. Lawson, David
(David Neale) II. Title. III. Series. [DNLM: 1. Cystic
fibrosis—Diagnosis—Congresses. 2. Cystic fibrosis—
Therapy—Congresses. W3 IN6866 9th 1984c / WI 820 I62
1984c]
RJ456.C9157   1984        616.3'7        84-5072
ISBN 0 471 90439 2

*British Library Cataloguing in Publication Data:*

International Cystic Fibrosis Congress
   *(1984 : Brighton)*
   Cystic fibrosis: Horizons.—(A Wiley medical
   publication)
   I. Title   II. Lawson, David
   616.3'7      RC858.C95

   ISBN 0 471 90439 2

# Preface

The Cystic Fibrosis Research Trust, London, are delighted, fifteen years after the 5th Congress held in Cambridge in 1969, once more to host an International CF Congress under the auspices of the I.C.F.(M.)A.

The morning sessions are devoted to well defined topics, chosen as the main growing points in research and patient care.

Invited speakers review the state of the art in each morning session, and submitted papers and discussion are related to this topic.

For all other topics, presentations are in poster form. The posters are on display throughout the Congress and ample time is allowed for discussion on site.

The afternoon sessions are somewhat experimental, and constitute an attempt to bring all posters into discussion in a series of plenary and sub-plenary sessions.

This volume contains the invited speakers' contributions in extenso, and each of these constitutes an authoritative presentation of the current state of knowledge in each field. All other contributions, whether oral or poster presentations, are here represented by abstracts.

# Contents

xii

# PRENATAL SCREENING AND HETEROZYGOTE DETECTION

David J.H. Brock

Human Genetics Unit, University of Edinburgh, Edinburgh, UK

## INTRODUCTION

Heterozygote detection and prenatal diagnosis of genetic disorders are traditionally based on the measurement of the product of a mutant gene. Despite over 40 years of intense investigation little is known about the molecular pathology of cystic fibrosis (CF). The chromosomal location of the gene is unknown, no genetic markers have been accepted as being closely linked to the CF locus, and there is profound disagreement on even the major areas of protein metabolism involved. In such a situation approaches to both heterozygote detection and prenatal diagnosis must be essentially pragmatic, and concentrate on analysis of enzymatic and protein systems where experimental findings or theoretical considerations suggest correlation with the CF gene. There is always a chance that such a shot-gun approach may yield results of clinical value, and furthermore that it may assist the process of unravelling the tangled web of metabolic systems in which lurks the expressed protein product of the mutant gene.

## HETEROZYGOTE DETECTION

The goals of heterozygote detection may be related either to a family or a population situation. In the former case the objective is to confirm or exclude heterozygosity in occasional individuals where carrying a single dose of the CF gene might prove disadvantageous. Examples are the siblings of affected individuals, men or women who wish to produce offspring from partners who have already borne affected children, or partners of affected women (and occasionally men) who are themselves CF homozygotes. In these situations the infrequency of carrier testing means that assay systems can be complex and technically laborious, and might even involve fibroblasts cultured from skin explants of the putative heterozygote. But, if on the other hand, heterozygote detection is to be linked to prenatal screening and used to segregate out from a large population all those

1

couples where both partners are heterozygotes, the test must be both technically simple and performable on a readily accessible tissue source. In effect this means rapid and automatable assay on serum, saliva, or urine samples.

A number of systems for heterozygote detection employing cultured skin fibroblasts have been reported in recent years. Breslow et al (1978) demonstrated that cells from obligate heterozygotes had survival times in the presence of low concentrations of dexamethasone which were intermediate between those of CF homozygotes and normal controls. However, at all concentrations of dexamethasone there was some degree of overlap between carriers and normals. Subsequently Breslow et al (1981) showed that if sodium transport into fibroblasts in the presence of ouabain was also measured, heterozygotes could now be distinguished from normal controls, although overlapping substantially with the values obtained with CF homozygotes. In principle the application of both tests simultaneously to cultured fibroblasts should be able to distinguish all three genotypes, and could thus form the basis for a carrier detection system.

Another test employing cultured fibroblasts was proposed by Shapiro et al (1979). They observed that when mitochondrial NADH dehydrogenase was measured, the pH profile of activity provided a substantial clue to the genotype. Amongst CF patients highest activity was found at pH 8.6, amongst heterozygotes the optimal activity was at pH 8.3, whilst amongst normal controls the maximal values were obtained at pH 8.0. Shapiro et al (1982) suggested that these observations were systematic and might form the basis of a heterozygote test, particularly since the Michaelis constant of the enzyme for NADH was different for the three genotypes. However, others have not been able to confirm these results (Sanguinetti-Briceno and Brock, 1982). The system does not seem to be transposable to the more accessible white blood cell or cultured lymphocyte systems.

A more practical carrier detection system, and one applicable to large populations, has been reported by Hosli and Vogt (1979). They produced data showing that gentle heat inactivation of plasma $\alpha$-mannosidase and acid phosphatase allows differentiation of normals from both CF heterozygotes and patients. The two enzymes retained nearly full activity (80-100 per cent) in normals, approximately half activity (40-60 per cent) in heterozygotes and lost virtually all activity in CF homozygotes (0-10 per cent). There was no overlap between the groups. However, a number of other workers

have been completely unable to reproduce these results
(Patrick and Ellis, 1979; Hultberg et al, 1981).  The
system does not appear to work outside the confines of
the Pasteur Institute.  Hosli and his colleagues
speculated on the reasons for this lack of
reproducibility (Ceder et al, 1983) and recently
Katznelson et al (1983) have reported on a "blind" trial
in which 45 plasma samples taken in Israel were all
correctly genotyped in the Pasteur Institute.  These
most intriguing results, coupled to the extreme
technical simplicity of the test, means that plasma
enzyme thermolability cannot yet be discounted.

One of the more durable biochemical systems purporting
to track the CF gene is that using high-resolution
polyacrylamide gel isoelectric focusing of serum
samples.  Wilson et al (1975) described a unique
protein doublet at a pI of 8.4 when carefully collected
serum samples were exposed to precisely controlled
isoelectric focusing in the presence of urea.   The
doublet, designated "cystic fibrosis protein" (CFP),
was demonstrated in both CF patients and heterozygotes
(Wilson et al, 1978).  Though this system has been
surrounded by considerable controversy, the presence of
CFP has been confirmed in a majority of serum samples
from CF heterozygotes and homozygotes as well as in a
small number of controls.   Wilson et al (1978) have
proposed isoelectric focusing as a general screening
method;  their argument is that since CF homozygotes
will be diagnosed clinically and by sweat test, other
individuals showing the CFP doublet can be labelled as
heterozygotes.  However, the diagnosis of CF is a matter
of considerable imprecision, so that the unambiguous
presence of CFP is not necessarily a test of
heterozygosity.  Furthermore, it is extremely difficult
to maintain high resolution isoelectric focusing over an
extended period of time, while a blind trial of the
method has produced unconvincing results (Brock et al,
1982).

In an attempt to obviate some of these difficulties,
Manson and Brock (1980) have used isoelectric focusing
as the first step in the production of a specific
antiserum against CFP.  Portions of acrylamide gel
corresponding to a pI of 8.2 to 8.5 were excised,
homogenised and injected into guinea pigs.  Absorption
of the resulting crude antiserum with serum samples
taken from individuals in whom CFP was definitely
absent resulted in an antiserum with apparent
monospecificity.  Tests of the antiserum by rocket
electrophoresis showed precipitin arcs which were
substantially greater in serum samples from CF
homozygotes than from CF heterozygotes, and which were
essentially absent in controls.  Quantitative

immunoprecipitation and immunoradiometric assays
(Figure 1) of serum samples from a panel of 14 CF
homozygotes, 29 heterozygotes and 23 controls allowed
correct assignments of genotype to be made on 94 per
cent of occasions (Bullock et al, 1982). Unfortunately
the technical problems involved in producing adequate
amounts of antiserum have yet to be resolved, so that
the suitability of this procedure for heterozygote
testing on a wide scale cannot be assessed. However,
the availability of a polyclonal guinea pig antiserum
makes the isolation of the antigen technically feasible,
and also provides the basis for a screening system for
the preparation of monoclonal antibodies from hybridoma
cells. Whether the antibody-defined CF-associated
antigen is the same as CFP remains to be established.

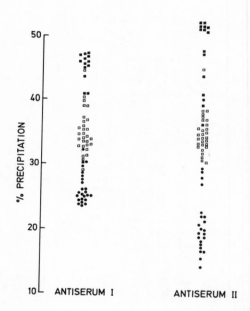

Fig. 1  Immunoradiometric assay of CFP with
percentage precipitation proportional to
antigen titre. Cystic fibrosis homozygote (■),
heterozygote (□) and normal (●) sera. The two
different antisera were obtained with an
interval of more than a year. Adapted from
Bullock et al (1982).

## PRENATAL DIAGNOSIS

Some years ago Nadler and his colleagues reported that
titration of trypsin-like activity in amniotic fluid
supernatant against the artificial substrate
4-methylumbelliferylguanidinobenzoate (MUGB) led to
significantly depressed values with CF homozygotes
(Nadler and Walsh, 1980). In both retrospective and
prospective studies affected fetuses had values more
than two standard deviations below the mean for normals,
and furthermore discrimination could be improved by
examination of the MUGB protease isoenzyme patterns
after isoelectric focusing. However, other laboratories
were unable to repeat these findings (Brock and
Hayward, 1983). In a recent review of experience in
prospective diagnoses, Nadler (1982) conceded that the
MUGB protease system led to an unacceptable level of
both false positives and false negatives. There now
appears to be a strong suspicion that such titration is
merely measuring the esterolytic component of albumin
and other plasma proteins (Schwartz, 1982).

It is known that CF is a disorder associated with
abnormal fluid and solute transfer across exocrine-
gland epithelial cells. Many of the organ systems
thought to be affected (e.g. sweat glands, pancreas,
bronchi) have their epithelial cell surfaces
specialised in the form of microvilli. There has been
a report that the number of microvilli on bile canali-
cular epithelium is reduced in CF (Dominick et al,
1976). Since amniotic fluid cells have a high content
of epithelioid-like cells prior to culture, it seemed
appropriate to investigate the prenatal diagnosis of CF
by measurement of amniotic fluid microvillar membrane
enzymes.

The most important enzymes of the microvillar membrane
are peptidases, glycosidases and phosphatases. In an
early study (Carbarns et al, 1983) it was noted that the
activities of two peptidases, $\gamma$-glutamyltranspeptidase
(GGTP) and aminopeptidase M (APM) were depressed in
amniotic fluid supernatant when the fetus had CF. This
finding was rapidly confirmed (Baker and Dann, 1983),
and the system extended to microvillar disaccharidases,
such as sucrase, lactase, maltase and trehalase (Van
Diggelen et al, 1983). For each of these enzymes
considerably depressed amniotic fluid values were found
in association with a CF fetus.

Brock et al (1983a,b) have now investigated the
potential of GGTP and APM assay more thoroughly. They
observed that activities in control amniotic fluids
declined with advancing gestation, and were not
normally distributed. Thus percentiles were needed to

define action lines.  The most impressive results were
obtained with GGTP assay.  At the 5th percentile of the
normal range the sensitivity of a positive test (low
GGTP value) was 78 per cent (7/9)while at the 10th
percentile it was 100 per cent (Figure 2).

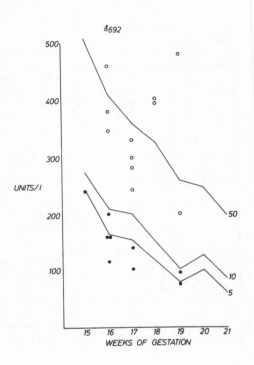

Fig. 2  Amniotic fluid GGTP activities with
percentile lines for 780 control fluids.  Fetus
with 1 in 4 risk of CF but normal outcome (O);
fetus with 1 in 4 risk of CF but affected
outcome (●).

Since the control range of amniotic fluid GGTP
activities had been constructed from 780 amniotic
fluids, it was possible to define the predictability of
a positive test indicating a CF fetus.  If prenatal
diagnosis were restricted to women with a 1 in 4 chance
of bearing an affected child, a positive result (GGTP
below the 5th percentile) gave a predictability of 5 : 1.

Further exploration of the potential of amniotic fluid
microvillar enzymes has focused on alkaline

phosphatase (ALP).  The alkaline phosphatases are a group of similar enzymes coded for by at least three distinct genetic loci (Mulivor et al, 1978).The placental isoenzyme is characterised by its heat stability and susceptibility to inhibition by phenylalanine.  Intestinal ALP is also inhibited by phenylalanine but may be differentiated by its heat lability.  A third genetic locus governs the universal isoenzyme (also called liver/bone/kidney), which is heat-labile, resistant to phenylalanine but markedly inhibited by homoarginine.  A combination of heat treatment and aminoacid inhibition can effectively separate these three major isoenzymes (Mulivor et al, 1978).

The activity of total amniotic fluid ALP shows a maximum at 18 weeks gestation, with a sharp decline on either side.  The proportions of phenylalanine-inhibitable and homoarginine-inhibitable activity remain very constant in second-trimester amniotic fluids.  About 50 per cent of total activity is retained in the presence of 2.5 mM phenylalanine and about 80 per cent with 10 mM homoarginine (Brock, 1983). According to the formula devised by Mulivor et al (1979), this means that about three-quarters of the total ALP activity is intestinal type and about one-quarter universal type.

When 21 amniotic fluids with a 1 in 4 risk of CF were tested in the system, they divided (with one exception) into two groups (Figure 3).  In samples where the outcome was an infant with CF there was residual ALP in the presence of phenylalanine of more than 80 per cent and in the presence of homoarginine of less than 65 per cent.  Samples where the outcome was a normal infant grouped around the mean for control fluids.  A single exception was an amniotic fluid from an affected pregnancy which had given misleading results in both GGTP  (Brock et al, 1983b) and disaccharidase (Van Diggelen et al, 1983) assays.  Figure 3 also shows the mean $\pm$  three standard deviations for 831 control fluids.  There were 17 with more than 80 per cent residual activity in the presence of phenylalanine and 41 with less than 65 per cent activity in the presence of homoarginine.  However, only 9 of 831 (1.1 per cent) control samples compared to 9 of 10 CF samples and 0 of 16 normal at-risk samples, had simultaneously more than 80 per cent residual activity in the presence of phenylalanine and less than 65 per cent activity in the presence of homoarginine.  This suggests a sensitivity for ALP isoenzyme assay of 90 per cent and a predictability for high-risk pregnancies of 28 : 1.

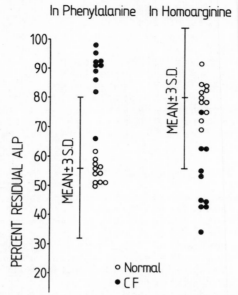

Fig. 3   Residual ALP activity in presence of
phenylalanine or homoarginine.   Solid bars
represent mean ±3standard deviations for 831
control fluids.   Symbols as in Fig. 2.

These results suggest that there is a profound deficiency of intestinal ALP in amniotic fluids when the
fetus has CF.   A more direct test of this hypothesis
has been made possible by the availability of a
monoclonal antibody with unique specificity for the
intestinal isoenzyme (Arklie et al, 1981).   Use of the
monoclonal in a coated-plate sandwich-type immunoassay
generated the results shown in Figure 4.     Results
correlated closely with those obtained by direct
enzymatic analysis of phenylalanine-inhibitable ALP.
The most plausible explanation for the low values of
intestinal ALP, as well as for GGTP, APM and
disaccharidases, is that in the CF fetus there is
impaired passage of the meconium from the gastrointestinal tract into the amniotic fluid.   This
assumption is supported by the finding of an extremely
sticky and viscid meconium in two fetuses aborted in
the second-trimester because of a presumptive diagnosis
of CF.

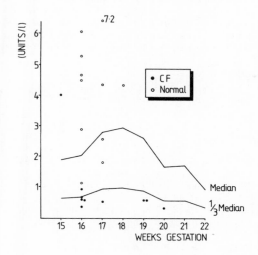

Fig. 4   Immunoassay of intestinal ALP using a
monoclonal antibody.   Solid lines represent
median and one third median of 124 control
fluids.   Symbols as in Fig. 2.

CONCLUSIONS

It will be apparent from this review that prospects for
reliable heterozygote detection in CF remain frustrat-
ingly elusive.   Because of the imprecision in clinical
diagnosis of the disorder itself, any proposed system
must be capable of distinguishing heterozygotes not only
from normals but also from affected homozygotes.   To be
really useful carrier detection should be applicable to
easily available tissues and also be technically simple.
Two systems which show signs of satisfying these
criteria are the thermolability of plasma hydrolases and
the immunoassay  of cystic fibrosis antigen.   Both have
yet to prove their reliability and reproducibility.

On the other hand there does now appear to be a real
prospect of making effective prenatal diagnoses of CF.
The assay of microvillar membrane enzymes in amniotic
fluid supernatant has shown promising results and been
reproduced in a number of different laboratories. For
the first time it has been possible to define the
sensitivity and predictability of diagnosis, and to
show figures that might prove acceptable to the mother
who has already borne an affected child. A prospective
trial currently in progress should shortly allow a
definitive assessment of the validity of this system.

## ACKNOWLEDGEMENTS

I thank the Cystic Fibrosis Research Trust for generous
financial support.

## REFERENCES

Arklie, J., Trowsdale, J., and Bodmer, W.F., 1981. A
    monoclonal antibody to intestinal alkaline
    phosphatase made against D98/AH-2 (HeLa) cells.
    Tissue Antigens, 17, 303-312.
Baker, S., and Dann, L.G., 1983. Peptidases in
    amniotic fluid: low values in cystic fibrosis.
    Lancet, 1, 716-717.
Breslow, J.L., Epstein, J., Fontaine, J.H., and Forbes,
    G.B., 1978. Enhanced dexamethasone resistance in
    cystic fibrosis cells: potential use for
    heterozygote detection and prenatal diagnosis.
    Science, 201, 180-182.
Breslow, J.L., McPherson, J., and Epstein, J., 1981.
    Distinguishing homozygous and heterozygous cystic
    fibrosis fibroblasts from normal cells by
    differences in sodium transport. New England Journal
    Medicine, 304, 1-5.
Brock, D.J.H., 1983. Amniotic fluid alkaline
    phosphatase isoenzymes in early prenatal diagnosis of
    cystic fibrosis. Lancet, 2, 941-943.
Brock, D.J.H., and Hayward, C., 1983. Prenatal
    diagnosis of cystic fibrosis by methylumbelliferyl-
    guanidinobenzoate protease titration in amniotic
    fluid. Prenatal Diagnosis, 3, 1-5.
Brock, D.J.H., Hayward, C., and Super, M., 1982.
    Controlled trial of serum isoelectric focusing in
    the detection of the cystic fibrosis gene. Human
    Genetics, 60, 30-31.
Brock, D.J.H., Hayward, C., and Gosden, C., 1983a.
    Amniotic fluid GGTP in prenatal diagnosis of cystic
    fibrosis: a word of warning. Lancet, 1, 1099.
Brock, D.J.H., Bedgood, D., and Hayward, C., 1983b.
    Prenatal diagnosis of cystic fibrosis by assay of
    amniotic fluid microvillar enzymes. Human Genetics,
    In press.

Bullock, S., Hayward, C., Manson, J., Brock, D.J.H., and
    Raeburn, J.A., 1982. Quantitative immunoassays for
    diagnosis and carrier detection in cystic fibrosis.
    Clinical Genetics, 21, 336-341.
Carbarns, J.B., Gosden, C., and Brock, D.J.H., 1983.
    Microvillar peptidase activity in amniotic fluid:
    possible use in the prenatal diagnosis of cystic
    fibrosis. Lancet, 1, 329-331.
Ceder, O., Hosli, P., Vogt, E., and Kollberg, H., 1983.
    Diagnosis of cystic fibrosis homozygotes and
    heterozygotes from plasma and fibroblast cultures.
    A three generation family study. Clinical Genetics,
    23, 298-303.
Dominick, H.C., Bassewitz, D.B., and Avens, P., 1976.
    Ultrastructure of the liver in cystic fibrosis. In:
    Proceedings of the Seventh International Cystic
    Fibrosis Congress, Paris, pp. 474-477.
Hosli, P., and Vogt, E., 1979. Detection of cystic
    fibrosis homozygotes and heterozygotes with plasma.
    Lancet, 2, 543-545.
Hultberg, B., Ceder, O., and Kollberg, H., 1981. Acid
    hydrolases in sera and plasma from patients with
    cystic fibrosis. Clinica Chimica Acta, 112, 167-
    175.
Katznelson, D., Blau, H., and Sack, J., 1983. Detection
    of cystic fibrosis genotypes. Lancet, 2, 622.
Manson, J.C., and Brock, D.J.H., 1980. Development of
    a quantitative immunoassay for the cystic fibrosis
    gene. Lancet, 1, 330-331.
Mulivor, R.A., Plotkin, L.I., and Harris, H., 1978.
    Differential inhibition of the products of the
    human alkaline phosphatase loci. Annals Human
    Genetics, 42, 1-13.
Mulivor, R.A., Mennuti, M., and Harris, H., 1979.
    Origin of the alkaline phosphatases in amniotic
    fluid. American Journal Obstetrics Gynecology,
    135, 77-81.
Nadler, H.L., and Walsh, M.M.J., 1980. Intrauterine
    detection of cystic fibrosis. Pediatrics, 66,
    690-692.
Nadler, H.L., 1982. Cystic Fibrosis Foundation.
    Heterozygote detection and prenatal diagnosis
    conference report, New York.
Patrick, A.D., and Ellis, R.B., 1979. Plasma
    hydrolases in cystic fibrosis. Lancet, 2, 1015-
    1016.
Sanguinetti-Briceno, N.R., and Brock, D.J.H., 1982.
    NADH dehydrogenase in cystic fibrosis. Clinical
    Genetics, 22, 308-311.
Shapiro, B.L., Feigal, R.J., and Lam, L.F.H., 1979.
    Mitochondrial NADH dehydrogenase in cystic fibrosis.
    Proceedings National Academy Sciences, 76, 2979-
    2983.

Shapiro, B.L., Lam,  L.F.H., and Feigal, R.J., 1982.
    Mitochondrial NADH dehydrogenase in cystic fibrosis:
    Enzyme kinetics in cultured fibroblasts. American
    Journal Human Genetics, 34, 846-852.
Schwartz, M., 1982.  A serine protease activity of
    human serum albumin towards MUGB:  implications for
    the use of MUGB reactivity in amniotic fluid in
    prenatal diagnosis of cystic fibrosis.  Clinica
    Chimica Acta, 124, 213-223.
Van Diggelen, O.P., Janse, H.C., and Kleijer, W.J.,
    1983.  Disaccharidases in amniotic fluid as possible
    prenatal marker for cystic fibrosis.  Lancet, 1,
    817.
Wilson, G.B., Fudenberg, H.H., and Jahn, T.L., 1975.
    Studies on cystic fibrosis using isoelectric
    focusing:  an assay for detection of cystic
    fibrosis homozygotes and heterozygote carriers in
    serum.  Paediatric Research, 9, 635-640.
Wilson, G.B., Arnaud, P., and Fudenberg, H.H., 1978.
    Improved method for the detection of cystic fibrosis
    protein in the serum using the LKB multiphor
    electrofocusing apparatus.  Paediatric Research,
    12, 801-804.

# IDENTIFICATION OF CF HETEROZYGOTES BY A LECTIN-LIKE FACTOR AND COFACTOR IN SERUM UTILIZING S-300 GEL FILTRATION.

Jack Lieberman, M.D. and W. Kaneshiro. Veterans Administration Medical Center and UCLA School of Medicine, Sepulveda, CA. 91343 U.S.A.

We have reported that the detection of a lectin-like factor in serum is a potential test for detecting carriers of the CF gene (J. Lab & Clin Med, 97:646, 1981). However, use of whole serum in a hemagglutination assay to measure lectin activity (with mouse-RBC and dextran-$SO_4$) was not entirely successful due to dietary and sampling variables that affect lectin activity. Since this lectin results from an IgM-bound cofactor, we explored use of an IgM peak isolated by S-300 Sephacryl filtration, instead of whole serum, for the assay. We were also able to detect free lectin-cofactor by adding normal pooled euglobulin to those serum fractions lacking IgM.

Of 43 CF parents (obligate heterozygotes), 41 (95%) had high lectin titers ranging between 1:64 to 1:1024 (median = 1:256). In contrast, 57 of 60 controls had low lectin titers ranging between 1:4 and 1:32, and 3 (5.0%) had high titers of 1:64 to 1:256 like those obtained from CF heterozygotes. Of 19 CF patients (homozygotes), 17 had elevated lectin titers between 1:64 and 1:4096. In CF patients we found that lectin activity could be reduced or totally removed by intravenous antibiotic therapy or high dose oral antibiotics.

Free lectin-cofactor was detected in the low MW fraction of serum from 42 of 52 heterozygotes and 14 of 16 CF patients. No one with normal lectin activity had free cofactor in their serum.

In urine, lectin activity was absent, consistent with the absence of IgM protein. Cofactor activity was also lacking when whole urine was tested; however, upon fractionation of the urine on G-25 Sephadex columns, cofactor was found in all 9 CF patients tested but in none of 15 obligate heterozygotes.

These studies confirm our previous observations of a lectin-like factor in the sera of both CF homozygotes and heterozygotes. The role of this factor in CF is yet to be determined. Finding cofactor in the low MW fraction of serum strengthens a positive test in heterozygotes, whereas its presence in urine is indicative of homozygosity. Use of the IgM fraction for assay of the CF-lectin in serum increases sensitivity and specificity of the test. Assay of a serum lectin and cofactor shows great promise as a screening test to detect the carrier state of the CF gene.

INTESTINAL DISACCHARIDASES IN AMNIOTIC FLUID AS MARKERS FOR THE PRENATAL DETECTION OF CYSTIC FIBROSIS;

W.J.Kleijer, H.C.Janse and O.P. van Diggelen.
Department of Clinical Genetics, Erasmus University,
Rotterdam, The Netherlands

Reduced activities of 4 disaccharidases - maltase, sucrase, trehalase and lactase - were previously shown in the amniotic fluid of pregnancies from which children affected with CF were born.(1). These studies have now been extended to 24 pregnancies at risk for CF. Several amniotic fluid samples were simultaneously studied by colleagues abroad (Boué, Paris; Schwartz, Copenhagen; Brock, Edinburgh).

The results for maltase and sucrase, which seem to be the most informative with respect to the fetal CF status, may be summarized as follows:

Reduced activities were found in 10 samples; 6 cases with values below the control ranges and 4 cases below the 5th percentile.
In this group 4 pregnancies ended with the birth of a CF patient, 2 were selectively terminated and 4 are· continuing.

Normal activities were found in 14 samples; i.e. above the 10th percentile of the control values.
In this group 2 pregnancies were studied retrospectively: 1 ended with birth of a CF child (reported previously by Brock) while in the other case CF is suspected (Schwartz). In 12 prospective studies 1 healthy child was born and 11 pregnancies are continuing.

By the time of this congress (June,1984) the outcome of all pregnancies will be known, which will enable an evaluation of the various attempted methods of prenatal detection of CF.

[1]Van Diggelen, Janse and Kleijer, Lancet i (1983) 817.

# ATTITUDES TOWARD PRENATAL DIAGNOSIS OF CYSTIC FIBROSIS AMONG PARENTS OF AFFECTED CHILDREN

M. Kaback, D. Zippin, P. Boyd, R. Cantor
Division of Medical Genetics,
Harbor/UCLA Medical Center
UCLA School of Medicine, Torrance, California

and

California Consortium of Cystic Fibrosis Centers:
N. Lewiston, B. Davis, R. Dooley, S. Giammona,
I. Harwood, B. Kagan, G. Kurland, A. Osher,
R. Rucker, R. Stiehm, and C. Wang

Supported by a grant from the March of Dimes
Birth Defects Foundation

INTRODUCTION

Over the past 15 years the option of fetal diagnosis in early pregnancy has become an important alternative in genetic (reproductive) counseling for many families. It is estimated that approximately 400,000 pregnancies have undergone mid-trimester amniocentesis for the purpose of assessing serious genetic disease or congenital defects in the fetus. Although, to date, few of the conditions identified in utero are amenable to any form of therapeutic intervention, such advances have been successfully employed in recent years for a few selected conditions and considerable progress in this regard is anticipated in the future.

For most, however, prenatal diagnosis provides a means for families at-risk for specified disorders in their offspring to gain accurate information upon which critical reproductive decisions can be made. Rather than facing the situation of "genetic roulette" which confronted such families in the past, requiring that they simply take their chances, prevent further reproduction, or take some other less-than-ideal option (e.g. artificial insemination by donor) many families, with the alternatives provided by prenatal diagnosis and elective pregnancy interruption, have been willing to attempt further pregnancies and, thereby to take the better-than-good odds that their fetus will be unaffected. In this way, literally thousands of families have been aided to have healthy children who they otherwise might not have been willing to even conceive or risk carrying to term.

Perhaps the most common and serious inborn error of metabolism in the western world is Cystic Fibrosis (CF). This debilitating disorder of infants, children, and young adults has evaded a basic clarification of its underlying defect. Considerable optimism has been generated intermittently over the past decade or two when various groups of investigators have reported discoveries apparently identifying clear and reproducible alterations in CF cells, body fluids, etc. Such findings raised great hopes for a prenatal detection method for CF and, in some instances, a means for CF heterozygote identification as well. Unfortunately, these early reports were not confirmed in other laboratories or failed to hold up under more extensive scrutiny and evaluation.

The prospect of prenatal diagnosis for CF is not, however, without considerable complexity, even if a definitive method were in hand. The wide spectrum of symptomology and severity, the highly variable course of the condition and the steadily improving prospect for minimizing serious complications and prolonging the life-quality of afflicted individuals, have made the limited options provided by a prenatal test clearly less-than-ideal. A definitive therapy, obviating all symptoms or even the prospect of a fundamental cure offer options which unquestionably have more universal appeal than selective abortion of fetuses afflicted with CF. Certainly, continued research to these ends must go forward. As an interim approach however, recognizing the futuristic possibilities of therapeutic or curative alternatives, prenatal diagnosis and the reproductive options it provides may be an important and widely adopted interim strategy for many families.

How critical an impact has the diagnosis of CF in a child and learning of the risk of recurrence in subsequent offspring had on the future reproductive plans of such families? Would prenatal diagnosis really be employed if it were available? Does the selective termination of pregnancies in which fetuses are found to have CF provide a potentially useful option to many? These are issues and questions about which there may be widespread opinions, but little if any definitive data. For this reason, the Cystic Fibrosis Foundation in the U.S., in conjunction with the March of Dimes Birth Defects Foundation co-sponsored a study targeted to families with children afflicted with CF, and aimed at gaining some insight into the aforementioned questions. The preliminary findings of that study comprise the basis of this report.

## STUDY DESIGN & SAMPLE STRATEGY

Throughout the State of California, 11 centers have been established for the care of children and young adults with CF. Such centers are located in tertiary medical facilites, almost all being part of a university/medical school complex. The patient populations served by this Consortium come from highly diversified socio-cultural backgrounds, both urban and rural in family lifestyle and covering the full spectrum of demographic variables. For these reasons, such a population is representative for assessing the spectrum of reproductive attitudes which may exist among families with children with CF. Approximately 1100 individuals with CF are followed currently by these centers. For the most part the centers act as providers and coordinators of care for the CF patients and their families; in some instances providing comprehensive "total" care and in others seeing the patients at defined intervals or in times of major crises.

As this study is primarily aimed at reproductive attitudes and further child-bearing decisions among such families, we elected to interview only those families in which the biological parents of the patient with CF were still residing together in the same household and where English was spoken by both parents. Most critically, since most of the issues raised were relevant only to families who were still of reproductive age, only families in which the mother of the CF child was 40 years of age or less were sought. Families whose children were seen anytime after January 1, 1977 were included if they met other eligibility criteria (even if their child was no longer living). The latter strategy was incorporated in order not to bias our sample toward families only with living children with CF as these may represent "milder" cases or younger ones in which a preselection against more severe experiences would result.

Ten of the 11 CF centers throughout California volunteered to participate in this study. Center records were reviewed with each

Director and his/her staff, and families believed to be eligible were so designated. A total 346 families, believed to meet eligibility requirements, were selected as the provisional study sample. A mailed communication from the center director which included consent forms and a separate 65-item self-administered questionnaire for each parent was included. A non-response within 4 weeks was followed by a second mailing and then, after a similar interval, multiple phone contacts (where necessary) were attempted. After 5 independent phone contacts were attempted (different times/different days), and in some instances a 3rd mailing, with no response or contact with the family, the household was regarded as unreachable. All data were collected between March and December of 1983.

RESULTS

Of the 346 provisional families selected, 79 households were unreachable (moved, wrong address, etc.) and 63 failed to meet study eligibility criteria (maternal age, language, both parents together). Thus, 204 eligible families were contacted and of these, 184 households responded. In six of these families, the father failed to respond; 178 did, and all 184 mothers completed the study instrument. Twenty eligible families failed to comply but 17 of these provided demographic data (by phone) which constitutes the nonrespondent sample. Overall then, responses were obtained from 362 parents of CF patients meeting all study criteria, and representing 184 of 204 (90%) of the eligible families contacted.

Demographic characteristics of this respondent cohort are provided in Table 1. These 184 families have produced 366 total offspring, 214 of which are afflicted with CF. Of these 214 CF patients, 193 (90.2%) were diagnosed by age 3 yrs (first affected child in the sibship) and the disorder was identified in 106 (50%) by 6 months of age.

Family Information

The number of children in these 184 families ranges from 1 child
(51 families) to 6 (1 family) with an average of 1.99 children per
family. There is a single CF-afflicted child in 157 of these
families, two CF-children in 24 families, and 3 children with the
disorder in 3 of the families. Twenty families have had one child
succumb with CF.

Analysis of these families by sibship size and the rank-order of
the CF-affected offspring in families with 2 or more children (n=
133), points to a major relevant finding in the study. With a
highly significant statistical value (z=3.5l; p < .0002), THE
CHILD WITH CF TENDS TO BE THE LAST CHILD BORN IN THE SIBSHIP. The
number of families who undertook additional pregnancies after
their first child with CF was identified is shown on Table 2. The
implications of this finding are quite clear and suggest that
couples stop having children after an offspring is identified with
CF and they are made aware of the likelihood of recurrence. This
conclusion is supported by subsequent findings in this report as
well.

In 22 of the 184 families (12%) another family member, in either
the mother's or father's families, had been diagnosed with CF
prior to the diagnosis of their child with the condition. This
substantiates the point that: FOR RELATIVELY COMMON AUTOSOMAL
RECESSIVE DISORDERS IN DESIGNATED POPULATIONS, THE VAST MAJORITY
OF CASES AT THE TIME OF DIAGNOSIS REPRESENT THE FIRST KNOWN CASE
ON EITHER SIDE OF THE FAMILY. This fact has important public
health implications. If any preventative strategy (e.g., carrier
screening and/or prenatal diagnosis of CF) is envisioned for
reducing the birth incidence of children afflicted with CF, then
waiting for a family to be identified as being at risk (by the
prior diagnosis of an affected family member) will have relatively
little impact on the overall disease incidence.

## Cystic Fibrosis Knowledge

Factual, genetic, and reproductively-relevant knowledge about CF among parents of CF patients was assessed by means of a 7-component set of questions. Of the 362 responding parents 52.1% accurately identified the approximate carrier rate for CF among North American Caucasians and 51.7% knew the estimated birth incidence among white newborns in the U.S. Given that both members of a couple are CF gene carriers, 85.9% knew the risk for CF in any pregnancy. Given that only one member of a couple carries the gene for CF, the risk for CF-affected offspring (0%) was known by 81.2% of respondents; and the risk that any child would be a carrier (50%) was correctly identified by 30.6% of parents. Ninety-nine percent knew that CF was not a contagious condition and 95.3% could correctly interpret a 25% risk statement. Approximately 65% of the parents answered 5 or more of the seven questions correctly, and 11% responded accurately on all items.

## Family Planning: Impact of Cystic Fibrosis

In addition to the 184 respondent families in which the mothers were 40 yrs. of age or less, responses were received from 27 other couples where the mothers were 41-45 yrs. old. For selected analyses these responses are included in this section, bringing the number of families to n= 211 and the total number of respondent parents to n= 414 (211 mothers and 203 fathers).

When asked if the identification of CF in their child caused them to CHANGE THEIR FAMILY SIZE, 102/211 or 48% of the families reported affirmatively, 11% were not sure, and 40% (n= 85) said "no". Of those who answered "yes" to this question, 60% of the families indicated that they had no further children and 36% indicated that they had fewer children than they would have liked. The remaining 4% (indicating a change in family plans) reported that they elected to have more children than they had planned originally (reproductive compensation?).

In 107 (51%) of these families, having a child with CF and learning of their risk led them to ALTER THEIR METHOD OR REGULARITY IN THE USE OF BIRTH CONTROL. When asked specifically about birth control methods, one or both members of 130 of the 211 couples (62%) indicated that they had undergone surgical sterilization. Of those 107 families which specifically indicated that the child with CF directly led to changes in their use of birth control, (67%) had surgical sterilization procedures performed on one or the other member. The remaining families, who indicated a change in birth control use, either began using birth control, changed to a more effective method, were "more careful" about birth control, or "abstained from sex".

Of the total respondent group (n=414) 54% favored the option of elective abortion by request and 38% were inclined toward abortion being available only in specific instances. Thirty-one individuals (7.6%) were against elective abortion under any circumstances. Of the group which supported abortion only in specific cases, 51% thought that it would be an acceptable basis for an abortion if it were established that the pregnancy would lead to a serious untreatable disease in the resultant child, while 25% of this group indicated uncertainty as to this indication. Twenty percent were not in favor of abortion under these circumstances.

PRENATAL DIAGNOSIS OF CF

OF ALL PARENTS RESPONDING, 78% FELT THAT THE DEVELOPMENT OF PRENATAL DIAGNOSIS FOR CF WOULD PROVIDE AN IMPORTANT REPRODUCTIVE OPTION FOR ALL OR MOST FAMILIES AT RISK FOR CF IN THEIR CHILDREN. A clear minority (8%) felt that it would be an important reproductive option for few or no families. When asked if they would have changed their family plans IF PRENATAL DIAGNOSIS FOR CF HAD BEEN AVAILABLE WHEN THEY BECAME AWARE OF THEIR RISK, 129 of

408 parents responding, (32%) indicated that their plans definitely would have been changed. Another 24% of respondents indicated uncertainty as to whether or not this would have changed their plans and 44% reported that this would not have influenced any further family planning.

Among the 184 couples where the mothers were 40 years of age or less, only 35 couples indicated that they would definitely have, probably have, or were undecided about having more children in the future. The remainder indicated that they would definitely not or would probably not have further children. Of these 35 families (nonsterilized and indicating undecided, probably, or definitely having more children in the future) APPROXIMATELY 75% INDICATED THAT THE DEVELOPMENT OF A PRENATAL TEST FOR CF IN THE NEXT 2 TO 5 YEARS WOULD INFLUENCE THEM TO HAVE MORE CHILDREN.

Overall, of the 414 parents responding to this survey instrument, 82% felt that fetal diagnosis for CF should be made available. Another 10% were uncertain as to the development of this methodology and 8% (34 individuals) were against this option. NO SIGNIFICANT ASSOCIATION WAS FOUND BETWEEN ATTITUDES AMONG RESPONDENTS TOWARD MAKING PRENATAL DIAGNOSIS OF CF AVAILABLE AND:

> -age
> -sex
> -prior death of a child with CF
> -CF knowledge
> -completed formal education
> -other family member with CF
> -Stated physical, emotional, or financial stress of caring
>  for their child with CF

SIGNIFICANT ASSOCIATIONS WERE FOUND BETWEEN ATTITUDES TOWARD PRENATAL DIAGNOSIS OF CF AND:

> -present religion

-self-scaled religiosity
-abortion attitudes
-number of children
-family income

As to religious preference, only Mormons were significantly less inclined toward prenatal diagnosis for CF being made available when compared to Protestants, Catholics, Jews, those of other religions, and those professing no religion. Importantly, even among the Mormon respondents (n=21), 57% were in favor of fetal tests for CF being made available. No significant differences were evident between the other parent groups (80% of 187 Protestants, 82% of 82 Catholics, and 100% of 17 Jewish respondents favored prenatal availability).

Scoring, themselves on a 4-point scale as to their religiosity, analysis of attitudes toward prenatal detection of CF in 407 respondents showed that 66% of the 93 parents who considered themselves very religious favored the availability of prenatal tests for CF. This attitude is significantly lower than the 84% of moderately religious, 90% of slightly religious, and 89% of not religious parents responding.

Parents with 5-6 children (n=20) were significantly less inclined (45% in favor; 35% against; 20% uncertain) toward the availability of prenatal diagnosis for CF than parents with 2-4 children (80% in favor) and parents with only 1 child (95% in favor).

As to abortion attitude and opinions on availability of prenatal testing for CF, highly significant differences were found between those favoring abortion on request, only in certain instances, or under no circumstances. Even among those completely against abortion who expressed opinions (n=30), 10 (33%) still favored prenatal test development; 40% were against, and 27% indicated uncertainty. Among the 218 respondents who favored abortion on request, 95% favored prenatal testing availability as did 73% of the 158 respondents who felt that abortion should be available only under specific circumstances.

### SUMMARY AND CONCLUSIONS

This study provides a detailed and unprecedented examination of reproductive attitudes and CF-related knowledge in parents of children and young adults with CF. Based on self-administered questionnaire responses from 362 parents of CF affected children (184 mothers and 178 fathers), data were obtained as to family constitution, reproductive (genetic) knowledge concerning CF, family planning issues, and attitudes toward abortion and the development of prenatal diagnosis for this disorder.

A number of important conclusions emerge from these analyses:

- The identification of a child in the family with CF has a major impact on the further reproduction of the couple. With high significance, the child with CF tends to be the last child born to the couple.

- Changes in family planning were reported by about 50% of the families, subsequent to the diagnosis of CF in their offspring. Of those who changed their family plans, 60% had no further children and 36% had fewer than they had hoped for.

  More than half of the families reported that changes in their use of or method of birth control resulted from their learning of their child's condition and its risk for recurrence. Sixty-seven percent of these families underwent surgical sterilization in one or the other parent

  In spite of varied opinions as to elective abortion in general, 81% of all parents favored the development of prenatal diagnosis for CF. More than 50% of families indicated that their family plans definately or probably would have changed had prenatal detection of CF been available to them.

While only 33 families in this study were undecided, possibly, or definately planning to have more children in the future, 70% of this group indicated that the development of a prenatal detection method would influence them to have more children.

In conclusion, it is evident that among this highly diversified parent cohort, a clear majority favor the development of a prenatal diagnostic method for CF. Even among subgroups where strong religious or personal imperatives exist against pregnancy interruption, the majority opinion is still in favor of or undecided about making such technology available. In light of the major reproductive impact which the diagnosis of CF in one of their children has had on most families, and the definitive steps which many have taken to avoid further child-bearing, the development of such an option seems not only desirable but clearly justified. Until a truly effective therapy, or even cure, can be established for CF, it would appear that prenatal diagnosis would be welcomed and utilized by many.

TABLE 1

DEMOGRAPHIC CHARACTERISTICS OF RESPONDENT POPULATION*

|  | Total | Male | Female |
|---|---|---|---|
| Number | 362 | 178 | 184 |
| **Age** | | | |
| Mean | 32.95 | 34.11 | 31.85 |
| St. Dev. | 5.28 | 5.27 | 5.07 |
| **Religion** | | | |
| Protestant | 46.4% | 46.3% | 46.4% |
| Catholic | 19.6% | 17.1% | 21.9% |
| Jewish | 3.1% | 3.4% | 2.7% |
| Mormon | 5.3% | 5.1% | 5.5% |
| Other | 3.6% | 4.0% | 3.3% |
| None | 22.1% | 24.0% | 20.2% |
| **Race** | | | |
| Caucasian--Not Hispanic | 95.5% | 96.0% | 95.1% |
| Caucasian--Hispanic | 3.1% | 2.8% | 3.3% |
| Black | .3% | .6% | ----- |
| Oriental | .3% | ----- | .5% |
| Other | .8% | .6% | 1.1% |
| **Education** | | | |
| Less than 12 Years | 5.8% | 5.6% | 6.0% |
| High School Graduate | 19.1% | 14.0% | 23.9% |
| Some College | 40.6% | 40.4% | 40.8% |
| College Graduate | 14.6% | 16.3% | 13.0% |
| Some Professional or Graduate School | 9.4% | 10.7% | 8.2% |
| Professional or Graduate Degree | 10.5% | 12.9% | 8.2% |
| **Family Income** | | | |
| Less than $15,000 | 12.8% | ---- | ---- |
| $15,000 to $30,000 | 36.1% | ---- | ---- |
| $31,000 to $45,000 | 25.6% | ---- | ---- |
| $46,000 to $60,000 | 16.1% | ---- | ---- |
| Above $60,000 | 9.4% | ---- | ---- |

* Includes only families where mother of CF patient is
  40 years of age or less.

TABLE 2

SUBSEQUENT PREGNANCIES IN 183 FAMILIES AFTER THE
DIAGNOSIS OF CYSTIC FIBROSIS IN THEIR CHILD

Number of Subsequent Pregnancies

|  | 0 | 1 | 2 | 3 | 4 | Total |
|---|---|---|---|---|---|---|
| Number of Families | 119 | 51 | 10 | 2 | 1 | 183 |
| % of Total | 65.0 | 27.9 | 5.5 | 1.1 | 0.5 | 100 |

# CHARACTERISTICS OF THE CF CELL

John A. Mangos, M.D. and R. Lee Boyd, Ph.D.

Department of Pediatrics
University of Texas Health Science Center
San Antonio, Texas

## INTRODUCTION

Cystic Fibrosis (CF) is the most common genetic disease which shortens the lifespan of Caucasians throughout the world. It is much less frequent among the Blacks and Orientals. It is transmitted in what appears to be an autosomal recessive mode of inheritance (Talamo, Rosenstein and Berminger, 1983). Because of the latter, it would be expected that the basic defect would express itself in all the cells of affected individuals. The expression of the basic defect could result in changes in the morphology, composition or function of the affected cells. Although scientists have searched for many years for the inherited molecular defect of CF, the identification of such a defect has not yet been achieved. If the basic defect had been known, a description of the "characteristics of the CF cell" would have been easy by focusing on the special areas of the various cells where the expression of the basic defect took place. Because the basic defect of CF is not known, the author of this paper has elected to focus on what is known about the morphological, compositional and functional characteristics of certain cells from patients with CF which are likely to be targets of the effects of the presumed inherited defect of this disease.

Investigations have been focused on specific cell types in CF because of one or more of the following reasons:

1. Some organs, such as the pancreas, lungs, sweat glands, and salivary glands, appear to be targets of CF and their cells have been studied in order to detect possible abnormalities.

2. Certain cells are easily obtainable, such as erythrocytes and leukocytes or buccal epithelial cells, and thus have been used for studies of CF.

3. Certain cells are easily cultured, such as skin fibroblasts and lymphocytes, and thus have been used extensively in CF research.

4. Certain cells, such as epithelial cells of the airways, have recently become the focus of investigative attention because of the demonstration of transport abnormalities across the tissues they form.

It is outside the focus of this presentation to discuss the morphological, compositional or functional characteristics of all the cells comprising the body of a patient with CF. Instead, a number of arbitrarily chosen cellular systems has been selected for review because of the reasons listed above. The cells which will be included in this presentation are:

1.  Epithelial cells:    These include the respiratory and digestive tract epithelia as well as the epithelia lining the ducts of exocrine glands.

2.  Secretory Cells  Since CF appears to be a generalized exocrinopathy, it is understandable that the secretory cells of exocrine glands have been investigated extensively.

3.  Cultured Skin Fibroblasts: Extensive studies have been conducted in CF research using cultured skin fibroblasts from patients and controls.

4.  Erythrocytes and Leukocytes:    These cells are easily obtained from patients and controls for various studies.  Lymphocytes have been used extensively for establishing long-term in vitro proliferating cell lines.

## EPITHELIAL CELLS

There are a number of organs which possess epithelial membranes comprised of different types of epithelial cells which have undergone structural and functional differentiation serving the specific functions of each organ. Such epithelial cells may be found in the airways, the gastrointestinal tract and the ducts of the exocrine glands.

Epithelial cells of the airways:   These cells line the nasal cavity and the remaining airways. They are ciliated and have the ability to propel mucus and other particulate matter.   The cilia beat rhythmically in a layer of aqueous fluid bathing the surface of the epithelium.   For many years, the "mucociliary clearance" was the main function attributed to these cells. The origin of the periciliary fluid and respiratory tract mucus was thought to be exclusively from the submucosal glands of the airways with some participation from the goblet cells, single mucus-secreting cells interspersed among the ciliated epithelial cells.  In recent years, however, it was pointed out, mostly through elegant electrophysiological studies, that the respiratory epithelial cells appear to be involved in the maintenance of the composition and volume of the periciliary fluid through processes of secretion and reabsorption of electrolytes and water translocation across the epithelial membranes lining the nose and the airways.

Morphological changes in CF:   In the trachea and large bronchi of an individual without CF the ciliated epithelial cell is the predominant cell type.   These cells are approximately 20 microns high, 6-10 microns in diameter and contain on the apical surface microvilli and cilia.  Each cell contains approximately 200 cilia which are 6-7 microns in length.   The cytoplasm contains abundant smooth endoplasmic reticulum, a well developed Golgi complex and abundant mitochondria, particularly in the sites of origin of the cilia. In CF, the ciliated epithelial cells of the airways do not present any abnormalities, particularly before widespread obstruction and infection occur. During the latter the airways epithelium may show denuded areas, epidermoid metaplasia of cells and goblet cell and basal cell hyperplasia. These epithelial changes are non-specific and provide no indication that detectable morphological abnormalities of the airway epithelial cells exist in CF. Most of the changes seen are identical to those occuring in other diseases where chronic airway obstruction and infection occur. Recently, Sturgess presented a detailed description of the characteristics of the bronchial mucosa in CF (Sturgess 1982).

Compositional changes in CF:   In spite of the fact that in recent years a number of abnormalities in the transport of sodium ions, in the permeability of chloride ions and in the pathways of chloride secretion have been identified in airway epithelial membranes from patients with CF, nothing is known about the intracellular ionic composition of the individual epithelial cells comprising these membranes. This area of cellular pathophysiology in CF needs further investigation, particularly now that technologies, such as ion-sensitive microelectrodes and x-ray microprobe analysis of such cells, have reached high levels of accuracy and reproducibility.

Functional changes in CF:     In the past few years, new methods of investigation of the ion movements across the airway epithelia using electrophysiological techniques along with methods for the study of submucosal gland secretion have brought about improved understanding of the homeostatic mechanisms regulating the fluid of the respiratory tract (Davis and Nadel, 1983). Active transport of chloride ions toward the airway lumen and of sodium ions toward the submucosa have been demonstrated in the dog trachea. In other species, variations of the same theme have been observed. More recently, the electrophysiology of the human nasal mucosa and of the mucosa of the tracheobronchial tree have been studied in situ in patients with CF and in control subjects. It was demonstrated that the luminal side of the respiratory epithelium is always negatively charged and that CF patients have consistently higher potential differences across the airway epithelium (Knowles, Gatzy and Boucher, 1981). This increased electronegativity of the CF airway epithelia was markedly decreased upon local application of amiloride, a blocker of sodium movements across cell membranes. The investigators postulated that increased transepithelial movements of sodium in the airways of patients with CF would result in dehydration of respiratory mucus and in depletion of periciliary fluid. These events could lead to inspissation of mucus, obstruction of the airways, secondary infection and, eventually, gradual destruction of the airways. In subsequent studies, the same investigators using nasal mucosal measurements concluded that in subjects with CF it appears that there exists an absolute decrease in luminal surface chloride ion permeability of epithelial cells (Knowles, Stutts, Spock, Fisher, Gatzy and Boucher, 1983 and Knowles, Gatzy and Boucher, 1983). They postulated that this decrease in chloride permeability may inhibit a potential path of chloride secretion leading to a "deficit" of luminal fluid. Thus, these electrophysiological studies suggest that decreased chloride secretion and increased sodium reabsorption cross the airway epithelia in patients with CF may be additively contributing factors in the relative "dessication" of the surface airway liquid in this disease. Further investigations in this area are needed in order to, hopefully, clarify the events leading to the pathophysiology of CF in the respiratory tract. One of the issues that needs to be specifically clarified is the ionic composition inside the epithelial cells comprising the airway mucosa in control subjects and in patients with CF. Furthermore, because of the relative inaccessibility of the airway epithelia for sampling of cells it would be extremely helpful if these epithelial cells could be cultured and studied in vitro. From unpublished reports, there appears that attempts to grow such cells are meeting with some success in 2-3 laboratories. In vitro availability of such cell lines from CF patients and controls will markedly enhance our efforts to elucidate the pathophysiology of CF, if the cell lines in vitro demonstrate detectable differences in cell function.

Other aspects of the function of these cells in CF, such as metabolic activity, possible secretory activity, ciliary beat, transmembrane transport of non-electrolytes and others, have not been studied yet. Another area that needs detailed studies in CF airway epithelia is the histochemical localization of key enzymes involved in the regulation of transport of ions and water across the epithelia. Furthermore, the duct of the submucosal glands of the airways has a "ciliated" portion covered with epithelial cells possessing numerous cilia. It has been proposed that the fine regulation of the ionic composition of the secretions produced by the submucosal glands of the airways may take place in this section of the duct and that this section may play an important role in the airway pathophysiology of CF (Sturgess 1982).

The ciliated epithelium and airway mucous gland system, both epithelial and submucosal, combine to form the mucociliary clearance system. This system is involved in clearance of inhaled particulate matter and microorganisms from the respiratory tract. Pathophysiological impairment of either of the components of the mucociliary system will, therefore, adversely affect clearance by the system. In addition to mucociliary clearance, pulmonary alveolar macrophages are important phagocytic cells which police the small airways and alveoli for removal of inhaled particulates and microorganisms. Pulmonary alveolar macrophages obtained by lavage of airways of CF patients have been shown to have no observable morphological or ultrastructural differences from those obtained from non-CF airways (Thomassen, Demko, Wood, Tandler, Dearborn, Boxerbaum and Kuchenbard, 1980). Moreover, the phagocytic capacity of the CF macrophages for Pseudomonas aeruginosa and Staphylococcus aureus was not different from that of non-CF macrophages. These authors have further shown an inhibitory effect of CF serum on the phagocytic capacity of the alveolar macrophages for Pseudomonas (Thomassen, Boxerbaum, Demko, Kuchenbrod, Dearborn and Wood, 1979 and Thomassen, Demko, Wood, Tandler, Dearborn, Boxerbaum and Kuchenbrod, 1980). The antiphagocytic effect was shown to be acquired upon chronic colonization in animals (Winnie, Klinger, Sherman and Thomassen, 1982). They, therefore, have suggested that chronic infection in CF may result from alteration of the lung fluid environment by a serum acquired extrinsic factor and does not appear to be related to an intrinsic cellular defect of the CF alveolar macrophage.

In CF patients with advanced airway disease there is extensive epidermoid metaplasia of the surface epithelium (Sturgess 1982). This is not a change specific to CF because it occurs with high frequency in diseases which cause airway epithelial damage other than that of CF. This epithelial change along with basal cell and goblet cell hyperplasia as well as submucosal gland hypertrophy observed in CF patients with long standing airway disease may actually play important pathophysiological roles. This topic along with other aspects of airway epithelial cell changes in CF have been recently reviewed (Sturgess 1982, Wood and Legris, 1982).

Epithelial cells of the digestive tract:    The digestive tract is lined by epithelial cells which vary in structure and function according to the area of the digestive tract they cover. If there is a generalized abnormality of transepithelial transport of monovalent ions, such as sodium and chloride, in CF one would expect to find expressions of this abnormality in all epithelial cells. The accessibility of the gastrointestinal mucosa is as difficult as that of the airways and makes sampling of epithelial cells from CF patients prohibitively difficult.   It was recently demonstrated in the author's laboratory that buccal epithelial cells can be obtained very easily by scraping the oral mucosa of the cheek and placing the cells in suspensions (Mangos 1983a). Furthermore, it has been shown that explants of oral mucosa from baboons and humans may be used for obtaining proliferating cell lines (Mangos 1983b). In a preliminary study of the concentrations of ionized calcium in the cytosol of these cells using calcium-sensitive microelectrodes, it was demonstrated that buccal epithelial cells from CF patients contained three times as much free-ionized calcium as did the same cells from controls (Table 1).

**TABLE 1.** The cytosolic ionized calcium concentration ($\mu M$) in 32 cells from 10 patients with CF and in 38 cells from 10 control subjects.

|  | Control | CF |
|---|---|---|
| $Ca^{++}$ | $0.68 \pm S.D.\ 0.11$ | $2.14 \pm S.D.\ 0.37$ |
|  | $p < 0.001$ |  |

These differences may be interpreted to suggest altered homeostatic handling of calcium by an epithelial cell in CF and raise the question whether or not similar functional alterations exist in other epithelial cells of patients with CF and particularly in secretory cells of exocrine glands where calcium ions play important role(s) in the stimulus-secretion coupling and other cellular functions.

The morphology and composition of the surface epithelial cells of the small and large intestines have been the topics of a number of excellent recent reviews (Neutra and Madara, 1982, Field 1982 and Hopfer 1982). While significant digestive dysfunction is present in CF patients which would raise the expectations to find morphological changes in the intestinal epithelium, no convincing data for structural, compositional or functional changes have been described yet in these epithelial cells. The histology of the small intestine is normal in CF (Antonowicz, Reddy, Khan and Shrachman, 1968 and Morin, Roy, LaSalle and Bonin, 1976). Increased mucus content of the goblet cells of the rectum and other histologic abnormalities of rectal biopsy material were proposed as a pathognomonic diagnostic aid for CF (Parkins 1963) twenty years ago. Recent studies do not agree with these earlier observations. Decreased peptide hydrolase activity and decreased tissue accumulation of phenylalanine and cycloleucine in biopsy specimens from the intestine of CF patients may be considered suggestive of intestinal epithelial cell functional abnormalities resulting in impairment of protein digestion. It is a common clinical experience that even the most meticulous pancreatic enzyme replacement therapy of CF patients does not reverse completely their steatorrhea and azotorrhea. This suggests that part of their malabsorption may be due to functional abormalities of the intestinal epithelium. Unfortunately, there are no experimental data explaining the nature of such cellular dysfunction.

Recently, electron microprobe x-ray microanalysis has been used for the studies of ion concentrations in the intercellular space of rabbit ileum (Neutra and Madara, 1982). It is hoped that such techniques will allow investigators to perform studies of the ionic composition of the intestinal epithelial cells in health and in CF.

Epithelial cells of the ducts of the exocrine glands: One of the two exocrine glands affected in a major way by CF is the pancreas. Unfortunately in most instances the exocrine pancreas of patients is completely destroyed and the chances for recovery of ducts or ductal cells for in vitro studies are nil. There are a number of hypotheses as to what the pancreatic ductal cell defects might be but are all based on indirect data obtained from analysis of duodenal fluid from CF patients with residual pancreatic function, as recently reviewed (Hadorn and Roscher, 1982). The other gland that is functionally affected in CF is the sweat gland.

The sweat gland is structured as follows: a proximal secretory coil is followed by an intermediate coiled duct segment which in turn is followed by the distal straight duct portion which opens in the epidermis. Spicer, et al. recently presented an excellent review of the morphology of the sweat gland in health and in CF (Spicer, Briggman and Baron, 1982).

Morphological changes in CF: Morphological studies using either light or electron microscopy have revealed no morphologic altertions in CF and whatever the basic defect of this hereditary disease might be appears to concern a molecular aberration unaccompanied by structural changes

(Spicer, Briggman and Baron, 1982). Because tight junctions appear to regulate paracellular ion flows, Briggman et al. compared the freeze-fracture morphology of tight junctions of eccrine sweat ducts from 11 controls and 7 CF patients (Briggman, Bank, Graves and Spicer, 1983). Exhaustive investigation of several parameters of freeze-fracture morphology revealed no significant differences between CF and control ducts, the sweat gland segment where the ion transport defect is presumed to be. It is of interest, however, that when the same morphological features were investigated in the secretory coils of the sweat glands, the segments presumed to function normally, significant differences in tight junction morphology were observed. It is reasonable to conclude that to this date no convincing morphological abnormality of the sweat gland duct epithelial cells has been presented. Na/K ATPase activity was compared by quantitative radioautography between normal and CF sweat ducts and no significant differences were found (Quinton and Tarmey, 1976 and Quinton 1981). Immunostaining for carbonic anhydrase showed no differences and amiloride fluorescence was comparably intense in both control and CF sweat ducts at the luminal apex of the epithelial cells (Spicer, Briggman and Baron, 1982).

Compositional changes in CF: There is no information about the composition of the epithelial cells lining the ducts of the sweat glands of control subjects and CF patients.

Functional changes in CF: There are no methods for the study of isolated duct cells from either controls or patients with CF. All the available information has been derived from in vitro microperfusion experiments, in vivo microcollections from single glands and in vivo and in vitro electrophysiological experiments. Based on the fact that the primary secretory fluid of the sweat gland is isotonic or slightly hypertonic to plasma in both CF and control subjects and that the fluid emerging from the sweat duct of patients contains much more sodium and chloride than that of controls, the investigations for the sweat gland dysfunction of CF have been focused on the sweat duct. The author first microperfused in vitro ducts from the sweat glands of patients with CF and controls and demonstrated defective reabsorption of sodium with no differences in water permeability in CF (Mangos, 1973a and 1973b). He attributed that dysfunction to a humoral factor contained in the sweat (Mangos 1967). Recently, on the basis of electrophysiological and analytical measurements, Quinton concluded that defective permeability to chloride ions also exists in the ducts of the sweat glands of patients with CF. He suggested that "impermeability of the duct to chloride" may be the basis of the electrolyte abnormality in the sweat duct epithelial as well as in the airway epithelia and possibly other epithelia of the patients with CF (Quinton 1983a and Quinton 1983b). This observation, along with the recent findings of Knowles, et al. (Knowles, Stutts, Spock, Fisher, Gatzy and Boucher, 1983 and Knowles, Gatzy and Boucher, 1983) suggest that defective permeability of epithelial cell membranes to chloride ions needs to be carefully investigated in CF in an effort to link this cellular dysfunction to the primary molecular defect of

CF. Such studies should include cellular energetics, localization and activities of various enzymes, membrane biosynthesis and function, ionic composition of the cells and ionic homeostatic mechanisms.

## SECRETORY CELLS OF EXOCRINE GLANDS

Efforts have been made to study the structure, composition and function of the secretory portions of exocrine glands, target organs of CF. In some instances, such as in the case of the pancreas and submandibular glands, the gland destruction and scarring are so severe in CF that meaningful structural, compositional and functional studies have not been possible. In other instances, extensive studies of the secretory segments of exocrine glands have been possible either in vivo or in vitro. Secretory acinar cells have been isolated from parotid glands of CF patients and controls and studied in vitro in the author's laboratory (Mangos and Donnelly, 1981 and Mangos 1981). Recently, Martinez reviewed the alterations in salivary gland structure and function in CF (Martinez 1982). It should be emphasized that the secretory cells of all exocrine glands are also of epithelial origin but have been differentiated into complex structures which support their secretory function.

Morphological changes in CF: The studies of the structure of the secretory segments of exocrine glands have been inconclusive in pinpointing morphological alterations that could be considered characteristic of CF. While the salivary glands have been reported to be enlarged in 92% of the CF patients, no other characteristic features were described in the morphology. When the author isolated parotid acinar cells from patients with CF and controls he noted that there were no gross differences in cell architecture by electron microscopy; the CF cells were larger than those from control parotids (mean diameter of 41 microns for CF cells versus 21 microns for control cells) and they appeared to have more abundant zymogen granules than the control cells; however, no morphometry of the cells was conducted to quantitate this observation. In the case of the sweat gland, there had been no morphological alterations in CF until the recent observation of some changes in the tight junctions of the secretory cells of the CF sweat glands by Briggman et al. (Briggman, Bank, Graves and Spicer, 1983). Significant differences were observed in the means of the number of strands, the distance and the depth between intersections for the tight junctions of the intercellular canaliculus of the secretory coil. The paradox is that by physiological studies, the secretory coil of the sweat gland is presumed to function normally in CF. In a recent study, the size of the submucosal glands of the airways of 21 patients with CF who died before 3 weeks of age was compared to that of 28 controls (Chow, Landau and Taussig, 1982). Using different methods of comparison no signficant differences in gland size were found. The absence of gland hypertrophy or hyperplasia at birth suggested that obstruction of the airways by mucus may not be primarily responsible for the increased susceptibility to respiratory tract infections in cystic fibrosis, but when present later in life may aggravate the situation.

Compositional changes in CF:    The availability of isolated cells from the
parotids of CF patients and controls permitted the first studies of cellular
composition of a secretory cell from an exocrine gland of a patient with
CF.    As shown on Table 2, the CF cells had the same ATP content and
oxygen consumption as the control cells; the amylase content was higher in
the CF cells than in the control cells; the sodium and calcium concentrations
were significantly higher and the potassium concentrations lower in the CF
cells than in the control cells.

**TABLE 2.**    Compositional differences between isolated parotid
acinar cells from CF patients and control subjects (Mangos and Donnelly,
1981 and Mangos 1981).

|  | **CONTROL** | **CF** |
|---|---|---|
| $[Na^+]$ (mEq/L of cells) | 28.3 ± 4.5 | 42.1 ± 4.9 |
| $[K^+]$ (mEq/L of cells) | 112.5 ± 10.2 | 84.1 ± 11.6 |
| $[Ca^{++}]$ (nanomoles/mg of cell protein) | 17.1 ± 3.1 | 28.7 ± 4.2 |
| [Amylase] | 198 ± 18 | 339 ± 30 |
| [ATP] (nanomoles per mg of cell protein) | 4.6 ± 1.6 | 5.9 ± 1.4 |
| [cAMP] (picomoles per mg of cell protein) | 2.3 ± 0.4 | 5.6 ± 1.2 |
| [cGMP] (picomoles per mg of cell protein) | 0.39 ± 0.12 | 0.17 ± 0.08 |
| $O_2$ Consumption ($\mu l \ O_2$ per hour per mg of cell protein) | 6.1 ± 1.4 | 6.4 ± 1.6 |

The increase in total calcium was most impressive but the available
methodologies at the time these experiments were conducted did not permit
the determination of the most important fraction of the calcium content of
the cells, the free, ionized cytosolic calcium.    It is known that while the
total calcium concentrations in various secretory cells are in the millimolar
range, the cytosolic ionized calcium concentrations are in the micromolar
range (Rubin 1982).    The ionized calcium is the biologically active fraction
which participates in the stimulus–secretion coupling, the translation of
autonomic receptor activation, the ionic homeostasis of the cells and other

important cellular functions.   Measurements of the concentrations of cytosolic ionized calcium in secretory cells have been accomplished in a number of laboratories, including that of the author, using calcium-sensitive microelectrodes.   However, because secretory cells are extremely difficult to obtain from CF patients, other cells have been sought for measurements of intracellular concentrations of ionized calcium in the cytosol and for studies of the possible relationships between ionized calcium handling and the regulatory mechanisms for other ions in these cells.  As described earlier in this paper the buccal epithelial cells have turned out to be easily and painlessly obtainable epithelial cells from CF patients and controls and appear to be an important tool for future studies of CF.  This cell system will be an exceptionally useful tool if current efforts to establish proliferating cell lines of buccal epithelial cells from CF patients and controls succeed.

Functional changes in CF:  Using the isolated parotid acinar cells from CF patients and controls the author was able to study various metabolic events in these secretory cells.   As shown in Table 3, there were significant differences in a number of functional parameters between cells from CF patients and those from control subjects.

**TABLE 3.**  Comparisons of functional responses between isolated parotid acinar cells from CF patients and from control subjects (Mangos 1981).

|  | CF Cells |
|---|---|
| Potassium efflux in response to cholinergic receptor stimulation | Decreased |
| Increase in intracellular cGMP content in response to cholinergic receptor stimulation | Reduced |
| Increase in intracellular cGMP content in response to beta adrenergic receptor stimulation | Increased |
| Increase in cell ATP content in response to cholinergic receptor stimulation | Same |
| Increase in $O_2$ consumption in response to cholinergic receptor stimulation | Same |
| Secretion of amylase in response to beta adrenergic receptor stimulation | Increased |
| Efflux of $^{22}Na$ across cell membrane | Reduced |
| $Ca^{++}$ uptake by cells | Reduced |

## CULTURED SKIN FIBROBLASTS

Skin fibroblasts have been used for the in vitro studies of many metabolic disorders. Since the first description of metachromatic staining of the cytoplasm of CF fibroblasts (Danes and Bearn, 1968) these cells have been used for numerous studies, the review of which is beyond the scope of this paper. A fairly extensive description of studies of fibroblasts in CF can be found in the recently published review chapter on CF (Talamo, Rosenstein and Berringer, 1983).

Morphological changes in CF:   It has become clear over the years that the CF fibroblast metachromasia is a non-specific effect which is difficult to reproduce and does not appear to represent a characteristic feature of CF. Extensive electron microscopical studies of the CF skin fibroblasts failed to reveal any characteristic changes (Spicer, di Sant'Agnese, Vincent and Ulane, 1980).

Compositional changes in CF:   Many studies comparing the composition of cultured skin fibroblasts from CF patients to that of cells from control subjects have been conducted in the past 15 years. Glycogen accumulation in the cytoplasm of CF cells has been reported but it did not appear to be a specific feature of CF (Pallavicini, Wiessman, Uhlendorf and di Sant'Agnese, 1976). The same could be said about the finding of accumulation of glycosaminoglycans in CF cells (Matalon and Dorfman, 1968). Extensive studies of the composition of the fibroblast membranes failed to show any differences between fibroblasts from CF patients and those from controls. Even after stimulation of protein synthesis such as the one occurring after exposure of the cells to dexamethasone, no differences could be found by 2-dimensional gel electrophoresis between CF cells and control cells. Many hydrolytic enzymes have been measured in CF skin fibroblasts (Talamo, Rosenstein and Berminger, 1983): normal activities of alpha-D-manosidase and beta-N-acetyl-glucosaminidase have been reported; while some abnormalites were noted in the carboxypeptidases A and B these enzymes are probably normal in CF skin fibroblasts; no differences of alkaline phosphatase intensity or activity have been demonstrated between CF and control fibroblasts; alpha-L-fucosidase has been found to be normal by some investigators while others have found elevated levels and isoenzymes with higher isoelectric points. Recent studies have demonstrated that CF skin fibroblasts had more cell-surface receptors for the sugar nucleotides UDP-galactose and UDP-glucuronic acid than control fibroblasts (Rudick, Rudick and Jones, 1983). Using two lectins, concomavalin A and wheatgerm agglutinin, the binding to membrane glycoproteins was studied and no differences between fibroblast from CF patients and controls were found (Harris and Bramwell, 1983). The sodium and potassium dependence of the Na/K pump and the Na and K composition of skin fibroblasts were compared and no differences were found (Reznick, Schneider and Mendosa, 1981). In the same study, however, the Na/K pump appeared to have a lower affinity for potassium in CF fibroblasts than in control cells.

With all the studies on the composition of the skin fibroblasts from CF patients and control subjects that have been conducted to this date it is interesting to note that reports of accurate determinations of the intracellular ionic composition which could permit the detection of differences characteristic for CF are very sparse.

Functional changes in CF:   Many investigators have attempted to discover secretory products of the fibroblasts that could be characterized as factors specific for CF.  The results so far are inconclusive and often confusing. Cell surface glycoproteins appear to be labelled normally and to be taken up and shed normally by CF skin fibroblasts (Owen 1978). The CF cells are able to synthesize complex carbohydrate side chains as shown by their ability to glycosylate a viral glycoprotein.    Normal methionine transport, normal composition and metabolism of linoleic and arachidonic acid and normal thymidine and uridine uptake have been found in CF skin fibroblasts (Talamo, Rosenstein and Berninger, 1983).  Lysomal enzyme secretion has been found to be normal in CF fibroblasts (Jessup and Dean, 1982) and the synthesis and isoenzyme profiles for alpha-L-fucosidase were not different between CF and control fibroblasts (Harris and Swallow, 1981).    Furthermore, the thermal lability of this enzyme was normal in CF fibroblasts (Scanlin and Glick, 1981).    A recent finding of potential importance has been the discovery that CF skin fibroblasts have reduced membrane Mg/Ca-ATPase activity (Ansah and Katz, 1980).    This, of course, raises the important question whether or not a subtle defect in the handling of calcium ions by CF skin fibroblasts may exist and may have significant functional implications. Shapiro et al. have demonstrated increased total calcium content of cultured CF fibroblasts, increases in calcium mitochondrial pool size and decreases in cellular NADH dehydrogenase activity in CF fibroblasts (Shapiro and Lam, 1982 and Shapiro, Lam and Feigal, 1982).

In relationship to increased calcium levels in CF fibroblasts, the levels of calmodulin and cAMP were studied in cultured skin fibroblasts. It was found that CF cells had increased content of calmodulin-like activity, increased content of cAMP synthesis in the presence of beta-adrenergic agonists and increased binding of a beta antagonist (Gnegy, Erickson and Markovac, 1981 and Markovac, Erickson and Hieber, 1981).

## ERYTHROCYTES AND LEUKOCYTES

Because of the ease of sampling and the expectation that the basic molecular defect would express itself in all somatic cells, early studies of CF were   focused   on   erythrocytes   and   later   on   lymphocytes and lymphoblasts.  The author expecting to find ion transport abnormalities in CF erythrocytes studied their monovalent cationic composition and the transport of sodium ions across the erythrocyte cell membrane and compared them to those of cells from normal controls twenty years ago (Lobeck 1966).  Both monovalent cationic composition and transmembrane transport of sodium of CF erythrocytes were found to be the same as in erythrocytes from control subjects. The subject of transmembrane transport abnormalities has come up a number of times in the past twenty years (Talamo, Rosenstein and Berninger, 1983). The author believes that there is no convincing evidence for such abnormalities at the present time. Inside-out vesicles of CF erythrocytes have been studied in terms of calcium uptake and were found to have much lower uptake than the same preparations from normal controls (Ansah and Katz, 1980). Abnormalities in the various ATPases in CF erythrocytes membranes have been suggested (Talamo, Rosenstein and Berninger, 1983). In a recent study, the zinc and copper content of CF erythrocytes were found to be significantly higher than in control erythrocytes, while the selenium content was found to be lower (Neve, Van Geffel, Hanocq and Molle, 1983). In another recent study, the erythrocyte superoxide dismutase and catalase activities in cells from CF patients and their parents were found to be significantly higher than in cells from age and sex matched controls while the peroxidation of lipids was reduced (Matkovics, Gyurkovitz, Laszlo and Szabo, 1982). In yet another study, the in vitro incorporation and transport of plasma nonesterified fatty acids into phospholipids of erythrocyte membranes from CF patients and controls were studied (Rogiers, Mandelbaum, Mozes, Vertongen, Dab, Crokaert and Vis, 1982). It was found that the in vitro turnover of palmitic and linoleic acids in the membrane phospholipids in CF erythrocytes is higher than in erythrocytes of health controls.

An interesting study of the insulin receptors of circulating CF and control monocytes demonstrated that the CF cells have higher numbers of insulin receptors and altered insulin affinity (Talamo, Rosenstein and Berninger, 1983). There have been several studies of the membrane composition of CF peripheral lymphocytes but no abnormalities characteristic of CF have been shown to exist (Talamo, Rosensteinm, Berninger, 1983). In cultured lymphocytes, less cAMP is produced in response to stimulation with isoproterenol in the CF cells than in control cells (Talamo, Rosenstein, Berninger, 1983). While there is an absolute decrease in the amount of alpha-L-fucosidase activity in CF lymphocytes, the isoenzyme patterns are normal and the enzyme subunit molecular weights are indistinguishable from those of controls. T-lymphocytes from CF patients appear to secrete a ciliary dyskinesia factor.

In recent years, the research work of P. Davis and her associates has demonstrated reduced beta adrenergic responses in lymphocytes, granulocytes and the cardiovascular system of patients with CF (Davis, Dieckman, Boat, Stern and Doershuk, 1983 and Davis and Kaliner, 1983). In the leukocytes, this defect appeared to be present in attenuated form in obligate heterozygotes for CF suggesting that it is inherited and not acquired as a result of disease. The numbers of beta adrenergic receptors and their binding capacity are the same in normal lymphocytes and in CF lymphocytes. The basal levels of cAMP were the same in both cell populations but the levels in response to isoproterenol ($10^{-8}$M) were significantly reduced in CF lymphocytes. Similar findings were observed in granulocytes. Davis et al. concluded that the lymphocyte and granulocyte

beta adrenergic defect in CF cannot be explained on the basis of
abnormalities of the beta receptors or of the adenylate cyclase itself. They
suggested that the receptor-cyclase coupling mechanism is a likely site for
this apparently heritable beta adrenergic defect in CF. In another study, the
granulocyte chemiluminescence was studied in cells from patients with CF
and controls (Graft, Mischler, Farrell and Busse, 1982). This
chemiluminescence is the result of activating the cellular respiratory burst
and oxidative metabolism. No differences were found between CF and
control granulocytes.

## DISCUSSION

The results of the studies reviewed in this paper point out that many
abnormalities in the morphology, composition or function of various cells
from patients with CF have been described. It seems that a whole new area
of cellular pathophysiology in this hereditary disease has emerged in the last
few years. The problem is that one cannot find a common thread that ties
all these interesting findings to a common morphological, compositional or
functional aberration that would be characteristic of CF and possibly related
to the basic defect of this disease. It seems that in the past few years
investigators of this disease have uncovered a number of interesting findings
of cellular pathophysiology in cells in situ or in cell cultures in vitro. Each
of these findings could be of extreme importance if we knew where it fits in
the various mechanisms regulating the intracellular composition and
comprising the cellular function. In other words, we are faced with some
knowledge of cellular pathophysiology of CF which cannot be explained
simply because our knowledge of the cellular physiology is still incomplete.
This situation is not new in CF research. In 1953 di Sant'Agnese discovered
the increase salinity of the sweat in CF (di Sant'Agnese, Darling, Perera and
Shea, 1953). The nature of the pathophysiology of the sweat gland could not
be explained until the body of knowledge on the physiology of this body organ
had been elucidated. It took investigators twenty years to elucidate the
physiology of the normal sweat gland in order to interpret the finding of
increased salinity of the sweat in CF as being due to defective reabsorption
of sodium from a duct with low permeability to water (Mangos 1973). It took
ten additional years to demonstrate that defective permeability of the
ductal cells to chloride ions may be the basis of defective reabsorption of
salt in the duct of the sweat gland in CF (Quinton, 1983). The search for the
explanation of this one feature of the organ pathophysiology of CF has been
difficult, tiring, often frustrating and perplexing and filled with
controversies and disappointments. It is fortunate that the investigators did
not give up their efforts but continued to carefully analyze the various
physiologic and pathophysiologic patterns and to pursue new leads. In the
course of the past thirty years, the CF-related research has contributed
immensely in many areas of physiology such as that of exocrine glands. We
have learned that progress in pathophysiology comes very slowly in spite of
immense efforts when the normal physiology and biochemistry are not
known.

Today, a similar situation exists in the area of cellular pathophysiology of CF. There are many exciting leads from past research. Each one of them could be the one to lead us, if appropriately followed, to the basic molecular defect of CF. The problem is that our knowledge of cell morphology, composition, function and biochemistry in the various cell systems involved in CF pathophysiology is so incomplete that we cannot follow the leads we have into the inner world of the cell. It is hoped that rapid advances in the studies of cell structure, composition and function will permit the investigators of this disease to unravel its mystery and, hopefully, devise new methods of therapy or prevention for the patients.

One of the most impressive findings of recent years has been the demonstration of increased electronegativity across the epithelia of the respiratory tract and the duct of the sweat gland in CF. It has been suggested that this is due to increased reabsorption of sodium in the airways which, if coupled with net transepithelial water fluxes, would tend to "dessicate" the airway fluid and thus affect the physicochemical behavior of mucus and the function of cilia in CF. However, such increased reabsorption of sodium could not explain the abnormality of handling of sodium and chloride by the duct of the sweat gland, where decreased reabsorption of sodium and chloride has been observed. The recent proposal that "decreased" permeability of the epithelial cell membrane of the airway epithelium to chloride ions may be an important component of the transport abnormality of CF in both airway epithelia and sweat ducts has more appeal in that it could explain the transepithelial transport abnormality in both organs. If, however, we are to accept defective chloride permeability of cell membranes as the universal abnormality of CF, many questions will remain unanswered: What happens in the gastrointestinal tract? Why is there no abnormality in the production of the cerebrospinal fluid in the choroid plexuses, a process known to depend on transcellular fluxes of chloride ions? Why are there no demonstrable abnormalities in the kidneys? Obviously, there is need for many additional studies in the areas of transepithelial transport of ions, particularly of chloride, if the recent observations are to become meaningful in understanding the pathophysiology of CF.

If the transepithelial transport abnormalities of CF are clarified at the organ in situ level or with organ explants in vitro, then one must assume that the cells demonstrating these abnormalities must also demonstrate abnormalities in their handling of monovalent ions resulting in compositional or functional changes. Unfortunately studies of these parameters of cell function cannot be studied with the cells in situ; there is need to isolate the appropriate cells and to study them in vitro. Furthermore, if proliferation of these cells can be accomplished under conditions of cell culture and if the in vitro proliferating cells maintain the presumed expressions of cell pathophysiology of CF, these in vitro cell systems may provide some of the most valuable tools in CF research. The same could be said about secretory cells from exocrine glands of patients with CF. In one set of such cells (the parotid acinar cells) compositional and functional cellular abnormalities have been demonstrated in CF. Over 90% of death of CF patients results from pulmonary insufficiency associated with overwhelming pulmonary infection by Pseudomonas aeruginosa. The reasons for this chronic colonization of CF patients by this ubiquitous, usually non-pathogenic, organism is not known; therefore, it is important to consider the characteristics of the CF cells which form the environment conducive for growth of the Pseudomonas. While no intrinsic morphological or compositional abnormality of the epithelial or glandular cells of the airways have been discernible, the mucous secretions in CF patients are different from those of normals. A relative decrease in the number of sialic acid producing cells and relative increase in the number of sulfated mucin producing cells was shown to be prominent histochemical features of lesions in CF (Lev and Spicer, 1965 and Spicer and Lev, 1966). The role of adherence of Pseudomonas to respiratory tract mucins in the pathogenesis of colonization and infection needs careful consideration. Adherence of Pseudomonas to mucin strands in airways of animals has been demonstrated (Ramphal and Pyle, 1983b and Boyd, Ramphal, Rice and Mangos, 1983). While the role of adherence to mucins may be protective in the normal mucociliary clearance system, in CF airways where the system becomes impaired, adherence to tenacious mucus in obstructed airways may potentiate colonization and proliferation of the Pseudomonas as suggested by Ramphal and Pyle (1983a). Moreover, the nature of the microorganism adapted to the environment of the CF respiratory tract may be an important consideration in the pathogenesis of the pulmonary involvement. A mucoid variant of Pseudomonas aeruginosa eventually becomes the predominant microorganisms colonizing the airways of CF patients, and the appearance of this variant in the sputum is associated with the precipitous deterioration of the patients' pulmonary function (Kulczycki, Murphy and Bellanti, 1978). Adherence of mucoid Pseudomonas to injured airways of animals was greater than adherence of non-mucoid Pseudomonas (Ramphal and Pyle, 1983b). Moreover, current work in the author's laboratory suggests that phagocytosis of mucoid variants by cultured pulmonary macrophages is delayed as compared to non-mucoid Pseudomonas. Increased adherence to mucus and delayed phagocytosis of mucoid Pseudomonas could account for the precipitous pulmonary involvement once the mucoid variants become established in the CF airways. Research is needed to determine the mechanisms for establishment of the environment conducive to growth and mutation of Pseudomonas to mucoid forms. This complex process involves many of the cellular systems addressed above. Since so little has been established as morphological or compositional differences intrinsic to CF cells, our attention directed to the physiology of the cellular systems may be the appropriate avenue to lead us to the basic defect in cystic fibrosis.

The following questions must be answered: Are these changes present in all secretory cells from exocrine glands of CF patients? What are the regulatory abnormalities that maintain this alteration of electrolyte homeostasis in these cells? Are these compositional and functional changes present in cells other than secretory, such as the circulating leukocytes or the cultured skin fibroblasts? What is the molecular basis for such a presumed alteration in cell regulation? These and many other questions call for research to answer them. The need is there. Every observation in cell pathophysiology of CF listed in this paper could potentially be the missing link that will allow us to locate the basic abnormality of CF. No lead should be left unexplored.

## REFERENCES

Antonowicz, I., Reddy, V., Khaw, K.T., Shwachman, H., 1968. Lactase deficiency in patients with cystic fibrosis. Pediatrics, 42, 492-498.

Ansah, T-A and Katz, S., 1980. Characterization of a plasma membrane enriched fraction of human skin fibroblasts derived from cystic fibrosis patients and age-matched controls. Proc. West Pharmacol. Soc., 23, 389-395.

Ansah, T-A. and Katz, S., 1980. Evidence for a $Ca^{++}$ transport deficiency in patients with cystic fibrosis. Cell Calcium, 1, 195-199.

Boyd, R.L., Ramphal, R., Rice, R., and Mangos, J.A., 1983. Chronic colonization of rat airways with Pseudomonas aeruginosa. Infect. and Immun. 39, 1403-1410.

Briggman, J.V., Bank, H., Graves, J.S. and Spicer, S.S., 1983. Freeze fracture morphology of the tight junctions of the eccrine sweat gland from patients with cystic fibrosis. Lab. Investig., 49, 62-68.

Chow, C.W., Landau, L.I., and Taussig, L.M., 1982. Bronchial mucous glands in the newborn with cystic fibrosis. Europ. J. Ped., 139, 240-243.

Danes, B.S., and Bearn, A.G., 1968. A genetic cell marker in cystic fibrosis of the pancreas. Lancet, 1, 1061-1064.

Davis, B. and Nadel, J.A., 1983. Control of airway secretions in cystic fibrosis, in Textbook of Cystic Fibrosis (Eds Lloyd-Still and Wright), pp 43-52. PSG, Inc., Boston, Bristol, London.

Davis, P.B., Dieckman, L., Boat, T.F., Stern, R.C. and Doershuk, C.F., 1983. Beta adrenergic receptors in lymphocytes and granulocytes from patients with cystic fibrosis. J. Clin. Inves., 71, 1787-1795.

Davis, P.B. and Kaliner, M., 1983. Autonomic nervous system abnormalities in cystic fibrosis. J. Chron. Dis., 36, 269-278.

di Sant'Agnese, P.A., Darling, R.C., Perera, G.A. and Shea, E., 1953. Abnormal electrolyte composition of sweat in cystic fibrosis. Pediatrics, 12, 549-555.

Field, M., 1982. Intestinal ion transport mechanisms and their regulation, in Fluid and Electrolyte Abnormalities in Exocrine Glands in Cystic Fibrosis (Eds Quinton, Martinez and Hopfer), pp 227-239. San Francisco Press, Inc., San Francisco.

Gnegy, M.E., Erickson, R.P. and Markovac, J., 1981. Increased calmodulin in cultured skin fibroblasts from patients with cystic fibrosis. Biochem. Medicine, 26, 294-298.

Graft, D.F., Mischeler, E., Farrell, P.M. and Busse, W.W., 1982. Chemiluminescence in adolescent patients with cystic fibrosis. Am. Rev. Resp. Dis., 125, 540-543.

Hadorn, B. and Roscher, A.A., 1982. Exocrine pancreatic function in cystic fibrosis, in Fluid and Electrolyte Abnormalities in Exocrine Glands in Cystic Fibrosis (Eds Quinton, Martinez and Hopfer), pp 182-192. San Francisco Press, Inc., San Francisco.

Harris, A. and Bramwell, M.E., 1983. Cystic fibrosis: a detailed analysis of fibroblast membrane glycoproteins. Clin. Chimica. Acta, 128, 41-51.

Harris, A. and Swallow, D. 1981. Alpha-L-fucosidase in cystic fibrosis: analysis of skin fibroblasts and liver. Clin. Chimica Acta, 116, 171-178.

Hopfer, U., 1982. Pathophysiological considerations relevant to intestinal obstruction in Cystic Fibrosis, in Fluid and Electrolyte Abnormalities in Exocrine Glands in Cystic Fibrosis (Eds Quinton, Martinez and Hopfer), pp 241-251. San Francisco Press, Inc., San Francisco.

Jessup, W. and Dean, R.T., 1982. Lysosomal enzyme secretion by cystic fibrosis fibroblasts is normal. Clin. Chimica. Acta, 126, 265-273.

Knowles, M.R., Gatzy, J. and Boucher, R., 1981. Increased bioelectric potential difference across respiratory epithelia in cystic fibrosis. New Engl. J. Med., 305, 1488-1492.

Knowles, M.R., Stutts, M.J., Spock, A., Fisher, N., Gatzy, J.T. and Boucher, R.C., 1983. Abnormal ion permeation through cystic fibrosis Respiratory Epithelium. Science, 221, 1067-1070.

Knowles, M.R., Gatzy, J and Boucher, R., 1983. Relative ion permeability of normal and cystic fibrosis nasal epithelium. J. Clin. Invest., 71, 1410-1417.

Kulczycki, L.L., Murphy, T.M., and Bellanti, J.A., 1978. Pseudomonas colonization in cystic fibrosis. JAMA, 240, 30-34.

Lev, R. and Spicer, S.S., 1965. A histochemical comparison of human epithelial mucins in normal and in hypersecretory states including pancreatic cystic fibrosis. Am. J. Pathol., 46, 23-47.

Lobeck, C.C., 1966. In Research on the Pathogenesis of Cystic Fibrosis (Ed P.A. di Sant'Agnese), pp 107-110. Wichersham Printing Co., Lancaster, Pennsylvania.

Mangos, J.A., 1983. Cytosolic [$Ca^{++}$] measurements in buccal epithelial cells from CF patients and controls. Abstract, In Proceedings of the 12th Annual Meeting of the European Working Group for Cystic Fibrosis, Athens, Greece, Oct 3-4, p 21.

Mangos, J.A., 1983. Unpublished observations.

Mangos, J.A. and McSherry, N.R., 1967. Sodium transport: inhibitory factor in sweat of patients with cystic fibrosis. Science, 158, 135-137.

Mangos, J.A., 1973a. Transductal fluxes of $Na^+$, $K^+$ and water in the human eccrine sweat gland. Am. J. Physiol., 224, 1235-1240.

Mangos, J.A., 1973b. Microperfusion study of the sweat gland abnormality in cystic fibrosis. Texas Rep. Biol. Med., 31, 651-663.

Mangos, J.A. and Donnelly, W.H., 1981. Isolated parotid acinar cells from patients with cystic fibrosis: functional characterization. J. Dent. Res., 60, 797-804.

Markovac, J., Erickson, R.P. and Hieber, V., 1981. Increased cAMP levels and beta-adrenergic agonist binding in cystic fibrosis. Biochem. Medicine, 26, 199-306.

Markovics, B., Gyurkovitz, K., Laszlo, A. and Szabo, L., 1982. Altered peroxide metabolism in erythrocytes from children with cystic fibrosis. Clin. Chimica Acta, 125, 59-62.

Martinez, J.R., 1982. Alterations in salivary gland structure and function in cystic fibrosis, in Fluid and Electrolyte Abnormalities in Exocrine Glands in Cystic Fibrosis (Eds Quinton, Martinez and Hopfer), pp 125-142. San Francisco Press, Inc., San Francisco.

Matalon, R. and Dorfman, A., 1968. Acid mucopolysaccharides in cultured fibroblasts of cystic fibrosis of the pancreas. Biochem. Biophys. Res. Comm., 33, 954-959.

Morin, C.L., Roy, C.C., LaSalle, R. and Bonin, A., 1976. Small bowel mucosal dysfunction in patients with cystic fibrosis. J. Pediatr. 88, 213-221.

Nere, J., Van Geffel, R., Hanocq, M. and Molle, L., 1983. Plasma and erythrocyte zinc, copper and selenium in cystic fibrosis. Acta Pediatr. Scand., 72, 437-440.

Neutra, M.R. and Madara, J.L., 1982. The structural basis of intestinal ion transport, in Fluid and Electrolyte Abnormalities in Exocrine Glands in Cystic Fibrosis (Eds Quinton, Martinez and Hopfer), pp 194-226. San Francisco Press, Inc., San Francisco.

Owen, E., 1978. Surface labeling of human skin fibroblasts of healthy and cystic fibrosis subjects. J. Mol. Med., 3, 203-108.

Pallaricini, J.C., Wiessman, U., Uhlendorf, W.B. and di Sant'Agnese, P.A., 1976. Glycogen content of tissue culture fibroblasts from patients with cystic fibrosis and other heritable disorders. Pediatrics 77, 280-286.

Parkins, R.A., 1963. The diagnosis of cystic fibrosis by rectal suction biopsy. Lancet 2, 851-855.

Quinton, P.M., 1981. Effects of some ion transport inhibitors on secretion and reabsorption in intact and perfused single human sweat glands. Pfluegers Archiv. Ges. Physiol., 391, 309-313.

Quinton, P.M. and Tormey, J.M., 1976. Localization of Na/K ATPase sites in the secretory and reabsorptive epithelia of perfused eccrine sweat glands: A question as to the role of the enzyme in secretion. J. Membr. Biol., 29, 383-399.

Quinton, P.M. and Bijman, J., 1983a. Higher bioelectric potentials due to decreased chloride absorption in the sweat glands of patients with cystic fibrosis. New Engl. J. Med., 308, 1185-1189.

Quinton, P.M., 1983b. Chloride impermeability in cystic fibrosis. Nature, 301, 421-422.

Ramphal, R. and Pyle, M., 1983a. Evidence for mucins and sialic acid as receptors for Pseudomonas aeruginosa in the lower respiratory tract. Infect. and Immun., 41, 339-344.

Ramphal, R. and Pyle, M., 1983b. Adherence of mucoid and non-mucoid Pseudomonas aeruginosa to acid-injured tracheal epithelium. Infect. and Immun., 41, 345-351.

Reznick, V.M., Schneider, J.A. and Mendoza, S.A., 1981. Na and K dependence of the Na/K pump in cystic fibrosis fibroblasts. Proc. Nat. Acad. Sci., 78, 7143-7146.

Rogiers, V., Mandelbaum, I., Mozes, N., Vertongen, F., Dab, I., Crakaert, R. and Vis, H.L., 1982. In vitro study of the incorporation and transport of nonesterified fatty acids into the phospholipids of the red blood cell membranes of cystic fibrosis patients. Pediatr. Research, 16, 761-768.

Rubin, R.P., 1982.  Calcium and cellular secretion.  Plenum Press, New York-London.

Rudick, V.L., Rudick, M.J. and Jones, P.M., 1983.  Glycosyl acceptors in intact and permealized normal and cystic fibrosis fibroblasts.  J. Cellular Physiol., 115, 143-150.

Scanlin, T.F. and Glick, M.C., 1981.  Alpha-L-fucosidase in cystic fibrosis. Clin. Chimica Acta, 114, 169-274.

Shapiro, B.L. and Lam, L.F.-H., 1982.  Calcium and age in fibroblasts from control subjects and patients with cystic fibrosis. Science, 216, 417-419.

Shapiro, B.L., Lam, L.F.-H. and Feigal, R.J., 1982.  Mitochondrial NADH dehydrogenase in cystic fibrosis:   enzyme kinetics in cultured fibroblasts. Am. J. Hum. Genetics, 34, 846-852.

Spicer, S.S. and Lev, R., 1966.  Histochemical methods for mucosubstances and their application in normal and pathologic states, in Research on Pathogenesis of Cystic Fibrosis (Ed di Sant'Agnese),  pp 26-50. Wickersham Printing Co., Harrisburg, Pennsylvania.

Spicer, S.S., Briggman, J.V and Baron, D.A., 1982.   Morphological and cytochemical correlates of transport in sweat glands of normal and cystic fibrosis subjects, in Fluid and Electrolyte Abnormalities in Exocrine Glands in Cystic Fibrosis (Eds Quinton, Martinez and Hopfer), pp 11-34. San Francisco Press, Inc., San Francisco.

Spicer, S.S., di Sant'Agnese, P.A., Vincent, R.A. and Ulane, M., 1980. Ultrastructural and cytochemical comparison of cultured normal and cystic fibrosis fibroblasts. Exp. Mol. Pathol., 33, 104-121.

Sturgess, J.M., 1982. Morphological characteristics of the bronchial mucosa in cystic fibrosis, in Fluid and Electrolyte Abnormalites of Exocrine Glands in Cystic Fibrosis (Eds Quinton, Martinez and Hopfer), pp 254-270. San Francisco Press, San Francisco.

Talamo, R.C., Rosenstein, B.J. and Berninger, R.W., 1983.  Cystic Fibrosis, in The Metabolic Basis of Inherited Disease (Eds. Stanbury, Wyngaarden, Fredrickson, Goldstein and Brown), pp 1889-1917.  McGraw-Hill, New York.

Thomassen, M.J., Boxerbaum, B., Demko, C.A., Kuchenbrod, P.J., Dearborn, D., and Wood, R.E., 1979.  Inhibitory effect of cystic fibrosis serum on Pseudomonas phagocytosis by rabbit and human alveolar macrophages. Pediatr. Res., 13, 1085-1088.

Thomassen, M.J., Demko, C.A., Wood, R.E., Tandler, B., Dearborn, D.G., Boxerbaum, B., and Kuchenbrod, P.J., 1980. Ultrastructure and function of alveolar macrophage from cystic fibrosis patients. Pediatr. Res., 14, 715-721.

Winnie, G.B., Klinger, J.D., Sharman, J.M. and Thomassen, M.J., 1982. Induction of phagocytic inhibitory activity in cats with chronic Pseudomonas aeruginosa pulmonary infection. Infect. and Immun., 38, 1088-1093.

Wood, R.E. and Legris, J., 1982. The role of fluid in electrolyte transport abnormalities in the pulmonary pathophysiology of cystic fibrosis, in Fluid and Electrolyte Abnormalities in Exocrine Glands in Cystic Fibrosis (Eds Quinton, Martinez and Hopfer), pp 289-298. San Francisco Press Inc., San Francisco.

AUTONOMIC SECRETORY RESPONSES OF CONTROL AND CF SUBMANDIBULAR ACINAR
CELLS.

M.A. McPherson, R.L. Dormer, J.A. Dodge and M.C. Goodchild,
Departments of Medical Biochemistry and Child Health, Welsh National
School of Medicine, Heath Park, Cardiff, U.K.

Our aim was to directly investigate whether the basic disturbance
in cystic fibrosis (CF) is due to abnormal autonomic regulation of
secretion in exocrine acinar cells.

We have studied control of secretion from human submandibular
acini and tissue fragments in vitro. Tissues were obtained from four
control (non CF) individuals and one CF patient. Control tissues were
from adult (age 26-48 yr) submandibular glands removed during operation for ductal calculi. The CF tissue was early (within 30 min)
post-mortem tissue from a two month old infant. Histology showed
well-differentiated acinar tissue. Viability was confirmed by
measurements of ATP concentrations and lactate dehydrogenase release.
Secretion was determined by measuring release of $^{14}$C glucosamine-
labelled mucins and amylase into the medium, in the presence or
absence of neurotransmitters. The results, which are summarized
below, are means of 3, with S.E.M.s $\leq$ 10% (control) or of 2 (CF).

| Secretion (% control) | MUCINS | | AMYLASE | |
|---|---|---|---|---|
| | IP | NA | IP | NA |
| | (10µM) | (10µM) | (10µM) | (10µM) |
| CONTROL CELLS | 229 | 185 | 386 | 328 |
| + propranolol 30µM | 87 | 118 | 110 | 155 |
| + phentolamine 30µM | 242 | 237 | 420 | 386 |
| CF CELLS | 118 | 288 | 92 | 277 |

Isoproterenol (IP) and noradrenaline (NA) both stimulated
secretion from control acinar cells. Their actions were mediated by
stimulation of β-adrenergic receptors, since they were blocked by a
β-blocker (propranolol) but not by an α-blocker (phentolamine). In
the CF cells, IP did not stimulate secretion of mucins or amylase,
indicating a complete lack of β-adrenergic responsiveness; although
the cells responded to noradrenaline, a mixed α- and β-agonist.

These studies are the first to characterise the type of receptor
controlling human submandibular mucin secretion in vitro. The
results suggest a switch from β- to α-adrenergic function in CF
exocrine acinar cells, which we postulate could be mediated by
alteration in a cytosolic $Ca^{2+}$-dependent regulator protein.

This hypothesis would provide an explanation for a heterozygote
advantage in CF and might explain many of the metabolic and
secretory abnormalities observed in this disease.

Supported by the Cystic Fibrosis Research Trust.

# CHANGES OF $Ca^{2+}$-, ENERGY- AND MEMBRANE-METABOLISM IN MITOCHONDRIA FROM CF CELLS.

vonRuecker, A.; Bertele, R.M.; Harms, H.K.; Shin, Y.S.; Endres, W.
Universitaets Kinderklinik, Munich, FRG (Director : Prof. H.B. Hadorn)

Probably a single gene accounts for the different biochemical abnormalities reported in literature on CF. Therefore it seems reasonable to assume that some basic event of cellular function is involved in CF, otherwise the diversity of results is hardly comprehensible. Our studies focussed on the important intracellular messenger $Ca^{2+}$. Intracellular $Ca^{2+}$ levels in CF cells have been shown to be elevated by various research groups including ours. $Ca^{2+}$ levels in fibroblasts were elevated by 36-77 % (n=64), in leukocytes by 38-46 % (n=21)(determined by isotope detection). By examining the endoplasmic reticulum and mitochondria,which store up to 98 % of intracellular $Ca^{2+}$, we have found that CF mitochondria take up about 2-3 times more $Ca^{2+}$ than control or heterozygote mitochondria ($P < .0005$, n=22, Student's t-test). On the other hand the isolated endoplasmic reticulum or microsomal fractions of CF cells did not accumulate more $Ca^{2+}$ than controls or heterozygote microsomal fractions.

With the help of ruthenium red, an inhibitor of energy-dependent mitochondrial $Ca^{2+}$ uptake, we could show that $Ca^{2+}$ influx and efflux are elevated in isolated CF mitochondria, resulting in net $Ca^{2+}$ increase. This may be the cause for a derangement of the important cytosolic $Ca^{2+}$ level in vivo. Studies of $Ca^{2+}$ uptake and energy metabolism in isolated mitochondria with various inhibitors (atractyloside, oligomycin) showed that ATP-transport (i.e. adenine nucleotide translocase) and ATP-hydrolysis (i.e. ATP-synthase) are significantly changed in CF versus controls. Furthermore the electron transfer activities of various respiratory enzymes (e.g. NADH-oxidase, succinate-cytochrome c reductase) are changed in CF mitochondria. Since all of these changes concern enzymes or functions associated with the mitochondrial inner membrane, a disorder of membrane metabolism (i.e. membrane lipids) was considered.

Preliminary examinations of membrane phospholipids in mitochondria from cultured cells (resolved on Silica Gel 60 TLC plates) demonstrated four phospholipid classes : phosphatidylcholine, phosphatidylethanolamine, cardiolipin and phosphatidylserine (from which phosphatidylinositol was not distinguishable). In CF mitochondria the relative amount of cardiolipin was about 43-54 % of the amount in controls. Furthermore an accompanying trend toward decreased amounts of all phospholipids in CF was observed (0.07 versus 0.05 µg/mg protein; n=2). These results suggest a disorder of the mitochondrial membrane at the level of membrane phospholipids in CF, possibly causing the changes of various membrane associated enzymes (cf. above) and functions (e.g. the regulation of intracellular $Ca^{2+}$ by mitochondria).

- This work was supported by the Deutsche Forschungsgemeinschaft.

$Ca^{2+}$, STIMULUS–SECRETION COUPLING
AND CYSTIC FIBROSIS

R.M. Case

Department of Physiology, University of
Manchester, Manchester M13 9PT, UK

## CYSTIC FIBROSIS AND SECRETION

Cystic fibrosis is a disease of secretory epithelia. Such epithelia
are capable of at least two distinct secretory processes: electrolyte and water transport and the secretion of macromolecules. These
processes I have described in detail at the preceding cystic
fibrosis congress in Toronto (Case 1980*b*). In principle, electrolyte secretion is the unidirectional transport of ions across an
epithelium accompanied by water in isotonic proportions. Macromolecular secretion comprises the synthesis, intracellular transport,
storage and discharge of a macromolecular product, usually a protein
(e.g. digestive enzymes, hormones) or glycoprotein (e.g. mucus).
Some epithelial cells are adapted specifically for one type of
secretion; others are capable of both.

To date, the only proven defect of secretory epithelia in CF is a
reduced $Cl^-$ permeability of the epithelial cells lining the sweat
gland duct (which is responsible for the elevated sweat $Na^+$ and $Cl^-$
concentrations in CF subjects) and possibly also the respiratory
tract (Quinton, 1984). Whether this is also a defect of other
epithelia primarily affected in CF (e.g. pancreas, gut, salivary
glands) is as yet unknown. In the sweat glands, macromolecular
secretion is virtually absent, whereas it is a prominent feature of
the respiratory tract (mucus) and pancreas (digestive enzymes). It
is the latter, of course, rather than the sweat glands, which become
necrotic in CF. Does this mean that there is also a basic defect in
macromolecular secretion or merely that a reduced $Cl^-$ permeability
somehow prevents proper excretion of mucus and digestive enzymes
from the respiratory tract and pancreatic ductal system respectively? We simply do not know.

## CYSTIC FIBROSIS AND CELLULAR $Ca^{2+}$ HOMEOSTASIS

Although the cellular bases of electrolyte and macromolecular
secretory processes are quite different, both are subject to control
by the same hormones and neurotransmitters. In general, such
stimuli evoke responses in target cells, including secretory cells,
by modulating the intracellular concentrations of either cyclic
3',5'-adenosine monophosphate (cAMP), or $Ca^{2+}$, or both. (The role
of cGMP as an alternative or additional intracellular mediator
remains elusive; see below).

TABLE 1.  Altered $Ca^{2+}$ homeostasis in CF

| | |
|---|---|
| ↑ $Ca^{2+}$ concentration in CF salivary secretions | Martinez 1982 |
| ↑ $Ca^{2+}$ concentration in isolated CF parotid cells | Mangos & Donnelly 1981 |
| ↑ $Ca^{2+}$ concentration in cultured CF fibroblasts and ↓ $^{45}Ca$ efflux from preloaded cells | Shapiro et al 1980 Roomans et al 1983 |
| ↑ $Ca^{2+}$ concentration in CF fibroblasts during ageing | Shapiro & Lam 1982 |
| ↑ accumulation of $Ca^{2+}$ by mitochondria from CF fibroblasts | Shapiro et al 1980 |
| ↑ content of the $Ca^{2+}$-binding protein, calmodulin, in CF fibroblasts | Gnegy et al 1981 |
| ↓ $Mg^{2+}+Ca^{2+}$-ATPase activity in CF red cells and fibroblasts | Katz 1980 |
| ↑ net $Ca^{2+}$ flux and/or retention in human leucocytes, rabbit tracheal epithelium and guinea-pig gastrointestinal epithelium exposed to CF plasma | Banschbach et al 1978 Bogart et al 1979 Morrissey & Mehta 1981 |
| ↑ $Ca^{2+}$ concentration in normal fibroblasts exposed to culture medium from CF fibroblasts | Ceder & Roomans 1983 |

The sequence of events initiated by activation of cell surface receptors which culminates in the appropriate physiological response of the target cell is usually referred to as stimulus-response coupling (stimulus-secretion coupling in secretory cells).  A few secretory processes seem to be regulated solely by changes in intracellular cAMP concentrations, the most relevant being secretin-stimulated $HCO_3^-$ secretion by the pancreatic ductal epithelium (Case, 1979).  Others are regulated principally by $Ca^{2+}$, and yet more by either or both messengers.  Which messenger is involved depends upon the nature of the stimulus or, more correctly, on the receptor which is activated, since some agents can elevate intracellular cAMP concentration by acting on one type of receptor (e.g. β-adrenergic, histamine $H_2$, vasopressin $V_2$, $5-HT_2$) and mobilise cell $Ca^{2+}$ by acting on a second set of receptors (α-adrenergic, $H_1$,$V_1$ and $5-HT_1$).

A number of observations indicate that cell $Ca^{2+}$ homeostasis may be disturbed in CF (Table 1).  Taken together these observations suggest that impaired cellular handling of $Ca^{2+}$, perhaps leading to enhanced accumulation of $Ca^{2+}$ by the cell, could be involved in the pathology of CF.  Therefore, the purpose of this article is to discuss factors involved in cell $Ca^{2+}$ homeostasis and review the role of $Ca^{2+}$ in stimulus-secretion coupling in the context of the pathophysiology of CF.  Because of the limitations on space, references will be restricted to reviews or recent research papers which lead into the literature.

## INTRACELLULAR $Ca^{2+}$ HOMEOSTASIS

The concentration of $Ca^{2+}$ in extracellular fluid is close to $10^{-3}$ M; approximately half of this $Ca^{2+}$ is ionised, the rest being bound to protein.  The *total* concentration of $Ca^{2+}$ within the cells is also

TABLE 2.  Some values of ionised Ca$^{2+}$ concentration in the cytoplasm of secretory cells

| | | Ca$^{2+}$ conc (M) | | |
|---|---|---|---|---|
| Cell | Technique | rest. | stim. | Reference |
| *Chironomus* sal gl | aequorin[2] | <5x10$^{-7}$ | | Rose & Loewenstein '76 |
| *Phormia* sal gl | electrode | 4x10$^{-7}$ | 7x10$^{-7}$ | O'Doherty '80 |
| *Calliphora* sal gl | electrode | < 10$^{-7}$ | > 10$^{-6}$ | Berridge '80 |
| Pancreatic acinus | electrode | 4x10$^{-7}$ | 1x10$^{-6}$ | O'Doherty & Stark '82 |
| Pancreatic acinus[1] | electrode | 4x10$^{-7}$ | | Streb *et al* '83 |
| Pancreatic acinus | aequorin | 2x10$^{-6}$ | 4x10$^{-6}$ | Dormer '83 |
| Pancreatic acinus | calculated[3] | 5x10$^{-8}$ | 1x10$^{-6}$ | Maruyama *et al* '83 |
| Platelet | quin-2[4] | 1x10$^{-7}$ | 3x10$^{-6}$ | Rink *et al* '82 |
| Adrenal medulla | quin-2 | 1x10$^{-7}$ | 4x10$^{-7}$ | Knight & Kesteven '83 |
| Hepatocyte | quin-2 | 2x10$^{-7}$ | 6x10$^{-7}$ | Charest *et al* '83 |

[1]Permeabilised cells; steady-state Ca$^{2+}$ concentration measured in incubation medium with external Ca$^{2+}$-electrode.
[2]Aequorin is a bioluminescent photoprotein, extracted from the jellyfish *Aequorea forskalea*, which emits light on binding Ca$^{2+}$.
[3]Calculated from information on the number of K$^{+}$-channels per cell and the regulation of this channel by Ca$^{2+}$; see text: 'The role of Ca$^{2+}$ in secretion'.
[4]Quin-2 is a synthetic, fluorescent Ca$^{2+}$-indicator.

close to 10$^{-3}$ M, slightly more in secretory and muscle cells. However, 99.99 % of all cell Ca$^{2+}$ is either bound to soluble proteins or to membrane proteins, or is sequestered within cytoplasmic organelles. Hence the concentration of *ionised* Ca$^{2+}$ in the cytosol (which can now be directly measured using a number of techniques) is close to 10$^{-7}$ M in a variety of cells (Blinks *et al*, 1982), including secretory cells (Table 2). The total, not free, cytosolic Ca$^{2+}$ is probably about 10$^{-4}$ M (i.e. the cytosol contains a Ca$^{2+}$-buffer system). The total Ca$^{2+}$ within organelles (endoplasmic reticulum, mitochondria and secretory vesicles) is in the millimolar range. However much of this is non-ionic (i.e. non-exchangeable) so that the free Ca$^{2+}$ concentration is probably about 10$^{-5}$-10$^{-4}$ M.

An enormous gradient for Ca$^{2+}$ entry into the cytoplasm therefore exists across the cell plasma membrane and across membranes of intracellular organelles. It is these gradients, together with the appropriate chemical properties of the Ca$^{2+}$ ion, which permit Ca$^{2+}$ its unique role as an intracellular mediator. During stimulation, entry of Ca$^{2+}$ into the cytosol from the extracellular space or from intracellular stores is accelerated so that cytosolic free Ca$^{2+}$ concentration rises up to 5-fold (Table 2). Since an average small cell contains about 10$^{-19}$ moles of free Ca$^{2+}$, the amount of Ca$^{2+}$ required for a 5-fold rise in concentration is minute.

Cell membranes are not totally impermeable to Ca$^{2+}$. Some Ca$^{2+}$ will therefore leak into the cytoplasm at all times. To counter this

TABLE 3.   Postulated and proven mechanisms involved in cell
           $Ca^{2+}$ homeostasis. (Modified from Case, 1980a)

$Ca^{2+}$ entry across the plasma membrane

          Passive entry
          Voltage-dependent $Ca^{2+}$ channels
          Voltage-independent $Ca^{2+}$ channels
          Pinocytosis

$Ca^{2+}$ uptake and release by intracellular membranes and proteins

          Inner surface of plasma membrane
          Sarcoplasmic and endoplasmic reticulum
          Mitochondria
          The nucleus
          The Golgi complex and secretory granules
          Other vesicular stores (e.g. lysosomes, non-secretory granules)
          $Ca^{2+}$-binding proteins (low affinity and high affinity)

$Ca^{2+}$ exit across the plasma membrane

          ATP-driven $Ca^{2+}$ pumps (i.e. $Ca^{2+}$-ATPases)
          $Na^+/Ca^{2+}$ exchange
          $Ca^{2+}/H^+$ exchange
          Exocytosis of granule contents

Not all mechanisms exist in all cells.  Thus $Na^+/Ca^{2+}$ exchange may be
restricted to electrically excitable cells; $Ca^{2+}/H^+$ exchange occurs in
prokaryotes and perhaps red cells


leak, and to remove $Ca^{2+}$ which enters during stimulation, a number
of $Ca^{2+}$-transport systems exist in cell membranes (Table 3).  These
systems maintain equilibrium.  If they fail, cytoplasmic $Ca^{2+}$
concentration will rise and, ultimately, cell death will ensue
(Farber, 1981).

Although total cell $Ca^{2+}$ concentration may be elevated in CF (Table
1), no measurements of cytosolic free $Ca^{2+}$ concentration have yet
been made.  Clearly this is crucial information.

## CHARACTERISTICS OF RESPONSES MEDIATED BY $Ca^{2+}$

From the foregoing discussion it is possible to draw up a list of
characteristics of cellular responses mediated by $Ca^{2+}$.  These
characteristics, which have been described in detail elsewhere,
(Case 1978), are analogous to those established by Sutherland and
colleagues in the case of cAMP.

1. The stimulus will elevate cytosolic free $Ca^{2+}$ concentration and
such elevation should occur before the simultaneously monitored
physiological response.  Although it is now possible to measure
cytosolic $Ca^{2+}$ concentration, only in muscle has it yet been possible
to show that an increase occurs before the cell response.

2. Experimental elevation of intracellular free $Ca^{2+}$ concentration
by non-specific means will mimic the action of the stimulus and/or
enhance submaximal stimulation.  This may be achieved in a number

of ways: (a) By direct injection of Ca$^{2+}$ through micropipettes inserted in the cell. This technique obviously has limited application (the response must be 'visible') but has been shown to cause neurotransmitter release and exocytosis in mast cells. (b) By accelerating Ca$^{2+}$ into the cell. One way of doing this is to expose the target tissue to a divalent cation-selective ionophore (A23187, ionomycin). In electrically excitable cells (see below), depolarisation will increase Ca$^{2+}$ entry. (c) By accelerating Ca$^{2+}$ release from intracellular stores. Calcium-ionophores may do this since they do not remain localised specifically in the plasma membrane. Other agents which may release intracellular Ca$^{2+}$ include caffeine (acting on sarcoplasmic reticulum) and inhibitors of oxidative phosphorylation (acting on mitochondria). (d) By hindering Ca$^{2+}$ exit across the plasma membrane. In cells possessing Na$^+$/Ca$^{2+}$ exchange channels, this may be achieved by removing extracellular Na$^+$. (e) By hindering Ca$^{2+}$ uptake into intracellular stores.

3. The effect of stimulus will be reduced by agents which either block Ca$^{2+}$ entry into the cell (see below) or the release of Ca$^{2+}$ from intracellular stores (e.g. trimethoxybenzoate compounds such as TMB-8), depending on the source of Ca$^{2+}$ used in coupling.

4. The stimulus will accelerate efflux of Ca$^{2+}$ from the cell. This can be most easily detected using $^{45}$Ca$^{2+}$ as a tracer, but also in some cases by using extracellular Ca$^{2+}$-sensitive electrodes. Where the extracellular space is an important source of Ca$^{2+}$ for coupling, it should also be possible to observe an increased influx of Ca$^{2+}$ into the cell.

5. Stimulation should alter (usually increase) the binding of Ca$^{2+}$ to regulatory proteins. To demonstrate this the site of regulation must be identified. As we shall see progress in this area in secretory tissues is slow.

## SOURCES OF Ca$^{2+}$ FOR STIMULUS-SECRETION COUPLING

Clearly, stimulus-evoked elevation of cytosolic free Ca$^{2+}$ concentration could, in theory, be achieved in a number of ways, namely by modulating the Ca$^{2+}$-permeability, Ca$^{2+}$-binding or Ca$^{2+}$-transporting properties of one or more of the membranes listed in Table 3. In practice it seems usually to be achieved either by accelerating Ca$^{2+}$ entry across the plasma membrane from the extracellular space, or by releasing Ca$^{2+}$ from an intracellular store, or by a combination of the two.

Most electrically-excitable cells possess voltage-dependent Ca$^{2+}$ channels which are 'opened' by depolarisation (e.g. after an action potential), thereby accelerating Ca$^{2+}$ entry and elevating intracellular Ca$^{2+}$ concentration. Such channels can be blocked by a variety of organic agents (e.g. verapamil, nifedipine) and by competing divalent and trivalent cations (e.g. Mg$^{2+}$, Co$^{2+}$, La$^{3+}$) (Rahwan, 1983).

Nerves and some endocrine cells (notably adrenal chromaffin cells and islet β-cells) possess such channels and in these cells accelerated $Ca^{2+}$ entry in response to appropriate stimuli plays an important role in stimulus-secretion coupling.

However, epithelial cells do not possess voltage-sensitive $Ca^{2+}$ channels and therefore this mechanism cannot be used. The suggestion by Sorscher and Breslow (1982) that clinical trials of $Ca^{2+}$-channel blockers be initiated in CF patients is therefore unfounded. Nonetheless, the extracellular space does seem to be an important source of $Ca^{2+}$ for stimulus-secretion coupling in a variety of epithelial cells (Table 4). How $Ca^{2+}$ entry is accelerated in such cells is unknown. Using patch-clamp techniques, Petersen and colleagues have been able to characterise two cation channels in the acinar cell plasma membranes of pancreas and salivary glands. One is specific for $K^+$; the other does not discriminate between monovalent cations. It is possible that a small $Ca^{2+}$ current, too small to be detected, may pass through the latter (see Case, 1984). An alternative mechanism for regulating $Ca^{2+}$ entry into epithelial cells is considered below.

It is also clear from Table 4 that a number of secretory cells, most noticeably pancreatic acinar cells, rely largely on mobilizing $Ca^{2+}$ from intracellular stores. In these cells $Ca^{2+}$ influx is hardly changed during stimulation and the secretory response is not related to the extracellular $Ca^{2+}$ concentration.

TABLE 4.  A comparison between various secretory tissues of the relative importance of intracellular and extracellular sources of $Ca^{2+}$ for stimulus-secretion coupling

| Target | Stimulus | Major source of $Ca^{2+}$ | | References |
| | | Extra-cellular | Intra-cellular | |
| --- | --- | --- | --- | --- |
| nerve | depolarization | ✓ | | Douglas '74 |
| adrenal medulla | ACh | ✓ | | Douglas '74 |
| mast cell | antigen | ✓ | | Douglas '74 |
| mast cell | 48/80 | | ✓ | Douglas '74 |
| islet β-cell | glucose | ✓ | ✓ | Wollheim & Sharp '81 |
| platelets | e.g. thrombin | | ✓ | Feinstein '80 |
| pancreatic acinus | ACh/CCK-PZ | | ✓ | Case '78 |
| parotid gland | β-adren | | ✓ | Butcher & Putney '80 |
| | ACh/α-adren | ✓ | ✓ | Butcher & Putney '80 |
| mandibular gland | ACh | ✓ | | Hunter et al '83 |
| insect sal gland | 5-HT | ✓ | ✓ | Berridge & Lipke '79 |
| sweat gland* | ACh/α-adren | ✓ | | Sato & Sato '81 |
| ileal mucosa* | e.g. 5-HT/ACh | ✓ | | Donowitz '83 |

*data are very incomplete for these epithelia

It is not yet possible to explain what determines whether the major
source of Ca$^{2+}$ for stimulus-secretion coupling is intracellular or
extracellular. Since different stimuli acting on the same cell (e.g.
the mast cell and parotid) use different sources, the choice cannot
depend upon the embryological origin of the cell (though, as
discussed above, cells or neural origin seem usually to use extracellular Ca$^{2+}$); nor does it depend on the size of the cell or the
nature of the secretory process (electrolyte versus macromolecular
secretion). The nature of the stimulus or, more correctly, the
receptor activated, is clearly an important, but not exclusive
factor.

Unlike endocrine cells, epithelial cells are polarised; their
receptors lie on the basolateral membrane while secretion occurs
across the luminal membrane. Since, as mentioned previously, the
cytosol has a large Ca$^{2+}$ buffering capacity (Rose & Loewenstein,
1976), it seems unlikely that Ca$^{2+}$ crossing the basolateral membrane
could directly influence secretory events at the luminal membrane.
Hence, even those epithelial cells which use extracellular Ca$^{2+}$
probably rely on an intracellular chain of events involving Ca$^{2+}$
stores.

## INTRACELLULAR Ca$^{2+}$ STORES

It is obvious that release of Ca$^{2+}$ from, and re-uptake into, intracellular stores play  an important role in regulating intracellular
Ca$^{2+}$ concentration and hence secretion. Many of the potential stores
listed in the middle section of Table 3 have been claimed as
reservoirs through which Ca$^{2+}$ is cycled during stimulus-secretion
coupling. It seems likely that Ca$^{2+}$ within the Golgi complex,
secretory granules and lysozomes is bound to secretory components
and is ultimately discharged from the cell during exocytosis. As
such it is probably non-labile and not involved in coupling, though
there have been occasional claims to the contrary. The same is
probably true of Ca$^{2+}$ in the nucleus.

The main debate centres on the relative importance of the inner
surface of the plasma membrane, the endoplasmic reticulum and mitochondria. The former may function as a store of 'trigger' calcium
which is released on stimulation and itself causes Ca$^{2+}$ release from
other internal stores.

Of the two major Ca$^{2+}$ reservoirs, the endoplasmic reticulum and
mitochondria, the former is more likely to be a stimulable store
since it has a high affinity for Ca$^{2+}$, but a relatively low
capacity (in most cells) and recent evidence from a number of
secretory cells (e.g. the pancreatic acinar cell; Streb et al, 1983)
supports this hypothesis. The mitochondria have a large capacity
but lower affinity for Ca$^{2+}$ and are therefore more likely to act as
internal Ca$^{2+}$ buffers.

## RELEASE OF Ca$^{2+}$ FROM INTRACELLULAR STORES

Stimuli which act inside a cell (e.g. steroid hormones, light) could presumably modulate the properties of both the plasma membrane and intracellular membranes directly. However, stimuli which evoke secretion bind to receptors on the outer plasma membrane and hence can only directly influence the properties of that membrane. If they are to modulate the properties of intracellular membranes, a link between the two membranes is necessary.

Direct connections, analogous to the T-tubules in skeletal muscle have been claimed in some cells (Henkart & Nelson, 1979). But even in skeletal muscle, despite much effort, it is still not certain how depolarisation of the T-tubule membrane evokes release of $Ca^{2+}$ from the sarcoplasmic reticulum at triads. The favoured mechanism suggests that charge transfer across the triad membrane is responsible. This mechanism cannot be involved in epithelial cells since they are not influenced by charge. A second mechanism, $Ca^{2+}$-induced $Ca^{2+}$ release, remains a possibility in smooth muscle and there is some evidence for it in some secretory cells. Such trigger-$Ca^{2+}$, released from the internal plasma membrane surface, might act either on the plasma membrane, to increase $Ca^{2+}$ entry through the non-specific cation channel (see above), or on the membranes of intracellular stores.

An increase in intracellular $Na^+$ concentration has often been implicated in the release of $Ca^{2+}$ from intracellular stores, especially mitochondria (Carafoli & Crompton, 1978). While a role for $Na^+$ cannot be excluded (especially in excitable cells), it is certainly true that in isolated pancreatic acinar cells which have been made "leaky" (by washing in $Ca^{2+}$-free media) secretagogue-induced release of $Ca^{2+}$ occurs without any possible change in internal $Na^+$ concentration (see Case, 1984).

Inorganic $PO_4{}^{3-}$ and the NAD/NADH ratio have also been implicated in the release of $Ca^{2+}$ from mitochondria *in vitro* (Carafoli & Crompton, 1978). Whether they act as such *in vivo* and in stimulus-secretion coupling is unknown.

Cyclic nucleotides are obvious candidates. In a great variety of cells, cGMP concentration increases in parallel with a rise in intracellular $Ca^{2+}$ concentration (Case, 1978; Rasmussen, 1981) perhaps because guanylate cyclase is activated directly or indirectly by $Ca^{2+}$. Thus, cGMP would seem a possible candidate for releasing $Ca^{2+}$ from intracellular stores. However, there is no evidence of such a role for cGMP in stimulus-response coupling. Indeed, it is still difficult to define any role for cGMP, though Rasmussen (1981) has suggested it may regulate the sensitivity of cellular response elements which are activated by $Ca^{2+}$.

The situation with regard to cAMP is a little clearer. Sometimes cAMP acts as a second messenger in its own right; other times it seems to enhance the $Ca^{2+}$ signal. In at least one instance, *Calliphora* salivary gland, cAMP has been clearly shown to mobilise $Ca^{2+}$ from an intracellular store (Berridge & Lipke, 1979). However this cannot be an essential role for cAMP since secretion in many cells is independent of changes in cell cAMP concentration.

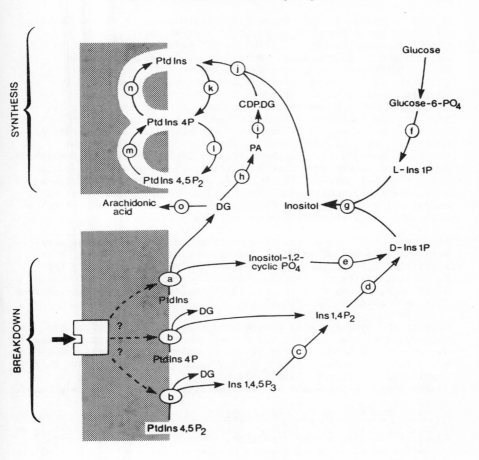

Fig. 1.   The metabolism of inositol phospholipids. For clarity, the synthetic processes have been separated from the break-down events that are stimulated by Ca$^{2+}$-mobilising stimuli. It is not clear yet whether each of these stimuli acts to hydrolyze each of the phosphoinositides. a – PtdIns phosphodi-esterase; b – polyphosphoinositide phosphodiesterase; c – Inositol trisphosphate (Ins1,4,5P$_3$) phosphomonoesterase; d – Inositol bisphosphate (Ins1,4,P$_2$) phosphomonoesterase; e – Inositol-1,2-cycle phosphate phosphodiesterase; f – Inositol-1-phosphate synthase; g – Inositol-1-phosphatase; h – Diacly-glycerol kinase; i – CTP phosphatidic acid cytidyl trans-ferase; j – CDP-diacylglycerol-inositol phosphatidate trans-ferase; k – PtdIns kinase; l – PtdIns4P kinase; m – PtdIns4,5P$_2$ phosphomonoesterase; n – PtdIns4P phosphomonoesterase; o – Diaclyglycerol lipase.   Modified from Berridge (1982) and reproduced with permission of the author and publisher (Churchill Livingstone).

A final hypothesis concerns phophastidylinositol (PtdIns). It has long been known that the response of a great variety of cells (including many secretory cells) to $Ca^{2+}$-mobilising stimuli is accompanied by an increased hydrolysis of PtdIns, to release inositol-1-phosphate leaving diacylglycerol in the membrane (Michell, 1982). More recent evidence suggests that the polyphosphoinositides, phosphatidylinositol-4-phosphate and phosphatidylinositol-4,5-bisphosphate, are the prime targets for hydrolysis (and that changes in PtdIns hydrolysis may, at least in part, reflect an equilibrium between PtdIns and the polyphosphoinositides (Fig. 1). Hydrolysis of polyphosphoinositides yields two water soluble products, inositol-1,4-bisphosphate and inositol-1,4,5-trisphosphate. Recent experiments show that inositol-1,4,5-trisphosphate, but not other inositol metabolites, releases $Ca^{2+}$ from a non-mitochondrial store (probably endoplasmic reticulum) in permeabilised pancreatic acinar cells in a manner indistinguishable from carbachol (Streb *et al*, 1983). How it does so remains to be determined.

If confirmed and expanded, this observation may explain how surface-acting agents can mobilise $Ca^{2+}$ from intracellular stores. Whether inositol-1,4,5-trisphosphate is also involved in regulating the $Ca^{2+}$-permeability of the plasma membrane remains to be determined. If it does, it may help to explain the existence of voltage-independent $Ca^{2+}$ channels in epithelia.

Whether the hydrolysis of phosphoinositides has other roles in stimulus response coupling is an open question. For example, the diacylglycerol produced from PtdIns hydrolysis may itself evoke secretion independent of $Ca^{2+}$ (Rink *et al*, 1983); furthermore this diaclyglycerol is rich in arachidonic acid, a precursor of prostaglandins and thromboxanes, whose synthesis it may therefore enhance.

## THE ROLE OF $Ca^{2+}$ IN SECRETION

Many, if not all, of the regulatory effects of intracellular $Ca^{2+}$ appear to be mediated by a small homologous group of high-affinity $Ca^{2+}$-binding proteins. Of these, the majority are localised in only one type of tissue. For example troponin C and parvalbumin are found in skeletal muscle, myosin light chains and leiotonin in smooth muscle and intestinal $Ca^{2+}$-binding protein in enterocytes. Each has a specific role to play. Thus, troponin C couples stimulation to response in skeletal muscle while leiotonin has the same function in smooth muscle. However one member of the group, calmodulin, is ubiquitus in distribution and seems capable of coupling stimulus to response in a variety of $Ca^{2+}$-mediated cell functions. On binding $Ca^{2+}$, calmodulin assumes a more helical conformation in which form it is able to activate a number of enzymes (Table 5).

The enzymic events involved in both macromolecular and electrolyte secretion are essentially unknown. The discharge of macromolecules is achieved by exocytosis which involves the migration of secretory granules towards, and eventual fusion with, the luminal plasma membrane. Either or both of these processes could presumably involve $Ca^{2+}$.

TABLE 5.  Some enzymes activated by Ca$^{2+}$ via
          calmodulin

Phosphorylase *b* kinase
Glycogen synthase kinase
Protein kinase
Myosin light chain kinase
Phospholipase A$_2$ (and perhaps other lipases)
NAD kinase (plants)
Adenylate cyclase (activation or inhibition)
Guanylate cyclase
Cyclic nucleotide phosphodiesterases
Ca$^{2+}$-ATPase

Inhibitory effects of Ca$^{2+}$ have also been observed for a number of
intracellular enzymes *in vitro*.  However, the concentrations of Ca$^{2+}$
required suggest these effects are probably not of physiological
significance.


Secretory cells possess an intricate terminal web beneath the
luminal cell membrane which contains actin, myosin, and actin-
associated proteins such as tropomyosin (Drenckhahn & Mannherz,
1983).  Compounds known to disrupt the functional organisation of
actin filaments and microtubules (e.g. cytochalasin B and colchicine)
interfere with secretion (Case, 1978).  It is therefore tempting to
suggest that an interaction between secretory granules and such
filaments, mediated by a Ca$^{2+}$-binding protein, is responsible for
movements of granules towards the cell membrane.

A number of possible roles for Ca$^{2+}$ in fusion can be envisaged (Case,
1978).  For example,  binding of Ca$^{2+}$ to the negatively charged
surfaces of granule and cell membranes may diminish electrostatic
repulsion between them and thereby facilitate fusion.  Alternatively,
activation of a phospholipase by Ca$^{2+}$ might promote the synthesis of
a fusogenic agent.

Exocytosis in pancreas, salivary glands and other secretory cells, is
accompanied by a rapid Ca$^{2+}$-dependent phosphorylation and dephosphorylation of cytosolic and secretory granule proteins (e.g.
Roberts & Butcher, 1983).  The significance of this altered phosphorylation in exocytosis remains unknown.  Perhaps it promotes the
interaction of secretory granules with cytoskeletal elements and/or
the luminal cell membrane.

Secretory cells are rich in calmodulin and evidence is beginning to
accumulate which suggests that calmodulin acts at some point(s) in
the chain of events leading to exocytosis.  A role for calmodulin
could be envisaged in a number of the Ca$^{2+}$-mediated processes just
described.  However evidence from the pancreatic β-cell suggests
that calmodulin is involved only in controlling intracellular Ca$^{2+}$
concentration and not in the process of exocytosis (Wollheim &
Sharp, 1982).

The role of Ca$^{2+}$ in fluid secretion is even less certain.  There is
no doubt that intracellular Ca$^{2+}$ can control the permeability of the

plasma membrane towards ions. The best known example is the $Ca^{2+}$-activated $K^+$ channel. Elevation of intracellular $Ca^{2+}$ concentration causes 'opening' of such channels in a variety of cells, including some secretory cells (Lew, 1983). The $K^+$ lost from the cell following activation of these channels may be taken up again linked to $Cl^-$ by means of a $Na^+/K^+/2Cl^-$ co-transport protein. Thus it has been proposed that such a linked system could supply $Cl^-$ for subsequent transport across the luminal cell membrane (Maruyama et al, 1983 and see Case, 1984). This may be true, but since neither $Ca^{2+}$-activated $K^+$ channels nor $Na^+/K^+/2Cl^-$ co-transport proteins are confined to secretory cells, they alone cannot play a unique role in electrolyte secretion.

In the salivary gland of *Calliphora*, secretion is evoked by 5-HT (Table 4). Stimulation of $5-HT_1$ receptors leads to the release of $Ca^{2+}$ from intracellular stores and to accelerated $Ca^{2+}$ influx. The resulting rise in cytosolic $Ca^{2+}$ concentration seems to regulate $Cl^-$ efflux across the luminal membrane and hence promotes secretion. Essentially the same situation may apply in those mammalian epithelia which use $Ca^{2+}$ as mediator. Whether the reduced $Cl^-$ permeability of sweat gland ductal epithelium is influenced by intracellular $Ca^{2+}$ concentration is unknown and it will remain so until the free $Ca^{2+}$ concentration is measured in these cells.

However it should be restated that a role for $Ca^{2+}$ is not obligatory in electrolyte secretory processes. $HCO_3^-$-secretion by pancreatic ductal cells seems to be regulated exclusively via cAMP. Perhaps phosphorylation of membrane proteins achieved either through cAMP-activated protein kinase or through $Ca^{2+}$-activated calmodulin is involved in modulating anion channels.

## CONCLUSIONS

Intracellular $Ca^{2+}$ plays a crucial role in a wide variety of cell functions, including secretion. Intracellular $Ca^{2+}$ homeostasis is a complex affair involving the participation of almost every component of the cell. Clearly any homeostatic imbalance will have far-reaching consequences. Such an imbalance appears to be a feature of a number of diseases including CF. Whether it is a primary cause of the symptoms in CF, or is secondary to pathological consequences of the disease, remains unknown.

## REFERENCES

Banschbach, M.W., Karam, A.G., Love, P.K. and Hilman, B.C., 1978. Cystic Fibrosis serum promotes [$^{45}$Ca] uptake by normal human leukocytes. Biochemical and Biophysical Research Communications, 84, 922-927.

Berridge, M.J., 1980. Preliminary measurements of intracellular calcium in an insect salivary gland using a calcium-sensitive microelectrode. Cell Calcium, 1, 217-227.

Berridge, M.J., 1982. 5-hydroxytryptamine stimulation of phosphatidylinositol hydrolysis and calcium signalling in the blowfly salivary gland. Cell Calcium, 3, 385-397.

Berridge, M.J. and Lipke, H., 1979. Changes in calcium transport across *Calliphora* salivary glands induced by 5-hydroxytryptamine and cyclic nucleotides. Journal of Experimental Biology, 78, 137-148.

Blinks, J.R., Weir, W.G., Hess, P., and Prendergast, F.G. 1982. Measurement of Ca$^{2+}$ concentrations in living cells. Progress in Biophsics and Molecular Biology, 40, 1-114.

Bogart, B.I., Conod, E.J., Gaerlan, P.F., Denning, C.R., and Conover, J., 1979. Biological activities of cystic fibrosis serum III CF serum induced uptake of $^{45}$Ca$^{++}$ by rabbit tracheal explants. Biochemical and Biophysical Research Communications,88, 1398-1404.

Butcher, F.R., and Putney, J.W. Jr., 1980. Regulation of parotid gland function by cyclic nucleotides and calcium, in Advances in Cyclic Nucleotide Research, Vol 13 (Eds. P. Greengard and G.A. Robison), pp 215-249. Raven Press, New York.

Carafoli, E. and Crompton, M., 1978. The regulation of intra-cellular calcium, in Current Topics in Membranes and Transport, Vol 10 (Eds. F. Bronner and A. Kleinzeller), pp 151-216. Academic Press, New York.

Case, R.M., 1978. Synthesis, intracellular transport and discharge of exportable proteins in the pancreatic acinar cell and other cells. Biological Reviews, 53, 211-354.

Case, R.M., 1979. Pancreatic secretion: cellular aspects, in Scientific Basis of Gastroenterology (Eds. H.L. Duthie and K.G. Wormsley), pp. 163-198. Churchill Livingstone, Edinburgh.

Case, R.M., 1980a. 'Cell Calcium' - a new international interdisci-plinary journal. Cell Calcium, 1, 1-5.

Case, R.M., 1980b. Epithelial transport processes involved in secretion and absorption, in Perspectives in Cystic Fibrosis (Ed. J.M. Sturgess),pp. 67-80. Canadian Cystic Fibrosis Foundation, Toronto.

Case, R.M., 1984. The role of Ca$^{2+}$ stores in secretion: a workshop discussion, in Secretion: Mechanisms and Control (Eds. R.M. Case, J.M. Lingard and J.A. Young). Manchester University Press, Manchester (in the press).

Ceder, O., and Roomans, G.M., 1983. Effects of culture medium on cystic fibrosis and normal fibroblasts studied by X-ray micro-analysis. Ultrastructural Pathology,4, 305-309.

Charest, R., Blackmore, P.F., Berthon, B., and Exton, J.H., 1983. Changes in free cytosolic Ca$^{2+}$ in hepatocytes following $\alpha_1$-adren-ergic stimulation. Studies on quin-2-loaded hepatocytes. Journal of Biological Chemistry 258, 8769-8773.

Donowitz, M., 1983. Ca$^{2+}$ in the control of active intestinal Na and Cl transport: involvement in neurohumoral action. American Journal of Physiology,245, G165-G177.

Dormer, R.L., 1983. Direct demonstration of increases in cytosolic free Ca$^{2+}$ during stimulation of pancreatic enzyme secretion. Bioscience Reports, 3, 233-240.

Douglas, W.W., 1974. Involvement of calcium in exocytosis and the exocytosis-vesiculation sequence. Biochemical Society Symposia, 39, 1-28.

Drenckhahn, D., and Mannherz, H.G., 1983. Distribution of actin and
    the actin-associated proteins myosin, tropomyosin, alpha-actinin,
    vinculin, and villin in rat and bovine exocrine glands. European
    Journal of Cell Biology. 30, 167-176.

Farber, J.L., 1981. The role of calcium in cell death. Life Sciences
    29, 1289-1295.

Feinstein, M.B., 1980. Release of intracellular membrane-bound
    calcium precedes the onset of stimulus-induced exocytosis in
    platelets. Biochemical and Biophysical Research Communications,
    93, 593-600.

Foder, B., Scharff, O., and Tønnesen, P., 1980. Activator-associated
    $Ca^{2+}$-ATPase in erythrocyte membranes from cystic fibrosis
    patients. Clinica Chimica Acta, 104, 187-193.

Gnegy, M.E., Erickson, R.P., and Markovac, J., 1981. Increased
    calmodulin in cultured skin fibroblasts from patients with cystic
    fibrosis. Biochemical Medicine, 26, 294-298.

Henkart, M., and Nelson, P.G., 1979. Evidence for an intracellular
    calcium store releasable by surface stimuli in fibroblasts (L
    cells). Journal of General Physiology, 73, 655-673.

Hunter, M., Smith, P.A., and Case, R.M., 1983. The dependence of
    fluid secretion by mandibular salivary gland and pancreas on
    extracellular calcium. Cell Calcium, 4, 307-317.

Katz, S., 1980. $Ca^{2+}$-transport and $(Mg^{2+}+Ca^{2+})$-ATPase activity in
    cystic fibrosis, in Perspectives in Cystic Fibrosis (Ed. J.M.
    Sturgess), pp 3-14. Canadian Cystic Fibrosis Foundation, Toronto.

Knight, D.E., and Kesteven, N.T., 1983. Evoked transient intra-
    cellular free $Ca^{2+}$ changes and secretion in isolated bovine
    adrenal medullary cells. Proceedings of the Royal Society of
    London, B218, 177-199.

Lew, V.L. (Ed.)., 1983. $Ca^{2+}$-activated $K^{+}$ channels. Collected papers
    and reviews. Cell Calcium, 4, 321-517.

Mangos, J.A., and Donnelly, W.H., 1981. Isolated parotid acinar
    cells from patients with cystic fibrosis. Morphology and
    composition. Journal of Dental Research, 60, 19-25.

Martinez, J.R., 1982. Alterations in salivary gland structure and
    function in cystic fibrosis, in Fluid and Electrolyte
    Abnormalities in Exocrine Glands in Cystic Fibrosis (Eds. P.M.
    Quinton, J.R. Martinez and U. Hopfer), pp 125-142. San Francisco
    Press, San Francisco.

Maruyama, Y., Petersen, O.H., Flanagan, P., and Pearson, G.T., 1983.
    Quantification of $Ca^{2+}$-activated $K^{+}$ channels under hormonal
    control in pig pancreas acinar cells. Nature, 305, 228-232.

Michell, R.H. (Ed.)., 1982. Inositol phospholipids and cell calcium.
    Collected papers and reviews. Cell Calcium, 3, 285-465.

Morrissey, S.M., and Mehta, J.G., 1981. Effect of cystic fibrosis
    and non-cystic fibrosis plasma on the movement and retention of
    $^{45}Ca^{2+}$ and $^{35}SO_4{}^{2-}$ in guinea-pig stomach and small intestine.
    Gut, 22, 788-792.

O'Doherty, J., and Stark, R.J., 1982. Stimulation of pancreatic
    acinar secretion: increases in cytosolic calcium and sodium.
    American Journal of Physiology, 242, G513-G521.

O'Doherty, J., Youmans, S.J., Armstrong, W.McD., and Stark, R.J.,
    1980. Calcium regulation during stimulus-secretion coupling:

continuous measurement of intracellular calcium activity. Science, 209, 510-513.

Quinton, P.M., 1984. The pathology of secretion in cystic fibrosis, in, Secretion: Mechanisms and Control (Eds. R.M. Case, J.M. Lingard and J.A. Young). Manchester University Press, Manchester. (in the press).

Rahwan, R.G., 1983. Mechanisms of action of membrane calcium channel blockers and intracellular calcium antagonists. Medicinal Research Reviews, 3, 21-42.

Rasmussen, H., 1981. Calcium and cAMP as Synarchic Messengers. Wiley, New York.

Rink, T.J., Sanchez, A., and Hallam, T.J., 1983. Diaclyglycerol and phorbol ester stimulate secretion without raising cytoplasmic free calcium in human platelets. Nature, 305, 317-319.

Rink, T.J., Smith, S.W., and Tsien, R.Y., 1982. Cytoplasmic free Ca$^{2+}$ in human platelets: Ca$^{2+}$ thresholds and Ca-independent activation for shape-change and secretion. FEBS Letters, 148, 21-26.

Roberts, M.L., and Butcher, F.R., 1983. The involvement of protein phosphorylation in stimulus-secretion coupling in the mouse exocrine pancreas. Biochemical Journal, 210, 353-359.

Roomans, G.M., von Euler, A.M., and Müller, R.M., 1983. Cystic fibrosis - ultrastructural and microanalytical studies. Scanning Electron Microscopy, 2, 697-712.

Rose, B., and Loewenstein, W.R., 1976. Permeability of a cell junction and the local cytoplasmic free ionized calcium concentration: A study with aequorin. Journal of Membrane Biology, 28, 87-119.

Sato, K., and Sato, F., 1981. Role of calcium in cholinergic and adrenergic mechanisms of eccrine sweat secretion. American Journal of Physiology, 241, C113-C120.

Shapiro, B.L., Feigal, R.J., and Lam, L.F-H., 1980. Intracellular calcium and cystic fibrosis, in Perspectives in Cystic Fibrosis (Ed. J.M. Sturgess), pp 15-28. Canadian Cystic Fibrosis Foundation, Toronto.

Shapiro, B.L., and Lam, L.F.-H., 1982. Calcium and age in fibroblasts from control subjects and patients with cystic fibrosis. Science, 216, 417-419.

Sorscher, E.J., and Breslow, J.L., 1982. Cystic fibrosis: A disorder of calcium-stimulated secretion and transepithelial sodium transport? The Lancet, 1, 368-370.

Streb, H., Irvine, R.F., Berridge, M.J., and Schulz, I., 1983. Release of Ca$^{2+}$ from a nonmitochondrial intracellular store in pancreatic acinar cells by inositol-1,4,5-trisphosphate. Nature, 306, 67-69.

Wollheim, C.B., and Sharp, G.W.G., 1981. Regulation of insulin release by calcium. Physiological Reviews, 61, 914-973.

CALCIUM AND CALMODULIN ARE INVOLVED IN THE DECREASED WATER
PERMEABILITY OF CELL MEMBRANES IN CYSTIC FIBROSIS.

C.S. Glaubensklee and W.R. Galey, University of New Mexico School of
Medicine, Department of Physiology, Albuquerque, New Mexico  87131.

Studies conducted in our laboratory (1,2) as well as others (3)
have suggested that calcium may be intimately involved in the
pathology of cystic fibrosis.  Further, our studies have shown that
the osmotic water permeability (Lp) of erythrocytes from patients
with cystic fibrosis is significantly lower than that of normal
individuals.  We have conducted experiments to test whether this
decrease in water permeability is related to the abnormal handling
of $Ca^{++}$ by the cells of Cystic Fibrosis (CF) patients.  In one series,
experiments both normal and CF erythrocytes were treated with the
calcium ionophores A23187 or X537A in the presence of 0.5 mM extracellular $Ca^{++}$.  It was observed that both treatments decrease the
water permeability of normal cells by ∿25% while cells from CF
patients showed no further significant decrease in the Lp.  This
suggests that a calcium-dependent decrease in water permeability is
already maximal in CF cells.  In a second series of studies, normal
and CF erythrocytes were treated with trifluoperazine, an inhibitor
of calcium binding to the intracellular calcium buffer, calmodulin.
While this agent inhibited water permeability in both, the inhibition
was less in the CF cells.  This observation reinforces the suggested
role of calcium in the regulation of membrane water permeability and
suggests that either the calcium buffering capacity of calmodulin is
reduced in CF cells or that its capacity to bind $Ca^{++}$ is saturated by
abnormally high intracellular $Ca^{++}$.  Further experiments showed that
membrane associated immuno-reactive calmodulin is decreased by
approximately 40% in cells from CF patients.  Measurements of cellular
calcium by atomic absorption spectroscopy showed most CF patients
to have increased cell calcium.  Increased cellular calcium was not
only related to decreased water permeability but also strongly
correlated (r=0.99) with elevated sweat electrolytes of CF patients.
We conclude that intracellular calcium and calmodulin activities are
involved in the decreased cell membrane water permeability found in
CF patients.

1) Schiffman, M., Gillon, J.J. & W.R. Galey.  Proc. 8th Int'l
   Congress Cystic Fibrosis, Canad. C.F. Foundation, Ontario, 1980.
2) Galey, W.R., M.J. Gillon & S. Murphy.  Pediatr. Res. II.
   1269-71, 1980.
3) Katz, S. Proc. 8th Int'l Congress Cystic Fibrosis, Canad. C.F.
   Foundation, Ontario, 1980.

GLYCOPROTEINS OF CF MUCUS

Ph. Roussel

Unité INSERM N°16, Place de Verdun, 59045 Lille, France

## INTRODUCTION

Cystic Fibrosis is a generalized exocrinopathy in which most of the clinical manifestations are initially due to obstruction of duct or organ passages by thick secretions or thick mucus (mucoviscidosis) affecting the respiratory tract, some salivary glands, the digestive and biliary tracts, the pancreas and the genito-urinary tract ; pancreatic insufficiency and respiratory infection may be considered as secondary effects (Talamo, 1983).

These abnormalities explain the efforts of the past 20 years devoted to the elucidation of a possible biochemical defect of mucus or of its main specific components, mucus glycoproteins, or mucins.

Mucus is widespread in Nature, from earthworm surface or eel skin to human mucosa. Like the superficial layers of skin, it occurs at the interface between the "milieu interieur" and the outside. This secretory product is synthesized by specialized cells of underlying mucosa and is organized as a layer which adheres to this mucosa and thereby protects it. However, unlike human skin, it has a rapid turnover, allows more exchanges between the outside and the mucosa (digestive absorption, transitory susceptibility to sperm penetration) and is quickly secreted in response to external stimulation of the mucosa.

The most characteristic part of mucus occurs as a gel, although in some secretions, such as bronchial or cervical secretions, mucus may be separated by centrifugation into a gel-phase and a sol-phase (Litt, 1976 ; Gibbons, 1978). The gel has rheological properties (Silberberg, 1982 ; Marriott, 1983) : it is viscous but its viscosity varies with the shear rate applied, which is characteristic of a non-newtonian fluid resembling a pseudoplastic material. It also exhibits elastic properties, being able to store energy and to dissipate this energy during flow.

These visco-elastic properties are indispensable to maintain the functions of the different forms of mucus : mucociliary clearance of the inhaled particles and microorganisms in the respiratory tree ; lubrication and protection of the mucosa in the gastro-intestinal tract ; regulation of sperm penetration through cervical mucus.

Different procedures are available which alter the rheological properties of mucus and permit its solubilization *in vitro* : disulphide bond-breaking agents or thiols, like N-acetylcysteine which has been used as a therapeutic aerosol in the treatment of bronchial hypersecretion ; treatment with proteolytic enzymes that break peptide linkages ; mechanical agitation ; treatment with chaotropic or dissociating agents (high molarity of urea or guanidinium chloride).

The physical properties of mucus which are essential for its function are closely related to its chemical composition. Mucus contains highly glycosylated glycoproteins, called mucus glycoproteins (or mucins), and non-mucin components that will be briefly reviewed before examining mucins and the problems raised by mucins in CF.

## "NON-MUCIN" COMPONENTS FROM MUCUS

Mucus, which is highly hydrated, has a small solid content (from 5-10%) (Potter, 1967) and has an electrolyte content (1% by weight) which resembles that of serum (Creeth, 1978). The large proportion of mucus glycoproteins in mucus has probably overshadowed the presence of other components such as proteins, lipids and serum-type glycoproteins, that differ from mucins by having a smaller number of carbohydrate chains containing mannose

and attached to the peptide by a linkage between N-acetylglucosamine and the amide group of asparagine (N-glycans) (Roussel,
1978). Occasionally polysaccharides and nucleic acids may also be
present. Although mucins are probably responsible for most of the
physical properties of mucus and for many of its functions, some
of the "non-mucin" components may exist in both the sol-phase and
the gel-phase of mucus and play important roles (Creeth, 1978).

    Proteins and serum-type glycoproteins may originate from
plasma transudation, be locally synthesized and secreted by mucosa, and may be derived from sloughed epithelial cells.
- The level of serum components such as albumin, serotransferrin,
immunoglobulins may increase in mucosal inflammation.
- Secretory immunoglobulin A are the main antibodies of exocrine
secretions. They are synthetized in the immunocytes of the submucosa as dimers linked by another polypeptide chain (J chain). In
order to cross the epithelium and to be secreted, they bind to a
receptor of the baso-lateral membrane of epithelial cells, are
internalized and secreted in the lumen with part of this receptor
(secretory component) (Kühn, 1982).
- A glycoprotein identical with lactotransferrin and synthesized
by serous cells and neutrophils occurs in salivary, respiratory
and gastric secretions ; it probably plays a defensive role
against bacteria.
- This is also the case for lysozyme, a small basic protein with
bacteriolytic activity secreted by serous cells.
- Many other proteins or glycoproteins such as proteolytic enzymes, various classes of protease inhibitors, proline-rich polypeptides, may be minor components of mucus.

    Until recently, only scant attention has been paid to
lipid that exists in exocrine secretions and that may affect the
physical and physiological properties of mucus. For a long time,
lipid has been described in respiratory mucus especially in CF
respiratory mucus (Potter, 1967), but it was considered to result
from cellular breakdown which is a feature of obstructive airway
diseases. Substantial quantities of lipid (about 20 per cent by
weight) have recently been characterized in gastric mucus

(Slomiany, 1983a) and in rat intestinal mucus. These lipids comprised neutral lipids, phospholipids, small amounts of glycosphingolipids and, interestingly glyceroglucolipids, a class of lipids that seems to be relatively specific for secretions. Lipids probably contribute to the rheological properties of mucus and to the protection of the gastric mucosa ; they may also modulate the cytolytic activity of the duodenal content.

Mucus from the gastro-intestinal or genito-urinary tracts and from non-infected respiratory secretion contains little nucleic acids. However purulent sputa, such as CF sputa, contain substantial amounts of DNA derived from the destruction of host cells, mainly leucocytes.

The presence of polysaccharide or proteoglycans has occasionally been reported.

### MUCINS

Mucus glycoproteins or mucins are macromolecules synthesized by mucous glands of the submucosa and/or by goblet cells of the epithelium surface (Neutra, 1982). They contain from 50 to 80 per cent carbohydrate consisting of different sugars, L-fucose (Fuc), D-galactose (Gal), N-acetyl-D-glucosamine (GlcNAc), N-acetyl-D-galactosamine (GalNAc) and sialic acid. They may also contain sulfate. In contrast to serum-type glycoproteins, that are N-glycosylated, and to proteoglycans, they contain neither mannose nor uronic acid.

The peptide part of these molecules is peculiar : threonine, serine and, to a lesser extent, proline, glycine and alanine, account for more than 65 per cent of the amino acid content.

Carbohydrate chains are attached to the peptide by O-glycosidic linkages between N-acetylgalactosamine and the hydroxyl group of threonine or serine (Figure 1) and can be released by alkaline-borohydride treatment (Carlson, 1977). Hundreds of oligosaccharide side-chains are attached to a central core protein and the general picture of a mucin molecule is that of a bottle-brush

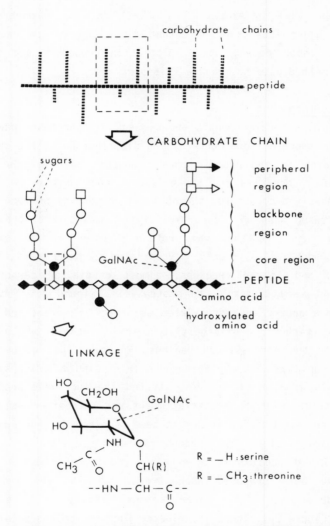

<u>Figure 1</u> : Schematic representation of the carbohydrate chains in a mucin molecule.

(Figure 1).

Mucins are very polydisperse and generally have a molecular weight (MW) in excess of $1 \times 10^6$ dalton. Moreover, even within a given secretion, important differences in MW have been observed. These depend on the isolation procedure and on the physical method used to measure this parameter.

General Conformation

Two general concepts about mucus glycoproteins have progressively emerged : one concerns the distribution of the carbohydrate chains on the protein core ; another one deals with the aggregating properties and the polymeric conformation of mucins, which probably accounts for the physical properties of mucus.

Based upon the susceptibility of mucins to proteases, it has been suggested that the protein core of mucins comprises different domains : highly glycosylated regions resistant to proteases and "naked" regions, almost devoid of carbohydrate chains and very sensitive to proteolysis (Figure 2). The naked regions are poorer in hydroxylated amino acids (serine and threonine) and richer in dicarboxylic acids (glutamic and aspartic acid) than the glycosylated regions. Moreover they contain some cysteine residues that may be engaged in disulphide bridges.

In 1963, Sheffner demonstrated the mucolytic properties of N-acetylcysteine on bronchial mucus and thereafter many mucin preparations from different origin have been found to be susceptible to thiol or other disulphide bond-breaking agents.

Based upon these observations, different models of mucins have been proposed where mucin subunits are linked by disulphide bridges of the naked regions directly or via a linker protein (Figure 2a). There is evidence for such polymeric structures in mucins from different secretions (gastro-intestinal, biliary, respiratory and ovarian-cyst mucin). Other models, where subunits would be linked end-to-end by disulphide bridges, have been proposed for cervical mucins (Figure 2b).

However there are exceptions to the disulphide-linked subunit models, for instance ovine submaxillary mucin. Moreover

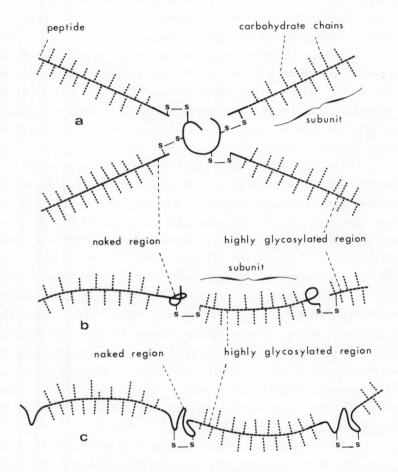

Figure 2 : Different models proposed for mucins : (a) windmill model of gastric mucins (Allen, 1983) ; (b) cervical mucins (Carlstedt, 1983) ; (c) respiratory mucins (Carlstedt, 1982).

some mucin preparations from the respiratory tract are not susceptible to thiol agents (Figure 2c) and, in this secretion, the
mucolytic effect of thiol may be due to the activation of
proteolytic enzymes still associated with mucins (Roussel, 1983).
Therefore, generalization of a polymeric structure based upon
interchain disulphide bridges has to be questioned.

Recently, tungsten replica of human bronchial mucins
have been examined by electron microscopy : they consist of long
threads with a length distribution broader than would be expected
for homogeneous material. This important heterogeneity in length,
which may be due in part to flexibility, remains a puzzling
problem (Slayter, 1983).

The possible role of disulphide bridges has been greatly
emphasized but other factors may be important for the formation
of polymeric structures from mucins subunits which may be linked
through non-covalent interactions. Mucins prepared without ion-
exchange chromatography are still non-covalently associated with
several peptides or proteins (Slayter, 1983). These associations
may be due to relatively strong hydrophobic interactions. Large
amounts of lipid are associated with respiratory or gastric mucin
preparations (Woodward, 1982 ; Slomiany, 1983a) and a few fatty
acid residues might be covalently linked to the carbohydrate
chains of gastric mucins (Slomiany, 1983b) although the bulk of
associated lipid is non-covalently attached to mucins. The group
of Slomiany has reported preliminary observations showing that
specific lipid classes were bound to the different domains of
mucins (Witas, 1983).

In conclusion mucin subunits may have a thread-like shape ; in the mucus they are probably coiled and their polymeric
conformation may be the result of several factors : direct or
indirect (via lipid or peptide) hydrophobic interactions and
possibly, but not necessarily, interchain disulphide bridges. In
solution, they probably have a roughly spherical conformation
(Harding, 1983).

## Carbohydrate chains

The structural elucidation of the various carbohydrate chains present in mucins reveals a still growing and remarkable diversity of carbohydrate chains (Van Halbeek, 1982).

The only common point of all carbohydrate chains is the N-acetylgalactosamine residue involved in the attachment of the chain to the peptide (Figure 1). Depending upon their species and organ origins, mucins may have a very wide diversity of carbohydrate chains from short chains (2 sugars), that may be sialylated, to long chains (more than 10 sugars), that may be sulfated. The diversity of chains is sometimes observed in the mucins secreted by the mucosa of a single individual.

Despite the complexity of the carbohydrate structures determined so far, different regions may be identified for each chain (Figure 1) : a core region comprising the sugars close to the N-acetylgalactosaminyl residue involved in the linkage to the protein, a backbone region which may be linear or branched, and a peripheral region (Hounsell, 1982). Various antigens may be expressed on these domains. The backbone regions may contain alternating sequences of galactose and N-acetylglucosamine and express I or i antigenic activities. The peripheral region may contain sulfate or sialic acid, and may express various blood group activities, H, A, B, Lewis[a], Lewis[b] or other antigens such as SSEA-1 or Sd[a]. This region may also contain structures that are organ-specific.

In other words a mucin molecule is very complex with regard to the number, structure and localization of the carbohydrate side chains. Moreover in certain secretions, mucins secreted by a single individual may represent a population of molecules with increasing acidity from neutral to sialylated and sometime sulphated molecules (Lamblin, 1977). Except for relatively simple models such as ovine submaxillary mucins where most of the chains are disaccharide units consisting of N-acetylgalactosamine and sialic acid, the structure elucidation of mucins molecule still represents a challenge !

The biosynthesis of the oligosaccharides of mucin occurs

in the Golgi apparatus of goblet cells or of mucous cells. This
biosynthesis involves sequential sugar additions to the peptide
backbone (Schachter, 1982). Each step requires a specific nucleotide sugar as sugar donor, and a specific glycosyltransferase that
recognizes the carbohydrate structure of the growing oligosaccharide acceptor. Several glycosyltransferases have been characterized, especially those involved in the synthesis of the different
types of core, and in the synthesis of some short carbohydrate
chains. Similarly the glycosyltransferases, that allow the synthesis of the peripheral structures responsible for blood-group A, B,
H, Lewis[a] or Lewis[b] activities, have been studied. The genetic
control of oligosaccharide biosynthesis depends upon the expression of the specific glycosyltransferases produced by a given
cell, for example blood group activities (Watkins, 1980). The
relative activities of the various glycosyltransferases, the relative amounts of the nucleotide sugars produced by a cell, and the
specificity of each glycosyltransferase may then also determine
which of several alternate biosynthetic pathways predominates.
However the knowledge of mucin biosynthesis is still very limited.

Mucins synthesized in mucin-producing cells accumulate in
mucous granules before being secreted into glandular ducts or at
the surface of the mucosa. Different factors such as cholinergic
agents, -adrenergic agents, secretin, prostaglandins or leukotrienes stimulate the secretion in certain mucosa (Jones, 1982 ;
Neutra, 1982 ; Lamont, 1983 ; Marom, 1983). Anti-inflammatory
drugs may inhibit the secretion. After being secreted the mucus
granules fuse with other granules or other secretory components
(proteins, glycoproteins, lipid, biliary pigments) to form the
mucus layer.

There are indications that the carbohydrate chain diversity of mucins represents an important defensive mechanism of the
mucosa : the carbohydrate chains of the mucins may protect the
underlying epithelium from bacterial adhesion.

## CF MUCINS

In CF, the earliest detectable lesion is dilation of the

lumen of the gland ducts and acini (Sturgess, 1982). Later on CF is characterized by mucous gland hypertrophy (enlargment of glands) and hyperplasia of goblet cells, even in areas where they normally are very scarce (such as bronchioles). Those modifications will generate hypersecretion of thick mucus responsible for meconium ileus at birth or for the respiratory problems, later on.

There is probably no definite alteration of the bronchial tree within the first months after birth and it is still unclear whether lung infection, a major concern in CF, precedes bronchial hypersecretion or not.

CF mucus appears to be dehydrated, this characteristic probably reflects abnormalities in water and ion movements of the exocrine glands or ducts (Quinton, 1983 ; Knowles, 1983).

Increased secretion of mucins has been observed in explants of post-mortem respiratory epithelium from CF patients as compared to explants of patients who died of non-respiratory diseases. This is probably related to hyperplasia.

Protein-bound carbohydrate of meconium from cystic fibrosis is lower than that of normal meconium. However mucins from cystic fibrosis meconium have a higher fucose content, than those from normal specimens (Clamp, 1979).

Increased sulfation of carbohydrate chains has been reported in bronchial mucins secreted by patients suffering from CF (Boat, 1978) or secreted by respiratory epithelial explants of CF patients (Boat, 1978 ; Frates, 1983). This may not be specific for CF (Lamblin, 1977) and may be associated with the severity of the disease (Chace, 1983). Longer carbohydrate chains have also been observed in respiratory and gastro-instestinal mucins (Lamblin, 1977 ; Wesley, 1983).

Fatty acid residues have been found covalently linked to gastric mucins, and recently it has been observed that CF gastric mucins were much more acylated than normal mucins (Slomiany, 1983b).

Bacterial infection of the respiratory tree especially by the mucoid variants of *Pseudomonas aeruginosa* is a major problem of CF. Since many adhesion phenomena between cells or mucus and bacteria probably involve interactions between cell or mucus carbohydrate chains and bacterial surface lectins, an inborn alteration of bronchial mucin carbohydrate chains inducing a specificity in bacterial adhesion and an alteration of the mucociliary clearance represents a tempting hypothesis to explain the increased risk of infection.

Owing to the very complex structure of mucins more work is necessary to clearly establish the basis of the abnormal character of CF mucus.

## REFERENCES

Allen A., 1983. Mucus. a protective secretion of complexity. TIBS, 8, 169-173.

Boat, T.F. and Cheng, P.W., 1978. Mucous glycoproteins in Cystic Fibrosis in Glycoproteins and Glycolipids in Disease Processes (Edr Walborg) pp 108-121. American Chemical Society, Washington D.C.

Carlson, D.M., 1977. Chemistry and biosynthesis of mucin glycoproteins, in Mucus in Health and Disease (Eds Elstein and Parke) pp 271-273. Plenum Press, New York and London.

Carlstedt, I., 1982. Normal respiratory mucin. Eur. J. Respir. Dis., 63, 493-495.

Carlstedt, I., Lindgren, H. and Sheehan J., 1983. The macromolecular structure of human cervical-mucus glycoproteins. 213, 427-435.

Chace, K.V., Leahy, D.S., Martin, R., Carubelli, R., Flux, M. and Sachdev, G.P., (1983). Respiratory mucous secretions in patients with cystic fibrosis : relationship between levels of highly sulfated mucin component and severity of the disease. Clin. Chim. Acta, 132, 143-155.

Clamp, J.R. and Gough, M., 1979. Study of the oligosaccharide units from mucus glycoproteins of meconium from normal infants and from cases of cystic fibrosis with meconium ileus. Clin. Sci., 57, 445-451.

Creeth, J.M., 1978. Constituents of mucus and their separation. Br. Med. Bull., 34, 17-24.

Frates Jr, R.C., Kaizu, T.T. and Last, J.A., 1983. Mucus glycoproteins secreted by respiratory epithelial tissue from cystic fibrosis patients. Pediatr. Res., 17, 30-34.

Gibbons, R.A., 1978. Mucus of the mammalian genital tract. Br. Med. Bull., 34, 34-38.

Harding, S.E., Rowe, A.J., Creeth, J.M., 1983. Further evidence for a flexible and highly expanded spheroidal model for mucus glycoproteins in solution. Biochem. J., 209, 893-896.

Hounsell, E.F. and Feizi, T., 1982. Gastrointestinal mucins. Structures and antigenicitics of their carbohydrate chains in health and disease. Med. Biol., 60, 227-236.

Jones, R., and Reid, L., 1982. Beta-adrenergic modulation of airway epithelial glycoprotein. Chest, 81, 25s-26s.

Knowles, M.R., Stutts, M.J., Spock, A., Fisher, N., Gatzy, J.T., and Boucher, R.C., 1983. Abnormal ion permeation through cystic fibrosis respiratory epithelium. Science, 221, 1067-1070.

Kühn, L.C., and Kraehenbull, J.P., 1982. The sacrifial receptor translocation of polymeric IgA across epithelia. TIBS, 299-302.

Lamblin, G., Lhermitte, M., Lafitte, J.J., Filliat, M., Degand, P. and Roussel, P., 1977. Etude comparative des mucines bronchiques purifiées à partir de l'expectoration de sujets atteints de mucoviscidose ou d'autres affections bronchiques chroniques. Bull. Eur. Physiopath. Resp., 13, 175-190.

Lamont, J.T., Ventola, A.S., Maull, E.A. and Szabo, S., 1983. Cysteinamine and prostaglandin F2$\beta$ stimulate rat gastric mucin release. Gastroenterology, 84, 306-313.

Litt, M., Khan, M.A. and Wolf, D.P., 1976. Mucus rheology : relation to structure and function. Biorheology, 13, 37-48.

Marom, Z., Shelhamer, J.H., Sun, F. and Kaliner, M., 1983. Human airway monohydroxyeicosatetraenoic acid generation and mucus release. J. Clin. Invest., 72, 122-127.

Marriott, C., 1982. Modification of the rheological properties of mucus by drugs, in Mucus in Health and Disease. II (Eds

82

Chantler, Elder and Elstein), pp 75-84. Plenum Press, New York and London.

Neutra, M.R., 1982. The functional structure of mucous cells. Chest, 81, 14s-19s.

Potter, J.L., Matthews, L.W., Spector, S. and Lemm, J., 1967. Studies on pulmonary secretions. Am. Rev. Respir. Dis., 96, 83-87.

Quinton, P.M., and Bijman, J., 1983. Higher bioelectric potentials due to decreased chloride absorption in the sweat glands of patients with cystic fibrosis. N. Engl. J. Med., 308, 1185-1189.

Roussel, P., Degand, P., Lamblin, G., Laine, A. and Lafitte, J.J., 1978. Biochemical definition of human tracheobronchial mucus. Lung, 154, 241-260.

Roussel, P., Houdret, N., and Lamblin, G., 1983. Mucin subunits linked by disulphide bridges ? TIBS, 8, 312.

Schachter, H., and Williams, D., 1982. Biosynthesis of mucus glycoproteins in Mucus in Health and Disease. II. (Eds Chantler, Elder and Elstein) pp 3-28. Plenum Press, New-York and London.

Sheffner, A.L., 1963. The reduction *in vitro* in viscosity of mucoprotein solutions by a new mucolytic agent, N-acetylcysteine. Ann. N.Y. Acad. Sci., 106, 298-310.

Silberberg, A., and Meyer, F.A., 1982. Structure and function of mucus, in Mucus in Health and Disease. II. (Eds Chantler, Elder and Elstein), pp 53-74. Plenum Press, New York and London.

Slayter, H., Lamblin, G., Houdret, N., Degand P. and P. Roussel, 1983. Complex structure of human bronchial mucus glycoproteins in Glycoconjugates, Proceedings of the 7th International symposium on Glycoconjugates (Eds Chester, Heinegard and Svensson) pp 562-563. Rahms i Lund, Sweden.

Slomiany, A., Slomiany, B.L., Witas, H., Zdebska, E., Galicki, N.I. and Newman, L., 1983a. Lipids of gastric secretion in patients with cystic fibrosis. Biochim. Biophys. Acta, 750, 253-260.

Slomiany, A., Witas, H., Aono, M., and Slomiany, B.L., 1983b. Covalently linked fatty acids in gastric mucus glycoproteins of cystic fibrosis patients. J. Biol. Chem., 258, 8535-8538.

Sturgess, J., 1982. Morphological characteristics of the bronchial mucosa in cystic fibrosis in Fluid and electrolyte abnormalities in exocrine glands in cystic fibrosis (Eds Quinton, Martinez and Hopper) pp 254-270. San Fancisco Press, San-Francisco, CA.

Talamo, R.C., Rosenstein, B.J., and Berninger, R.W., 1983. Cystic Fibrosis in The Metabolic Basis of Inherited Disease (Eds Stanbury, Wyngaarden, Frederickson, Goldstein and Brown), pp 1889-1917. McGraw-Hill Book Co., New York.

Van Halbeek, H., Dorland, L., Vliegenthart, J.F.G., Hull, W.E., Lamblin, G., Lhermitte, M., Boersma, A., and Roussel, P., 1982. Primary structure determination of fourteen neutral oligosaccharides derived from bronchial mucus glycoproteins of patients suffering from cystic fibrosis employing 500-MHz [1]H-NMR spectroscopy. Eur. J. Biochem., 127, 7-20.

Watkins, W.M., 1980. Biochemistry and genetics of the ABO, Lewis and P blood group systems. Advances in Human Genetics, 10, 1-136.

Wesley, A., Forstner, J., Qureshi, R., Mantle, M., and Forstner, G., 1983. Human intestinal mucin in cystic fibrosis. Pediatr. Res., 17, 65-69.

Witas, H., Sarosick, J., Aono, M., Murty, V.L.N., Slomiany, A. and Slomiany, B.L., 1983. Lipids associated with rat small-intestinal mucus glycoprotein. Biochem. Biophys. Acta, 120, 67-76.

Woodward, H., Horsey, B., Bhavanandan, V.P., and Davidson, E.A., 1982. Isolation, purification and properties of respiratory mucus glycoproteins. Biochemistry, 21, 694-701.

HOME INTRAVENOUS THERAPY: A MANAGEMENT OPTION FOR THE PATIENT WITH CYSTIC FIBROSIS.

Karen Wery, RN PNA, Cynthia Drysdale, MSSW, Robert Stone, M.D., Mary T. O'Neill, RN PNA, Children's Hospital Medical Center of Akron, Akron, Ohio.

Home intravenous (IV) therapy may be a useful clinical tool in the management of patients (pts) with Cystic fibrosis (CF), offering an alternative and/or adjunct to hospital care.

The evolution of aminoglycoside, broad spectrum penicillin, and third and fourth generation cephalosporins has had a major impact on the life expectancy and ultimate outcome of treatment in pts with CF. Indications for IV antibiotics include positive cultures for Hemophilus influenzae or Pseudomonas, that are resistant to oral antibiotics or in conjunction with negative pt response to oral antibiotics (increasing cough, fever, dyspnea), or in weight loss. Traditionally, IV antibiotics have been utilized in the hospital as part of an overall "tune-up", including postural drainage, nutritional and psychosocial supports.

Home IV therapy has been utilized by 11 CF pts at Children's Hospital Medical Center of Akron during the past 2 years. The program is offered to all CF pts over 6, who initially qualify on the basis of a careful evaluation by the CF team, including a comprehensive medical and psychosocial overview. Disease status is a primary indicator, as well as the willingness of a candidate to experiment with the program. For some pts, the availability of a watchful, trained, and supportive assistant (parent, older sibling, or spouse) may be paramount to the ultimate success of the project. The demands of time, skill, hygiene and proximity to a hospital or a reasonable medical alternative are key components. A teaching program is implemented covering the reconstitution, doseage, and administration of medication. This involves the care and maintenance of the heparin lock (IV site), disposal of used equipment, and signs and symptoms of medication reaction or infection, and thrombophlebitis. Pts must sign an informed consent prior to hospital discharge.

Pts and/or parents who successfully engage in the home IV therapy program gain physical and emotional independence from hospital confinement, and increased self-esteem. The pt for whom the program is unsuccessful may have experienced anxiety surrounding administration of medication, and negative repercussions based on "bringing the sickness" into a heretofore healthy environment. Finally, the demands of the program may exacerbate the already burdensome regimen for the pt or caregiver.

Home IV therapy programs are by no means considered a panacea. One cannot, however, dispute the fact that they are a cost saving mechanism whereby hospital perdiem charges are eliminated, as well as ancillary service charges.

# THE NUTRITIONAL STATUS AND THE PULMONARY ABNORMALITIES AS A FUNCTION OF AGE IN CYSTIC FIBROSIS AND HEALTHY CHILDREN.

H.J. Neijens, A. Breeman, M. Sinaasappel, H.J. Degenhart,
K.F. Kerrebijn and H.K.A. Visser
Dept. paediatrics, Erasmus University and University Hospital
Rotterdam / Sophia Children's Hospital, Gordelweg 160, 3038 GE
Rotterdam, the Netherlands.

Little data are available about the abnormalities in the nutritional status and respiratory function and their interrelationship as a function of time in cystic fibrosis (CF) patients.

Therefore, the nutritional status (assessed by weight, height, arm circumference, skinfold thickness, creatinine/height index, serum albumin, -transferrin and lymphocyte count) was studied in 60 pre- (0-12 years) and postpubertal (18-25 years) CF patients. The prepubertal patients were divided in four age cohorts (0- 2; 3-5; 6-9; 10-12 years). The patients were selected at random from the outpatient clinic of the Sophia Children's Hospital. The same measurements were performed in healthy children, matched for age and sex. These were compared to the data in CF patients (Wilcoxon, paired test). The findings in the CF children were related to the degree of malabsorption, the food intake and the pulmonary condition, the latter as characterized by the forced vital capacity (FVC), the forced expiratory volume in 1 second ($FEV_1$) and the chest X-ray score.

In the CF children the nutritional variables, except height, serum transferrin and lymphocytes count, tend to decline from the age of 9 years on. In the 10-12 and the 18-25 old CF patients a significant lower skinfold thickness ($P<0.001$), arm circumference and creatinin/ height index ($P<0.05$) were found than in the healthy subjects, indicating fat and muscle wasting. In the CF patients over 18 years of age weight corrected for height was significantly lower ($P<0.05$) than in the healthy children of the same age. The serum albumin had lower values in the 10-12 ($P<0.01$) and in the 18-25 age CF patients ($P<0.05$), although they were still within the normal range. A decline in FVC and $FEV_1$ was already present at the age of 6 in most CF children. The variables of the nutritional status were found to be highly correlated with those of the pulmonary variables ($P< 0.001$) but not with fat malabsorption or food intake.
It is concluded that a decrease in the respiratory condition precedes a decrease in the nutritional status while both are related. This suggests the respiratory pathology is an important determinant of the nutritional status.

THE MANAGEMENT OF PSEUDOMONAS CHEST
INFECTIONS - THE WAY FORWARD

N. Høiby

Statens Seruminstitut, Department of
Clinical Microbiology at Rigshospitalet
Copenhagen, Denmark

## INTRODUCTION

In the majority of patients with Cystic Fibrosis (CF) the history
of the disease is determined by the severity of the pulmonary
infection and inflammation. The accumulated evidence indicates that
bacteria, notably Pseudomonas aeruginosa, remain the most important
cause of exacerbations of respiratory symptoms in CF patients.
Consequently, chemotherapy against P. aeruginosa is one of the
keystones of the treatment for Cystic Fibrosis. There is, however,
no consensus of opinion on the most appropriate chemotherapeutic
regimen. The disagreement concerns the administration of antibiotics,
and whether treatment should be given depending on symptoms alone
or in conjunction with laboratory results indicating an infection.
However, most doctors would probably agree that to settle the
question of the "best" therapeutic approach, one has to understand
the nature and pathogenesis of the chronic lung infection caused
by P. aeruginosa in CF lungs.

## THE NATURE AND PATHOGENESIS OF THE CHRONIC
## P. AERUGINOSA LUNG INFECTION IN CF

CF patients contract chronic P. aeruginosa infection at any age. The
mean age of the onset of the infection in the Danish CF centre was
9-10 years (Szaff et al. 1983). The mean duration of the infection
was 3-4 years, but some of our patients have suffered from chronic
P. aeruginosa lung infection for more than 10 years. A few of our
patients have succumbed due to chronic P. aeruginosa infection of
a shorter duration in the past, however, due to the currently
available efficient anti-pseudomonas antibiotics this is not
observed any more. Before the P. aeruginosa infection becomes
chronic, most of the patients experience intermittent colonization
by non-mucoid strains, which subsequently become mucoid when the
infection becomes chronic (Høiby 1982).

The toxins of some P. aeruginosa strains, e.g. exotoxin A, proteases
etc., probably contribute to the pathogenesis of the chronic infection only during the first few months. Later on, when the antibody
response developes, at least the proteases seem to be neutralized
by the antibodies, and free proteases are not detectable in sputum
of CF patients at that stage of the infection. Immune complexes

isolated from sputum of such patients, however, contain P. aeruginosa proteases (Döring et al. 1983). The chronic P. aeruginosa infection in CF patients is therefore characterized by an antibody response which eventually, is directed against most of the antigens and toxins of P. aeruginosa. The P. aeruginosa strains isolated from such patients seem in a peculiar way to be adapted to the host and the host's immune response because they are nearly always mucoid strains which frequently are deficient in O-antigens (polyagglutinable) (Hancock et al. 1983). During the last 6 to 8 years evidence has ac-cumulated that the inflammatory response in the lungs, which is dominated by neutrophils, and the tissue damage is rather caused by immune complex formation in the lungs that by action of toxins (Høiby and Schiøtz 1982). In accordance with these results it is not surprising that the pulmonal pseudomonas infection in CF patients is a localized infection which does not spread outside the lungs, i.e. the mechanism of tissue damage is quite different from that in acute overwhelming pseudomonas infections seen in burn patients or patients suffering from leukemia.

### STRATEGIES OF ANTIBIOTIC TREATMENT OF P. AERUGINOSA LUNG INFECTION IN CF PATIENTS

One of the major drawbacks of antibiotic chemotherapy against P. aeruginosa lung infection in CF patients is that no orally admini-stered efficient antibiotics exist at the present time. Systemic therapy can only be given parenterally, in most cases by the intraveneous route. This means that most patients require hospita-lization although out-patients intravenous medications have been administered in some CF patients (Høiby et al. 1982).

TABLE 1.  Comparative activity against P. aeruginosa from 80 patients and dosages of some antibiotics

| Antibiotic | Geometric mean of MIC ($\mu$g/ml) | Daily dose of intraveneous therapy(mg/kg) | Daily dose of aerosol therapy (mg) |
|---|---|---|---|
| Tobramycin | 0.9 | 10 - (20) | 200 |
| Gentamicin | 2.9 | 5 | 200 |
| Netilmicin | 4.7 | 5 - (12) | |
| Ceftazidime | 0.4 | 150 | |
| Cefsulodin | 1.2 | 150 | |
| Azlocillin | 7.3 | 300 | |
| Carbenicillin | 9.9 | 500 | 1000 - 2000 |

An alternative route of administration is the aerosol treatment which has been used successfully in some clinics (Hodson et al. 1981). Table 1 shows the in vitro activity of anti-pseudomonas antibiotics

and the dosages used for intraveneous administration or for aerosol
treatment.

The aerosol antibiotic therapy has been used in Cystic Fibrosis since
1946 (Mearns 1979). In the 1950's and 1960's neomycin was the drug
of choice but one of the consequences of this treatment was that
several patients suffered from loss of hearing as a side effect.
Because of the risk of ototoxity with neomycin treatments, some of
the newer aminoglycosides such as gentamicin and tobramycin are
preferable for aerosol treatment. Hearing tests should, however, be
carried out at intervals. Aerosol treatment with a combination of
carbenicillin and gentamicin against P. aeruginosa infection has
proved efficient in a double-blind randomized cross-over trial
(Table 2) (Hodson et al. 1981).

TABLE 2.   Respiratory function: Group data of CF patients
           with P. aeruginosa infection treated with aerosol
           carbenicillin and gentamicin

| Treatment period | Mean $FEV_1$ (ml) | Mean FVC (ml) | Mean PEFR (l/min) |
|---|---|---|---|
| Antibiotic aerosol[1] | 1566 | 2656 | 323 |
| Placebo aerosol[2] | 1300 | 2314 | 283 |
| Significance[3] | $p<0.001$ | $0.02>p>0.001$ | $p<0.001$ |

[1] 17 patients each had 6 monthly recordings-total 102 assessments.

[2] 16 patients each had 6 monthly recordings and 1 had 4
monthly recordings-total 100 assessments.

[3] Student's unpaired $t$ test.
From Hodson et al. 1981. Reproduced by permission of The
Lancet.

This strategy of treatment is well suited for antibiotic therapy at
home of CF patients who are showing deterioration of lung function
and require frequent hospital admission for intraveneous therapy of
chronic P. aeruginosa lung infection. However, like with other kind
of anti-pseudomonas chemotherapy eradication of the bacteria is not
accomplished by aerosol treatment and despite the aerosol treatment,
some patients will require hospitalization for intraveneous therapy
(Hodson et al. 1981).

Intraveneous antibiotic therapy is the cornerstone in P. aeruginosa
treatment. High doses given as bolus injections are necessary because penetration of the drugs to sputum is not very efficient and
surprisingly low levels are detectable in CF sputum (Permin et al.
1983). The short-time bacteriological results are more favourable
when a combination of a beta-lactam antibiotic with aminoglycoside
is used as compared to monotherapy (Høiby et al. 1982, Szaff et al.
1983).However, in nearly all cases P. aeruginosa will re-occur in

sputum of the patients within a few months (Table 3). Temporary
eradication of P. aeruginosa is more easily obtained early in the
chronic lung infection during the first few courses of chemotherapy
and when the antibody response is rather low (Høiby et al. 1982).

TABLE 3.    Eradication and re-occurrence of P. aeruginosa
            in the lungs of CF patients after anti-pseudomonas
            chemotherapy

| | Period of the study | | | |
| | 1971-1975 (51 patients, 132 courses of chemotherapy) | | 1976-1980 (58 patients, 427 courses of chemotherapy) | |
| Time after completion of chemotherapy | % of patients[1] free of P. aeruginosa | % of treatments free of P. aeruginosa | % of patients[1] free of P. aeruginosa | % of treatments free of P. aeruginosa |
|---|---|---|---|---|
| Immediately after[2] | 68 | 36 | 79 | 35 |
| 1 month | 15 | 4.5 | 21 | 4.7 |
| 2 months | 2.5 | 0.8 | 10 | 1.9 |
| 3 months | 2.5 | 0.8 | 7 | 0.9 |
| 4 months | 0 | 0 | 1.7 | 0.2 |

[1]After one or more of the treatments.

[2]$\leq$ 24 h.

From Szaff et al. 1983. Reproduced by permission of Acta
Paediatrica Scandinavica.

Although not demonstrable by all authors, the bulk of evidence
supports the beneficial clinical role of anti-pseudomonas chemotherapy in CF patients (Høiby et al. 1982). The short-time effects
of anti-pseudomonas chemotherapy on lung function, WBC and ESR are
shown in Table 4. The effect on the lung function is detectable
also in rather advanced stages of the disease and it is in most
cases still detectable 1-3 months after completion of chemotherapy.
Therefore based on such observations, the Danish CF Centre decided
to treat the patients with chronic P. aeruginosa infection regularly
with 2-week courses every 3 months. The result of that regimen was
favourable as reflected by an increase of 5-year survival from the
time of onset of P. aeruginosa infection from 54 % to 82 % (p<0.05)
(Fig. 1). Furthermore, the lung function also improved significantly
(Szaff et al. 1983). The intensive "maintenance" chemotherapy against
P. aeruginosa infection, therefore, improves survival and quality
of life of CF patients although permanent eradication of P. aeruginosa is not accomplished.

TABLE 4.  Efficacy on non-bacteriological parameters of
14-day courses of ceftazidime in combination
with tobramycin in 11 CF patients with chronic
P. aeruginosa lung infection

| | Before treatment (median) | After treatment (median) | Increased | Decreased | Statistics |
|---|---|---|---|---|---|
| Leucocytes $10^9$/l | 15.4 | 8.6 | 1/11 | 10/11 | p<0.01 |
| Neutro- phils $10^9$/l | 9.0 | 2.8 | 1/11 | 10/11 | p<0.01 |
| Lympho- cytes $10^9$/l | 3.9 | 3.4 | 3/11 | 8/11 | N.S. |
| Peak expiratory flow rate[1] | 67 % | 101 % | 6/8 | 2/8 | p<0.05 |
| Forced vital capacity[1] | 49 % | 71 % | 7/8 | 0 | p<0.02 |
| Forced expiratory volume 1 sec.[1] | 30 % | 52 % | 8/8 | 0 | p<0.01 |

[1]In 8 patients. One patient was too ill and 2 were too
young to co-operate. The values are in percentage of
predicted values of normal persons of the same height
and sex.
From Høiby et al. 1982. Reproduced by permission of the
authors.

## SIDE EFFECTS AND OTHER PROBLEMS OF INTENSIVE CHEMOTHERAPY ATAINST P. AERUGINOSA INFECTION

The drawbacks of intensive chemotherapy are the high cost, development of allergy towards antibiotics, development of resistant P.
aeruginosa strains and increased risk of cross-infection among the
patients if they are treated in the same center (Høiby et al. 1982,
Zimakoff et al. 1983). None of these drawbacks are negligible. The
average cost of antibiotics used for four 2-week courses during 1
year is about 4.000-5.000 US$ per patient, and there is no reason
to believe that new antibiotics under development will be cheaper.
The dosages of carbenicillin and gentamicin used by Hodson et al.
(1982) are also expensive (11 US$ per day). This kind of treatment,
therefore, depends upon the heavy economical support of the society
for treatment of the individual patient. The problem of drug allergy
in CF patients is pertinent since many of the patients will develope
allergy towards one or more of the beta-lactam antibiotics (Høiby et
al. 1982). Both type 1 and type 3 allergic reactions may be seen,
but it is a surprising experience, that subsequent skin tests may
not demonstrate the type of allergy and some of the patients may

even tolerate repeated treatment with drugs which previously induced
allergic reactions (Høiby et al. 1982). One may speculate whether
some of the allergic reactions are not due to antibodies against
drugs but rather due to reactions between antibodies and bac-
rial antigens which are released due to the bacteriolytic action of
the drugs in patients undergoing intensive chemotherapy.

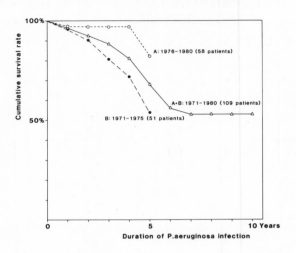

Fig. 1.    Survival (life table method)   of 109 CF patients
with chronic P. aeruginosa infection. The patients enter
the calculations at the onset of the infection. Group A
(58 patients) was treated with regular chemotherapy 3-4
times per year. These patients contracted the chronic
infection in the period 1976-80. Group B (51 patients)
was only treated with chemotherapy during clinical
deteriorations of the lung disease. Group B patients
contracted the chronic infection in the period 1971-75.
Data from Szaff et al. 1983.

Several reports have demonstrated the development of resistance in
P. aeruginosa against beta-lactam antibiotics, and also in some
cases against aminoglycosides during courses of chemotherapy (Høiby
et al. 1982). In most cases, however, after completion of chemotherapy when the selective pressure stops there is a decrease of antibiotic resistance of the P. aeruginosa strains isolated from the
patients (Høiby et al. 1982). If frequent intensive chemotherapy is
used in a patient, and in a clinic, the problem of resistant strains
may become severe. In the Danish CF Clinic we have seen a development and spread of a tobramycin resistant P. aeruginosa strain among
our CF patients during 1983. Unfortunately, this strain was also
resistant against most of the beta-lactam antibiotics available.
If, therefore, intensive anti-pseudomonas chemotherapy is used in
a CF center measures should be undertaken to avoid cross-infection
in the ward and in the out-patient clinic i.e. patients harbouring

multi-resistant P. aeruginosa strains should be isolated from other
CF patients.

## SUMMARY OF THE RESULTS OBTAINED WITH CURRENT STRATEGIES OF ANTI-PSEUDOMONAS CHEMOTHERAPY IN CF PATIENTS

The results obtained with the intensive anti-pseudomonas chemotherapy
given at regular intervals with respect to survival and quality of
life of the patients are encouraging. In most cases this regime
requires hospitalization but this may, to some extent, be avoided by
the use of aerosol antibiotics given at home. P. aeruginosa is,
however, not permanently eradicated by any of the regimens currently
used. Repeated courses of "maintenance" chemotherapy is therefore
not a permanent solution in CF patients and the cost and the side
effects of this "maintenance" chemotherapy are considerable.

## FUTURE TREATMENT POSSIBILITIES OF CHRONIC P. AERUGINOSA LUNG INFECTION IN CF PATIENTS

Most clinicians hesitate to treat the P. aeruginosa lung infection
in CF patients until it has become chronic and/or obvious clinical
signs of infection are present. It has, however, been shown that the
bacteriological results are more favourable if patients are treated
early in the infection (Høiby et al. 1982). It would be a logical
step to treat the patients very early i.e. at the onset of the
colonization. This approach has been very successful with respect
to Staph. aureus and H. influenzae infection in the Danish CF Centre,
where oral drugs can be used (Høiby et al. 1982). Such approach to
treat P. aeruginosa infection could be carried out either by intravenous therapy or preferably by aerosol therapy. However, it would
be greatly aided if orally administered efficient anti-pseudomonas
drugs were available. The drug companies should therefore be en-
couraged to develop oral drugs with anti-pseudomonas activity.

The P. aeruginosa lung infection in CF patients is a chronic infection which may run for more than ten years. No other chronic infections (for instance tuberculosis or leprosy) are treated with
short-time antibiotic chemotherapy. It would therefore be a logical
step to try to adopt some of the experience obtained in the field
of anti-tuberculosis or anti-leprosy chemotherapy for the treatment
of P. aeruginosa infection in CF patients. That would imply the use
of combination chemotherapy for many months even after eradication
of the bacteria from the sputum. Such an approach could be evaluated
in a few patients, and if the results were favourable, controlled
randomized studies could be carried out.

Based on the hypothesis that the chronic P. aeruginosa lung infection
is an immune complex disease several other theoretical treatment
possibilities exist. If the antibodies or immune complexes are
removed by plasmapheresis this might temporarily stop the inflammatory process. This has been tried without convincing success in our
center. It may be because the offending antigen (P. aeruginosa) is
not removed at the same time, and so the immune system is still

stimulated and new antibodies and immune complexes are formed.
Bronchial lavage has also been tried and reported efficient by some
authors (Kulczycki 1981). This approach may lead to removal of antibodies, antigens and immune complexes from the secretions but not
from the lung tissue and bronchial wall. Inhalation with steroid
hormones (Beclomethasone) has been attempted in our patients, with
no convincing effect possibly because it is impossible to get the
drug out into the peripheral airways where the inflammatory process
takes place (Schiøtz et al. 1983). Systemic treatment with steroids
and other anti-inflammatory drugs has not been tried systematically
in CF patients with chronic pseudomonas infection, so data about
the value of this possible therapeutic approach are not available.

Suppression of the antibody response by cytostatic drugs might also
be a possibility although it is not tempting to depress the antibody
response in patients in whom the airways are so vulnerable to various
bacterial species. A more tempting approach would be to block some
of the mediators of the inflammatory response. The existence of an
inhibitor of $C_1$-esterase is already known and an inhibition of the
whole complement cascade (which is not yet possible) would presumably
diminish the inflammatory response and thus the tissue damage considerably. Also protease inhibitors could result in less tissue
damage. Alpha-1-antitrypsin preparation is now commercially available
and is claimed to diminish the chronic inflammation in the lungs of
patients with alpha-1-antitrypsin deficiency. The administration of
protease inhibitors which support the patient's own inhibitors in
neutralizing the proteases of the inflammatory exsudate may prove
beneficial.

All these alternative possibilities are of course examples of symptomatic treatment, none of them can at present match proper antibiotic treatment, and none of them will be able to substitute
research into the factors that explain why CF patients are so
susceptible to pulmonary infections.

## ABSTRACT

Current anti-pseudomonas chemotherapy in CF patients consists of
aminoglycosides and beta-lactam antibiotics given as combination
therapy intraveneously for 2 weeks. Alternatively, some clinics
treat the patients at home with aerosolized antibiotics. The lung
function and the inflammatory parameters improve considerably
during courses of chemotherapy. Treatment with anti-pseudomonas
chemotherapy on a regular basis every 3 months improve the 5-year
survival of CF patients from the time of the onset of the chronic
P. aeruginosa infection from 54 % to 82 % and the lung function also
improves significantly. However, some drawbacks of the intensive
"maintenance" chemotherapy are obvious. The cost is considerable,
some of the patients will develop allergy to the drugs used and
some of the patients will be colonized by resistant strains of P.
aeruginosa. Future research should be carried out concerning the
possibility of early intensive chemotherapy before the P. aeruginosà
infection becomes chronic, and of prolonged chemotherapy with combination of antibiotics for many months after the infection has

become chronic. Other possibilities of treatment which are based on
the experimental and clinical evidence of immune complexes as the
main courses of the tissue damage in the lungs of CF patients during
the chronic P. aeruginosa infection are discussed.

## REFERENCES

Döring, G., Buhl, V., Høiby, N., Schiøtz, P.O. and Botzenhart, K.,
    1983. Detection of proteases of Pseudomonas aeruginosa in immune
    complexes isolated from sputum of cystic fibrosis patients. Sub-
    mitted for publication to Journal of Infectious Diseases.
Hancock, R.E.W., Mutharia, L.M., Chan, L., Darveau, R.P., Speert, D.
    P. and Pier, G.B., 1983. Pseudomonas aeruginosa isolates from
    patients with cystic fibrosis: A class of serum-sensitive, non-
    typable strains deficient in lipopolysaccharide O side chains.
    Infection and Immunity, 42, 170-177.
Hodson, M.E., Penketh, A.R.L. and Batten, J.C., 1981. Aerosol car-
    benicillin and gentamicin treatment of Pseudomonas aeruginosa
    infection in patients with cystic fibrosis. Lancet,ii, 1137-1139.
Høiby, N., 1982. Microbiology of lung infections in cystic fibrosis
    patients. Acta Pædiatrica Scandinavica, Supplement 301, 33-54.
Høiby, N. and Schiøtz, P.O., 1982. Immune complex mediated tissue
    damage in the lungs of cystic fibrosis patients with chronic
    Pseudomonas aeruginosa infection. Acta Pædiatrica Scandinavica,
    Supplement, 301, 63-73.
Høiby, N., Friis, B., Jensen, K., Koch, C., Møller, N.E., Støvring,
    S. and Szaff, M., 1982. Antimicrobial chemotherapy in cystic
    fibrosis patients. Acta Pædiatrica Scandinavica, Supplement, 301,
    75-100.
Kulczycki, L.L., 1981. Experience with 632 bronchoscopic bronchial
    washings (BBW) done on 173 cystic fibrosis (CF) patients during a
    16-years period (1965-1980). 1,000 Years of Cystic Fibrosis
    Collected Papers (Ed.: Warren J. Warwick), pp 95-112. University
    of Minnesota.
Mearns, M.B., 1979. Aerosol therapy in cystic fibrosis. Pädiatrische
    Fortbildungskurse für die Praxis,48, (Ed. E. Rossi), pp 76-93.
    Karger, Basel.
Permin, H., Koch, C., Høiby, N., Christensen, H.O., Friis-Møller,
    A. and Møller, S.,  1983. Ceftazidime treatment of chronic
    Pseudomonas aeruginosa respiratory tract infection in cystic
    fibrosis. Journal of Antimicrobial Chemotherapy, 12, Supplement A,
    313-323.
Schiøtz, P.O., Jørgensen, M., Flensborg, E.W., Færø, O., Husby, S.,
    Høiby, N., Jacobsen, S.V., Nielsen, H. and Svehag, S.-E., 1983.
    Chronic Pseudomonas aeruginosa lung infection in cystic fibrosis.
    Acta Pædiatrica Scandinavica, 72, 283-287.
Szaff, M., Høiby, N. and Flensborg, E.W., 1983. Frequent antibiotic
    therapy improves survival of cystic fibrosis patients with chro-
    nic Pseudomonas aeruginosa infection. Acta Pædiatrica Scandinavica,
    72, 651-657.
Zimakoff, J., Høiby, N., Rosendal, K. and Guilbert, J.P., 1983.
    Epidemiology of Pseudomonas aeruginosa infection and the role of
    contamination of the environment in a cystic fibrosis clinic.
    Journal of Hospital Infection, 4, 31-40.

SUPPLEMENTAL NUTRITION IN CYSTIC FIBROSIS: Improved growth, body
protein accretion and dynamic aspects of protein turnover.
Shepherd, R.W., Holt, T.L., Cooksley, W.G.E., Thomas, B.J.,
Ward, L.C., Royal Children's Hospital; Dept of Medical Physics,
Qld Inst Technology; Depts of Child Health & Biochemistry,
University of Queensland, Brisbane, Australia.

Previous studies of nutritional growth retardation in cystic fibrosis
(CF) have demonstrated a nutritional deficit similar to that of
protein-energy malnutrition but with paradoxically increased myofibrillar protein catabolism (MPCat). To investigate potential
benefits of protein energy supplementation and further assess protein
turnover, we studied changes in body composition, whole body protein
synthesis (WBPSyn), catabolism (WBPCat) and MPCat before and after
supplementation in 10 undernourished CF children and in eight healthy
controls. Enteral supplements were with a peptide formula that
increased protein-energy intakes 20-40% over ad libitum oral intake
for a minimum of six months delivered either as an oral supplement
or nocturnal intragastric feeding. Body composition was assessed by
anthropometry, total body $^{40}K$ (TB$^{40}$K) and creatinine excretion;
WBPSyn and Cat by $N^{15}$glycine turnover and N balance; net protein
deposition was measured as WBPSyn-WBPCat and MPCat by urinary 3-
methylhistidine excretion. Compared with controls, CF children had
significantly reduced body mass, body fat and muscle mass and
significantly less net protein deposition with excessive MPCat.
With supplements, catch-up weight gain ($p<0.05$), and growth ($p<0.02$)
occurred with increased fat ($p<0.01$), TB$^{40}$K ($p<0.01$) and muscle mass
($p<0.01$). Increased net protein deposition occurred, related to the
marked increase in WBPSyn ($p<0.01$) and moderate increase in WPBCat
($p<0.05$) in all patients studied, and normalization of the high
rate of MPCat observed in five of six patients.

|  | Mass | Fat | Muscle | TB$^{40}$K | TBPSyn | TBPCat | Net Dep | MPCat |
|---|---|---|---|---|---|---|---|---|
|  | %std | | | (g) | | g Kg$^{-1}$ 24 hr$^{-1}$ | | |
| C | 100±1 | 14±1 | 30±1 | | 4.7±0.3 (n=5) | 3.2±0.9 | 1.5±0.6 | 0.53±0.04 (n=8) |
| CF | 78±3 | 8±1 | 22±2 | 60±7 | 4.2±0.4 (n=4) | 3.3±0.7 | 0.9±0.2 | 0.76±0.16 (n=6) |
| CF(s) | 84±3 | 11±1 | 25±1 | 70±8 | 6.5±0.9 | 4.4±0.9 | 2.1±0.4 | 0.51±0.26 |

We conclude that undernutrition in CF is partly related to a state
of chronic catabolic stress and that improved intake can cause net
protein accretion with improved growth by increasing synthesis in
excess of catabolism.

# NUTRITIONAL REHABILITATION IN MALNOURISHED PATIENTS WITH CYSTIC FIBROSIS: EFFECT ON THE COURSE OF THE DISEASE.

E.V. O'Loughlin, D. Forbes, H. Parsons, B. Scott, D. Cooper, D.G. Gall
Department of Pediatrics, University of Calgary and Divisions of
Gastroenterology and Nutrition, and Pulmonology, Alberta Children's
Hospital, 3330 Hospital Drive N.W., Calgary, Alberta.  T2N 4N1  CANADA

Cystic fibrosis patients with normal nutritional status appear to have a better prognosis than those who are malnourished. Whether or not improved nutrition in the malnourished patient alters the course of the disease is unclear. This study examined the effect of nutritional rehabilitation in CF patients with severe disease. METHODS:  Patients of less than 90% ideal body weight (IBW) were entered into the study. During an initial 6 month period we attempted to increase caloric intake by oral supplementation. If weight gain was not achieved, patients were advanced to nocturnal nasogastric feedings (NG) with a semisynthetic formula in addition to regular diet. Anthropometric measurements, biochemical parameters, pulmonary function tests(PFT's), days of hospitalization,episodes of pneumonia and patient well being were followed. RESULTS: 12 malnourished patients (6 males, 6 females; age 7-27 years) with mean IBW 76.7% predicted, were studied over 7-16 months. Steatorrhea was present in 8. Oral supplementation was initiated in 11 patients (mean duration 6.1 months); only 2 patients gained weight, 1 patient died and 2 withdrew. NG feedings were commenced in 6 because of failure to gain with oral supplementation, One patient commenced NG feeding without prior oral supplementation because of severity of disease. Weight gain was achieved in 6 of 7 patients with NG supplementation (mean 6.2 months). In all, 8 patients successfully gained weight, mean % IBW increased from 76 to 89%.
Weight gain was associated with a significant ($p<.05$) increase in lean body mass ($23.9\pm3.0$ vs $26.7\pm3.2$ kg), total body fat ($3.2\pm0.7$ vs $7.3\pm1.1$ kg) and height velocity ($0.28\pm0.05$ vs $0.49\pm0.09$ cm/month). There was a significant ($p<.05$) decrease in episodes of pneumonia requiring hospitalization ($1.6\pm0.3$ vs $1.1\pm0.4$ / 6 months) and improvement in patient well being. Number of days in hospital, biochemical parameters and PFT's were unchanged. Table ($\overline{X}\pm SE$, % predicted) presents PFT's obtained 0 to 6 months before and 6 months after nutritional rehabilitation.

| MONTHS | FEV | $FEV_1$ | $FEV_{25-75}$ | RV/TLC |
|--------|-----|---------|---------------|--------|
| -6 | $56\pm7$ | $41\pm6$ | $17\pm3$ | $240\pm11$ |
| 0 | $60\pm7$ | $40\pm6$ | $16\pm3$ | $270\pm19$ |
| 6 | $60\pm6$ | $37\pm5$ | $12\pm2$ | $270\pm15$ |

CONCLUSION: We were unsuccessful in achieving weight gain in the majority of patients with oral supplementation but weight gain was readily achieved with NG supplementation. While pulmonary function was unchanged, nutritional rehabilitation after 6 months was associated with increased height velocity, lean body mass, adipose tissue and patient well being and decreased episodes of pneumonia.

FUTURE DIRECTIONS IN SUPPLEMENTAL
NUTRITION

Dr. D.B.A. Silk MD FRCP

Co-Director, Department of Gastroenterology
and Nutrition, Central Middlesex Hospital
Acton Lane, London, NW10

Cystic fibrosis is common in white European and North
American populations with a birth incidence of around
1:2000 (Bearn 1973) and where intensive birth screening
has been undertaken the incidence may be as high as
1:1200 (Stephan 1973).    It is a multi-system disorder
with its main impact on the respiratory tract, leading
to repeated chest infections, and on the gut where the
main problem is exocrine pancreatic insufficiency.   In
the neonate this latter defect leads to acute intestinal
obstruction due to meconium ileus, a complication which
was encountered in   5% of a large series of cystic
fibrosis patients studied in France (Chazalette,
Dutau, Chevalir, et al 1977).   Other clinical problems
in the disease include rectal prolapse and ileal atresia
and in older patients nasal polyps, diabetes and hepatic
cirrhosis.

Nutritional disturbances are common in cystic fibrosis
(CF) and on occasions may be the presenting feature.
The nutritional disturbances may arise as a consequence
of malabsorption or result from inadequate nutrient
intake in the presence of increased metabolic demands
that may occur in the presence of severe respiratory
disease.   It follows from what we understand of the
natural history of the disease that both factors may be
combined in many cases.

## NUTRITIONAL STATUS IN CYSTIC FIBROSIS

Although much has been written about the nutritional
status in CF,  Berry, Kellogg, Hunt et al 1975 reported
one of the first detailed surveys in a large group of
patients.   The findings showed that CF patients
maintained weight approximately one standard deviation
below the mean until the age of eight years, after which
there was a progressive decline in growth rate compared
to normal.   Poor growth was associated with low
concentrations of serum albumin and urea nitrogen.

99

Similar growth characteristics were found by Sproul and
Huang eleven years previously (1964).    Similar findings
were later reported by Yassa, Prosser and Dodge in
1978 and in particular both height and weight of their
patients decreased progressively with age in the older
children.    There is general agreement that with the
onset of puberty and the corresponding growth spurt in
normal children, the CF child tends to fall away from
standard growth curves.    This increase in the relative
degree of underweight is partly explained by the delayed
puberty which is common in CF and partly by clinical
deterioration (Berry, Kellogg, Hunt et al 1975).    As
height like weight is on average about one standard
deviation below the population mean during childhood,
children with CF appear not only short for their age,
i.e. stunted, but also underweight for their height,
i.e. wasted.    Although wasting may be a prominent
clinical feature in early infancy before diagnosis
adequate nutritional supplementation usually leads to an
improvement in muscle wasting and if it re-appears in
later life it usually is associated with uncontrolled
respiratory infection, with or without the presence of
permanent lung damage (Kraemer, Rudeberg, Hadorn and
Rossi 1978).

## NUTRITIONAL INTAKE

Patients with CF have been characterised in the
literature as having voracious appetites despite
remaining remarkably underweight for height and age
(Hubbard and Mangrum 1982).    Review of the literature
shows that the voracious appetite is usually noticed
during infancy (Shwachman 1975;   Dodge and Yassa 1980).
Although in older CF patients caloric and protein
intakes above recommended daily allowances (RDA) may
be found (Hubbard and Mangrum 1982), mean intakes of
calories and protein corrected for age and height are
usually about 80 - 89% of RDA (Dodge and Yassa 1980;
Chase, Long, and Lavin 1979).    At first sight such
figures could be taken to imply a modest reduction only
in nutritional intake.    However, the findings do not
take into account loss of nutrients in the stool
occurring as a consequence of malabsorption nor do the
findings take note of increases in requirements that
occur in response to episodes of pulmonary infection
that are such a hallmark of CF.

## SPECIFIC NUTRITIONAL DEFICIENCIES

The evidence for specific nutritional deficiencies in
patients with CF has recently been reviewed (Chase, Long
and Lavin 1979).

## PROTEIN

It is well established that despite adequate pancreatic
replacement therapy, patients with pancreatic
insufficiency due to CF excrete increased amounts of
faecal nitrogen (Lapey, Kattwinkel, di Sant'Agnese
et al 1974).   The increased faecal nitrogen is accounted
for by both unhydrolysed proteins and amino acids of
dietary origin.   The faecal amino acids are derived in
part from intraluminal bacterial degradation of intact
proteins and to defects in active absorption of neutral
amino acids (Milla, Kilby, Rassam et al 1983).

## FATS

An enormous range of steatorrhoea has been found in CF
patients with untreated pancreatic insufficiency
(Lapey, Kattwinkel, di Sant'Agnese et al 1974).
Although pancreatic supplements decrease fat excretion
the efficacy of pancreatic supplements, even when given
with $H_2$-receptor antagonists, is disappointing (Cox,
Isenberg, Osher et al 1979) and most, if not all CF
patients with pancreatic insufficiency still have
steatorrhoea on treatment.   The variability of
steatorrhoea in CF patients is likely to be due to the
variable retention of a very small fraction of the
total pancreatic secretory capacity for lipase and
colipase and in this context Forstner, Gall, Corey
et al (1980) have shown that colipase correlates much
better than lipase with the degree of steatorrhoea and
may be a more accurate measure of physiological capacity
for fat digestion in CF patients.

Medium chain triglycerides (MCTs) are less dependent on
pancreatic enzymes for absorption since they are much
more rapidly hydrolysed by pancreatic lipase and may be
absorbed directly by the mucosal cell (Isselbacher 1967).
A significant reduction in steatorrhoea has been shown
to be obtained in children with CF by substituting MCT
or LCT (Kuo and Huang 1965).   Forstner et al (1980)
have not only confirmed this but have shown added
benefits of administering MCT with pancreatic
supplementation.

## ESSENTIAL FATTY ACIDS

CF patients have been shown to have abnormal fatty acid
composition of blood and tissue lipids.   The
predominant alteration of fatty acid composition is a
deficiency of the essential fatty acid linoleic acid
with increases in palmitoleic acid and oleic acid
(Hubbard 1980).   These alterations are not reversed
when pancreatic enzyme supplements are administered in

sufficient quantities to significantly reduce
steatorrhoea (Hubbard, Dunn, di Sant'Agnese 1977).    The
evidence that there might be a relationship between the
observed abnormalities of fatty acid metabolism,
particularly in relationship to the control of
prostaglandin synthesis, to the pathophysiology
underlying the clinical manifestations of CF, have been
reviewed (Hubbard 1980;  Chase, Long and Lavin 1979).
Although a number of attractive hypotheses have been
suggested, it is pertinent to remember that there are
patients with the pulmonary lesions of CF who not only
have normal exocrine pancreatic function but also
normal fatty acid composition of their blood and tissue
lipids (Hubbard 1980).   Moreover, if an altered membrane
structure was related to the basic defect in CF one
would hope to be able to detect this abnormality in
fibroblasts.   Current studies have shown that protein
and glycoprotein components (Baig, Cetorelli and
Roberts 1975) and lipid components (Riordan, Alon and
Buchwald 1979) of plasma membranes from fibroblasts
from patients with CF are no different than similar
analysis from normal individuals.

### VITAMINS

It is not clear whether patients with CF require
specific supplementation with water soluble vitamins.
In a recent study (Congden, Bruce, Rothburn et al 1981)
vitamin B1, B2 and B6 status was found to be adequate
and there was little evidence of folic acid deficiency.
In some of the patients vitamin C stores were considered
to be inadequate despite daily supplements with 50 mg
of the vitamin.   Patients with CF have been reported
as having low levels of vitamin B12 and impairment of
B12 absorption, the latter improving following
ingestion of pancreatic supplements (Deren, Arora,
Toskes et al 1973).   Recent studies have shown that
orally administered vitamin B12 is bound by R protein
in the stomach at acid pH and remains bound at the
nearly neutral pH of the small intestine until the R
protein moiety is degraded by the synergistic action
of trypsin and chymotrypsin together possibly with
elastase (Allen, Beetharam, Podell et al 1978).    It
therefore seems likely that intrinsic factor - vitamin
B12 binding occurs in the small intestine and not
stomach and only after vitamin B12 is released from the
R protein vitamin B12 complex by the action of
pancreatic proteases.   It follows therefore, that in CF
patients with pancreatic insufficiency vitamin B12
deficiency is likely to develop if pancreatic
supplements are not administered and that small
supplements of vitamin B12 may well be required from

time to time.  Vitamin A levels in CF patients are low
even in the presence of conventional supplements
(Congden et al 1981).  Serum 25-OH cholecalciferol
levels have been shown to be low in some patients
whether or not they were receiving a daily supplement
of 400 IU vitamin D (Congden et al 1981).  Vitamin E
levels are nearly always low unless supplements are
given (Harries and Muller 1971).  Vitamin K
deficiency with bleeding secondary to hypothrombinaemia
may also occur in CF and vitamin K supplements may well
be required.

### TRACE ELEMENTS

There is some confusion in the literature as to whether
the zinc status of CF patients is reduced or normal
(Halsted and Smith 1970;  Palin, Underwood and Denning
1976).  One of the reasons for the uncertainty is that
most authors have measured plasma zinc levels which are
poor indicators of zinc deficiency.  There is work to
suggest that low plasma zince levels may be associated
with growth retardation which in turn can be reversed
if zinc supplements are given (Halsted and Smith 1970;
Dodge and Yassa 1978).

The extent of dietary iron absorption in CF patients is
dependent upon iron stores being increased when iron
stores are low and normal in CF patients with normal
iron stores (Heinrich, Bender-Gotze and Gabbe 1977).

Selenium is an important trace element and its major
role is as an integral part of the enzyme glutathione
peroxidase, which protects lipids in membranes from
oxidation.  It has been suggested that selenium
deficiency could account for most, or perhaps all of
the clinical features of CF.  Plasma selenium
concentration is the measurement of choice in detection
of selenium deficiency (Kingsnorth 1984).  Since levels
are  usually normal in patients with CF (Lloyd-Still
and Ganther 1980;  Castillo, Landon,    Eckhardt et al
1981) selenium supplementation would appear to be
contra-indicated in CF patients, particularly since at
least one fatality has occurred in a young child with
CF who was receiving oral selenium supplements
(Hubbard, Barbero and Chase 1980).

It should be appreciated that in addition to zinc, iron
and selenium, deficiency syndromes have been described
for iodine, cobalt, copper, chromium, molybdenum,
manganese and vanadium (Silk 1983), so that more work
needs to be done in the area of trace element
metabolism in cystic fibrosis.

## DANGERS OF PROTEIN CALORIE MALNUTRITION IN CYSTIC FIBROSIS

There is now very strong evidence to show that protein
calorie malnutrition has a deleterious effect on immune
function, particularly on humeral and cellular immunity
as well as on certain aspects of phagocytic function
(Dowd and Heatley 1984). In CF patients infection and
decreased immunocompetence frequently co-exist and for
most patients establishment of the primary causative
factor is virtually impossible, (Raeburn 1977).    As
mentioned above, specific nutritional deficiencies do
exist in CF patients and there is an association between
a number of these deficiencies and impaired immune
function.   This is so for zinc (Dowd and Heatley 1984),
piridoxine (Axelrod and Trakatellis 1964), vitamin C
(Neumann, Lawlor, Stiehm et al 1975), and vitamin A
(Bhaskaram and Reddy 1975). · There have been a number
of attempts to return tests of immune function to normal
by nutritional repletion.  In several studies oral and
intravenous nutritional supplementation has proven
beneficial (Mullin and Kirkpatrick 1981;  Law, Dudrick
and Abdou 1973).   Since immunity is impaired in CF
patients (Raeburn 1977) and the hallmark of the disease
is repeated and severe respiratory infections, there is
a sound rational basis for believing that more effort
should be directed towards improving the nutritional
status of CF patients.

## NUTRITIONAL SUPPORT IN CYSTIC FIBROSIS

When one reviews the literature concerning nutritional
support in CF patients it becomes evident that
nutritional status can be improved and normal rates of
weight gain achieved by simply being aware of the need
to monitor nutritional intake and to supply simple
nutritional supplements.   One interesting factor is
that in the face of an awareness about nutritional
intake there may be a betterment of pancreatic enzyme
replacement therapy (Parsons, Dumas, Beaudry et al 1980).

Although the lifespan of CF patients is improving
(Phelan and Landau 1979;  Crozier 1974), problems with
pulmonary infection become increasingly important.
Nutritional intake and growth characteristics of CF
patients declines with age (Berry et al 1975).   One of
the main reasons for this is likely to be the frequent
episodes of anorexia associated with acute exacerbations
of pulmonary infection.   As malnutrition, infection and
decreased immunocompetence frequently co-exist (Dowd
and Heatley 1984), there is every reason to believe
that nutritional management of CF patients might play
an important role in effecting the course of pulmonary
disease and longterm outcome of CF patients (Kraemer

et al 1978).    It is for this reason that several
attempts are currently being made to improve absorbed
intake of calories, nitrogen and specific nutrients
with specific nutritional support programmes.    A
chemically defined "elemental" diet consisting of a
partial enzymic hydrolysate of whole protein, a glucose
polymer mixture and medium chain triglycerides has been
administered either as the sole means of nutritional
intake or as a supplement to the normal diet in at least
three different studies (Allan, Mason and Moss 1973;
Berry et al 1975;   Yassa, Prosser and Dodge 1978).
Increased rates of weight gain and improvement in growth
characteristics have been seen in some of the patients
treated, but very little in the way of demonstrable
effects on lung function or radiological appearances
were found.    On the basis of their experiences Yassa
et al (1978) concluded that the expense and impalatabil-
ity of the diet outweighed its  minimal beneficial
effect on growth (Yassa et al 1978).    A more recent
study of nutritional supplementation which has aroused
much interest is the one reported by Shepherd,
Cooksley and Cooke (1980) in which twelve patients were
given intravenous nutrition (130% recommended daily
allowance) for three weeks, using intralipid amino acids
and glucose.    There was a weight gain observed which
persisted after the intravenous therapy was stopped and
the gain in weight was still continuing at six months.
In addition, significantly fewer pulmonary infections
were observed in the six months post therapy,
sustained and significant improvements were noted in
clinical score and pulmonary function and there
appeared a marked improvement in well-being and ad
libitum nutrient intake.    The implications of this
study are that in problem patients with CF, specific
nutritional support can favourably affect growth,
clinical status and the course of chronic pulmonary
disease.

## THE FUTURE OF NUTRITIONAL SUPPORT IN CYSTIC FIBROSIS

While the study of Shepherd et al (1980) is of great
interest because it suggests beneficial effects of
nutritional support not only in the short, but also in
the long term, it should be emphasised that the study
was uncontrolled and the parenteral rather than the
enteral route was used.    Parenteral nutrition is
inconvenient to the patient, it is expensive and not
without serious side effects (Silk 1983).    It has
seemed to us therefore, that the continuing aim in CF
patients should be to provide nutritional support via
the enteral rather than parenteral route, particularly
since gastrointestinal function is clearly sufficient

to at least permit the absorption of pre-digested
nutrients.    The possible long term benefits of the
parenteral nutrition study, particularly on the natural
history of the chronic pulmonary disease, should we
believe, not be ignored and our future aims are to
determine whether specific nutritional support
administered via the enteral route has any significant
short and long term effects on the natural history of
pulmonary disease in CF patients.    Our present aims of
nutritional support are as specific as this as Berry
and co-workers (1975) have already shown under
controlled trial conditions that specific nutritional
support has significant benefits on nutritional status
of CF patients.

## ENTERAL NUTRITION IN CYSTIC FIBROSIS

There is no evidence, nor for that matter any reason,
for believing that intake of normal food in the presence
of pancreatic supplements should be discouraged in CF
patients.    The objective of any nutritional support
programme designed to assess efficacy as far as the
natural history of chronic pulmonary disease is
concerned would be to enhance nutritional intake by
supplementing normal diet by administering nutritional
formulations that meet the nutritional needs of the
patients.

Diet formulation.   In patients with CF nutrient
assimilation is impaired on account of the co-existing
exocrine pancreatic insufficiency.   It follows that
when optimum absorption is required, nutrients should be
presented to the gut in a pre-digested form and indeed
to ensure that maximal possible absorption is achieved
the pre-digested nutrients should ideally be presented
in the form in which they are absorbed fastest in the
normal clinical setting.    It should be appreciated from
the outset that the old term "elemental" diet is a
misnomer.  Used initially to describe the early free
amino acid and glucose containing diets, it has later
been used to describe all the other diets containing
pre-digested nutrients that are far from "elemental"
in design.  Recent work shows that the products of
luminal protein digestion are absorbed in the form of
small peptides as well as free amino acids and moreover
it appears that peptide rather than free amino acid
transport is the major mode of absorption of protein
digestion products (Silk 1981).  As intestinal perfusion
studies show that amino acid nitrogen is absorbed
faster from partial enzymic hydrolysates of whole
protein than from equivalent equimolar amino acid
solutions, there seems reason to believe that partial
enzymic hydrolysates of whole protein constitute the

most  suitable peptide based nitrogen source for use
in cystic fibrosis (Silk, Fairclough, Clark et al 1980).
Our recent studies have shown that absorption
characteristics of partial enzymic hydrolysates of
whole protein are affected both by the type of starter
protein studied and the type of hydrolysis procedure
used to produce it, so at present no firm recommendations
can be made about these (Keohane, Brown, Grimble et al
1982).   Absorption characteristics are also affected by
the peptide chain length (Keohane, Grimble, Brown et al
1983) and most recent data suggests that optimum
absorption occurs if partial enzymic hydrolysates of
whole protein are formulated to contain peptides with a
chain length of 2-3 amino acid residues (Rees, Grimble,
Keohane at al 1984).

The carbohydrate energy source of most of the
commercially available enteral diets consist of a
partial amylase hydrolysate of corn starch.   The
intestinal assimilation of these starch hydrolysates has
now been characterised (Jones, Brown, Loran et al 1983)
and there is evidence to show that hydrolysates
consisting predominantly of high molecular weight
glucose polymers with a low osmolality are relatively
well assimilated even in the absence of luminal amylase
activity (Jones, Brown, Grimble et al 1981) so that
these should probably constitute the carbohydrate
fraction of the energy source.

As outlined above, medium chain triglycerides are
better assimilated in cystic fibrosis than long chain
triglycerides so that MCTs rather than LCTs should
form the basis of the lipid fraction of the energy
source in diets for use in cystic fibrosis.   Particular
care in cystic fibrosis must be made to include the
essential fatty acid linoleic acid, not only to prevent
the development of essential fatty acid deficiency, but
to avoid the possible     deleterious effects that
essential fatty acid deficiency may have in the
pathogenesis of the pulmonary lesion in CF (see above).

Proprietary pre-digested "elemental" diets.  In the UK
at present there are at least three potentially suitable
diets available.   All are in powder form and require
blending before administration.  Flexical contains
rather an unsuitable hetergeneous peptide nitrogen
source.   Vivonex contains free amino acid as nitrogen
source and consequently is relatively hypertonic as
compared to the others.  Although there are no clinical
files to substantiate it, it probably contain
insufficient linoleic acid for long term use in cystic
fibrosis.   Nutranel is the best of the available diets
at present.  Approximately 20% of its energy content is

in the form of fat and of this 50% consists of MCTs.
The carbohydrate energy source consists of a heterogeneous glucose polymer mixture and the nitrogen source
consists of quite a balanced partial enzymic hydrolysate
of whole protein.  We are currently studying a pre-
digested diet called Reabilan.  This has the advantage
of being produced in liquid form, the nitrogen source
consists of small peptides produced by a rationally
designed hydrolysis procedure.  35% of the total energy
content is in the form of lipids and of this a
significant proportion is in the form of MCTs.  This
diet has an added attraction as far as CF patients are
concerned, because a high proportion of fatty acid
distribution of lipid energy source is in the form of
linoleic acid and in addition also contains significant
proportions of its fatty acid distribution as gamma
linolenic acid, the precursor of linoleic acid.

We consider it preferable to use the commercially
produced diets rather than formulating our own diet in
the diet kitchen.  This is so because there is now
controlled data to show that the incidence of diarrhoea
is higher when "home-brew" rather than commercial diets
are used for enteral feeding (Keighley, Mogg, Bently
et al 1982).   Care is still needed to ensure that the
powdered diets are prepared for clinical use under
reasonably sterile conditions as problems with infection
have been well documented during the blending process
(Casewell 1979).

Techniques of administration.  In our experience it has
proved very difficult to precisely document and control
intake of enteral diets if they are administered as an
oral supplement.  Many patients have found that most of
the proprietary pre-digested diets mentioned above are
not nearly as palatable as the manufacturers claim and
excessive nursing time is taken up cajoling patients to
ingest the desired quantities.  At present therefore,
we have preferred to attempt to administer enteral
diets in CF patients via a naso-gastric tube.  We know
from previously published data that naso-gastric
feeding does not result in a diminution of appetite for
normal food (Hall, Manning and Symes 1983) so that on
theoretical grounds we could provide enteral nutritional
support via the naso-gastric route continuously over
twenty four hours.  Special problems exist however, in
CF patients, particularly with those admitted to
hospital on account of recurrent pulmonary infections,
as aggressive chest physiotherapy is required which
makes naso-gastric feeding extremely difficult.  For
this reason our current trial protocol is based on the
use of nocturnal enteral nutrition as a means of
increasing nutritional intake.  Patients receiving

specific nutritional support receive twelve hours of
nocturnal naso-gastric feeding while in hospital,
followed by twelve hours of nocturnal enteral feeding
for a month following hospital discharge.

The patients are intubated with a fine bore naso-gastric
feeding tube.    Some problems may well be encountered
in patients with nasal polyps and the frequency of this
problem is currently being assessed.    The enteral diet
is administered from 1.5 - 2 litre diet containers by
gravity infusion.

Use of starter regimes.  Upper abdominal symptoms
including distention, discomfort, colicky pains as well
as diarrhoea are said to frequently occur if full
strength enteric feeding regimes are introduced too
quickly (Silk 1980).    A number of factors have been
implicated in the pathogenesis of these side effects.
These include intolerance to high osmotic loads of
nutrients administered during enteral feeding, lactose
intolerance, use of contaminated feeds and concomitant
antibiotic therapy (Silk 1983).    It has been generally
believed that the incidence of these side effects can be
minimised by gradually introducing full strength
enteric feeds over a three to four day period by means
of "starter regimes".

Our most recent controlled studies have however, shown
that starter regimes are unnecessary (Keohane, Attrill,
Love et al 1984).    We therefore routinely now
recommend that full strength enteral feeding regimes be
prescribed from the outset.    Diarrhoea, when it occurs
appears related to concomitent oral or parenteral antibiotic therapy (Keohane et al 1984).    The incidence of
this complication during enteral feeding of CF patients
is currently being assessed.

CONCLUSION

In this article I have attempted to review the evidence
that protein calorie malnutrition does occur in
patients with CF.    There is reason to believe that this
has an adverse effect on the outcome of recurrent
pulmonary infections.    The conclusion that can be
reached from the literature is that there are certainly
grounds for believing that specific forms of
nutritional support are indicated to improve the
nutritional status of these patients and since there is
reason to believe that such nutritional support might
have a beneficial effect on the natural history of the
chronic pulmonary disease of CF, this hypothesis should
continue to be tested under controlled trial conditions.

## REFERENCES

Allan, J.D., Mason, A., and Moss A.D., 1973.
Nutritional supplementation in the treatment of cystic
fibrosis of the pancreas. American Journal of
Diseases of Childhood, 126, 22-26.

Allen R.H., Beetharam, B., Podell, E. and Alpers, D.H.
1978.    Effect of proteolytic enzymes on the binding
of  cobalamine to R protein and intrinsic factor.
Journal of Clinical Investigation, 61, 47-56

Axelrod, A.E. and Trakatellis, A.C. 1964.
Relationship of pyridoxine to immunological phenomena.
Vitamins and Hormones, 22, 591-607

Baig, M.M., Cetorelli, J.J. and Roberts R.M., 1975.
Plasma membrane components of skin fibroblasts from
normal individuals and patients with cystic fibrosis.
Journal of Pediatrics, 82, 72 -76

Bearn, A.G. 1973.   Genetics of Cystic Fibrosis, in
Clinics of Gastroenterology (Ed. McConnell), 2, 515

Berry, H.K., Kellogg, F.W., Hunt, M.M., Ingberg, R.L.,
Richter, L. and Gutjahr, C. 1975.    Dietary
supplement and nutrition in children with cystic
fibrosis.    American Journal of Diseases of Children,
129, 165-171

Bhaskaram, C.R. and Reddy, V.    1975.    Cell mediated
immunity in iron and vitamin deficient children.
British Medical Journal, 111, 522

Casewell, M.W. 1979.    Nasogastric feeds as a source of
Klebsiella infection for intensive care patients.
Research and Clinical Forums. 1, 101-105

Castello, R., Landon, C., Eckhardt, K., Morris, V.,
Levander, O. and Lewiston, N.    1981.    Selenium and
vitamin E status in cystic fibrosis.    Journal of
Pediatrics, 99, 583-591

Chase, H.P., Long, M.A. and Lavin, M.H. 1979.    Cystic
fibrosis and malnutrition.    Journal of Pediatrics,
95, 337-347

Chazalette, J.P., Dutan, G., Chevalier, G., Filliat, M.
and Galabert, G. 1977.    Study of the medium and
long term survival of 28 cases of meconium ileus.
In:  Proceedings of the VIIth Internation Cystic
Fibrosis Congress.

Congden, P.J., Bruce, G., Rothburn, M.M., Clarke, P.C.N.
Littlewood, J.M., Kellfher, J. and Losowsky, M.S.
1981.    Vitamin status in treated patients with
cystic fibrosis.    Archives of Disease in Childhood,
56, 708-714

Cox, K., Isenberg, J., Osher, A. and Dooley, R. 1979
The effect of cimetidine on maldigestion in cystic
fibrosis.   Journal of Pediatrics, 94, 488-492

Crozier, D.N. 1974.   Cystic fibrosis, a not so fatal
disease.   Pediatric Clinics North America, 21, 935-
960

Deren, J.J., Arora, B., Toskes, P.P., Hansell, J. and
    Sibruga, 1973.    Malabsorption of crystallin vitamin
    B12 in cystic fibrosis.    New England Journal of
    Medicine, 288, 949-950
Dodge, J.A. and Yassa, J.G. 1978.    Zinc deficiency
    syndrome in a British youth with cystic fibrosis.
    British Medical Journal. 1, 411
Dodge, J.A. and Yassa, J.G. 1980.    Food intake and
    supplementary feeding programmes.    In.
    Proceedings of the 8th International Congress of
    Cystic Fibrosis, Toronto, Canadian Cystic Fibrosis
    Foundation 125-126
Dowd, P.S. and Heatley, R.V. 1984.    The influence of
    undernutrition on immunity.    Clinical Science,
    66, 241-248
Forstner, G., Gall, G., Corey, M., Durie, P., Hill, R.
    and Gaskin, K. 1980.    Digestion and absorption of
    nutrients in cystic fibrosis.    In.    Proceedings
    of the 8th International Congress of Cystic
    Fibrosis, Toronto, Canadian Cystic Fibrosis
    Foundation, 137-148
Hall, M.J., Manning, A.P. and Symes, C. 1983.    Effect
    of supplemental enteral nutrition on anthropometric
    measurements, nitrogen balance and pre-existing oral
    intake.    Gut, 24, A496
Halsted, J.A. and Smith, J.C. 1970.    Plasma zinc in
    health and disease.    Lancet, 1, 322-324
Harries, J.T. and Muller, D.P. 1971.    Absorption of
    different doses of fat soluble and water miscible
    preparations of vitamin E in children with cystic
    fibrosis.    Archives of Disease in Childhood. 46,
    341-344
Heinrich, H.C., Bender-Gotze, C.H. and Gabbe, G. 1977.
    Absorption of inorganic iron-($59Fe^{2+}$) in relation to
    iron stores in pancreatic insufficiency due to
    cystic fibrosis.    Klinische Wochenschrift, 55,
    587-594
Hubbard, V.C., Dunn, G.D. and di Sant'Agnese, P.A.
    1977, Abnormal fatty acid composition of plasma
    lipids in cystic fibrosis:   a primary or secondary
    defect?    Lancet, 2, 1302-1304         .
Hubbard, V.S., Barbero, G. and Chase, H.P. 1980.
    Selenium and cystic fibrosis.    Journal of Pediatrics,
    96, 421-427
Hubbard, V.S. 1980, Nutrient requirements of patients
    with cystic fibrosis. In: Proceedings of the 8th
    Congress of Cystic Fibrosis, 149-160
Hubbard, V.S. and Mangrum, P.J. 1982, Energy intake
    and nutrition counceling in cystic fibrosis.
    Journal of the American Dietetic Association,
    80, 127-131
Isselbacher, K.J. 1967.    Mechanisms of absorption of
    long and medium chain triglycerides.    In:   Medium

Chain Triglycerides. (Ed. Senior) pp 21-34

Jones, B.J.M., Brown, B.E., Grimble, G.K. and Silk,
    D.B.A. 1981. The formulation of energy dense
    enteral feeds - the use of high molecular weight
    glucose polymers. In Proceedings of the 3rd
    European Congress of Parenteral and Enteral
    Nutrition p 75

Jones, B.J.M., Brown, B.E., Loran, J.S., Edgerton, D.,
    Kennedy, J.F., Stead, J.A. and Silk, D.B.A. 1983.
    Glucose absorption from starch hydrolysates in the
    human jejunum. Gut, 24, 1152-1160

Keighley, M.R.S., Mogg, B., Bently, S. and Allan, C.
    1982. 'Home Brew' compared with commercial
    preparations for enteral feeding. British Medical
    Journal, 1, 163-164

Keohane, P., Brown, B., Grimble, G. and Silk, D.B.A.
    1982. Effect of protein composition and hydrolysis
    procedures on intestinal handling of protein
    hydrolysates in man. Clinical Science, 62, 47

Keohane, P.P., Grimble, G.K., Brown, B.E. and Silk,
    D.B.A. 1983. Nitrogen absorption from protein
    hydrolysate in man - significance of peptide chain
    length composition. Gastroenterology, 84, 1206

Keohane, P.P., Attrill, H., Love, M., Frost, P. and
    Silk, D.B.A. 1984. The significance of 'Starter
    regimes' and diet osmolality - a controlled trial.
    British Medical Journal (in press)

Kingsnorth, A.N. 1984. Trace elements in adult total
    parenteral nutrition. British Journal of Parenteral
    Therapy, 5, 8-22

Kraemer, R., Rudeberg, A., Hadorn, B. and Rossi E. 1978.
    Relative underweight in cystic fibrosis and its
    prognostic value. Acta Paediatrica, 67, 33-37

Kuo, P.T. and Huang, H.N. 1965. The effect of medium
    chain triglycerides upon fat absorption and plasma
    lipid and depot fat of children with cystic fibrosis
    of the pancreas. Journal of Clinical Investigation,
    44, 1924-1933

Lapey, A., Kattwinkel, J., di Sant'Agnese, P.A., and
    Lastor, L. 1974. Steatorrhoea and azotorrhoea and
    their relation to growth and nutrition in
    adolescents and young adults with cystic fibrosis.
    Journal of Pediatrics, 84, 328-334

Law, D.K., Dudrick, S.J. and Abdon, N.I. 1973.
    Immunocompetence of patients with protein-calorie
    malnutrition: the effects of nutritional repletion.
    Annals of Internal Medicine, 79, 545-550

Lloyd-Still, J.D. and Ganther, H.E. 1980. Selenium
    and glutathione peroxidase in cystic fibrosis.
    Paediatrics, 65, 1010-1015

Milla, P.J., Kilby, A., Rassam, U.B., Ersser, R. and
    Harries, J.T. 1983. Small intestinal absorption of
    amino acids and a dipeptide in pancreatic

insufficiency. <u>Gut</u>, 818-824

Mullin, T.J. and Kirkpatrick, J.R. 1981. The effect
of nutritional support on immune competency in
patients suffering from trauma, sepsis and malignant
disease. <u>Surgery</u>, 90, 610-614

Neumann, C.G., Lawlor, G.J., Stiehm, E.R., Swendseid,
M.E., Newton, C., Herbert, J., Animann, A.J. and
Jacob, M. 1975. Immunologic responses in malnourished children. <u>American Journal of Clinical Nutrition</u>
28, 89-104

Palin, H.D., Underwood, B.A. and Denning, C.R. 1976.
The effect of oral zinc supplementation on plasma
levels of vitamin A and retinol-binding protein in
cystic fibrosis. <u>Pediatric Research</u>, 10, 358

Parsons, H., Dumas, A., Beaudry, P. and Pencharz, 1980.
Dietary conselling and nutritional supplementation in
the treatment of cystic fibrosis and its effect on
growth. In: <u>Proceedings of the 8th International</u>
<u>Congress of Cystic Fibrosis Foundation</u> pp 161-165

Phelan, P. and Landran L. 1979. Improved survival of
patients with cystic fibrosis. <u>Medical Journal of</u>
<u>Australia</u>, 1, 261-270

Raeburn, J.A. 1977. Nutrition and immunity in cystic
fibrosis. <u>Proceedings of the Nutrition Society</u>,
36, 77-83

Rees, R.G., Grimble, G.K., Keohane, P.P., Higgins, B.E.,
West, M., Spiller, R.C. and Silk, D.B.A. 1984.
Peptide chain length of protein hydrolysates
influences jejunal nitrogen absorption. <u>Gut</u>,
(in press)

Riordan, J.R., Alon, N. and Buchwald, M. 1979. Plasma
membrane lipids of human diploid fibroblasis from
normal individuals and patients with cystic fibrosis.
<u>Biochimica et biophysica acta</u>, 574, 39-47

Shwachman, H. 1975. Gastrointestinal manifestations of
cystic fibrosis. <u>Pediatric Clinics North America</u>
22, 787-805

Shepherd, R., Cooksley, W.G.F. and Cooke, W.D. 1980
Improved growth and clinical, nutritional and
respiratory changes in response to nutritional therapy in cystic fibrosis. <u>Journal of Pediatrics</u>, 7,
351-357

Silk, D.B.A., Fairclough, P.D., Clark, M.L., Hegarty,
J.E., Maws, T.C., Addison, J.M., Burston, D.,
Clegg, K.M. and Matthews, D.M. 1980. Use of a
peptide rather than free amino acid nitrogen source
in chemically defined "elemental" diets. <u>Journal</u>
<u>of Parenteral and Enteral Nutrition</u>, 4, 548-553

Silk, D.B.A. 1980. Enteral nutrition. <u>Hospital</u>
<u>Update</u>, 6, 761-776

Silk, D.B.A. 1981. Peptide transport. Clinical
Science, 60, 607-615

Silk, D.B.A. 1983. In: <u>Nutritional Support in</u>
<u>Hospital Practice</u>. Blackwell Scientific
Publications, Oxford. pp 51-67
Sproul, A. and Huang, N. 1964. Growth patterns in
children with cystic fibrosis. <u>Journal of</u>
<u>Pediatrics</u>, 65, 664-676
Stephan, U. 1973. In: <u>Fundamental problems of</u>
<u>Cystic Fibrosis</u>. (ed. Mangos) Inter-
continental Medical Book Corporation, New York
p 281
Yassa, J.G., Prosser, R and Dodge, J.A. 1978.
Effect of an artifical diet on growth of
patients with cystic fibrosis. <u>Archives of</u>
<u>Disease in Childhood</u>, 53, 777-783

# PHYSICAL ACTIVITY AND SELF-TREATMENT IN PATIENTS WITH CYSTIC FIBROSIS

Monica Blomquist, Hans Gilljam, Birgitta Strandvik,
Lars-Gösta Wiman, Departments of Physiotherapy, Paediatrics and
Lung Medicine, Karolinska Institutet, Huddinge University Hospital,
Stockholm, Sweden

To make patients with Cystic Fibrosis (CF) more independent of other
people we introduced self-treatment, consisting of forced expiratory
technique with postural drainage, percussion, and ventilation with
chest compression. Since physical activity has been shown to improve
the patients' pulmonary function and general condition, we reinforced
the program with intensified exercise. To evaluate these different
components, the study was designed in two parts; phase I with increased physical activity and conservative physiotherapy treatment for 6
months and phase II with the same physical activity and self-treatment for another 6 months. No help of physiotherapists or parents was
allowed during phase II.

Twelve patients, 6 boys and 6 girls, 14-25 years old (mean 20 years),
participated in the study. Their clinical score was 65-91 (mean and
median 78). The patients were followed clinically at monthly check-
ups and every 6 month with chest X-rays, spirometry, and exercise
testing with arterial blood gas analysis. The physical activity was
adjusted to personal interest and capacity, and prescribed twice a
day, for a minimum of 15 minutes each time and until the pulse reached
at least 75% of that at maximal working capacity.

The clinical conditions, evaluated by chest X-rays, infection frequency, and including clinical score according to Shwachmann, were
unchanged throughout the whole study. No significant improvement was
noticed in forced vital capacity (FVC), forced expiratory volume (FEV)
and $FEV_{1.0}$, or in maximum expiratory flow rate ($MEF_{50}$). However, after
phase I, most patients improved their $PO_2$ during rest ($p<0.01$).
During exercise $PO_2$ increased significantly in phase I ($p<0.01$) and
throughout the whole study period ($p<0.05$). Although $PCO_2$ showed a
tendency to decrease, these changes were not significant.

In conclusion, we found that exercise improved the blood gas values
without significant changes in the roentgenological findings or pulmonary function. During self-treatment the condition was mainly unchanged, indicating that self-treatment, combined with regular physical activity, could replace conservative physiotherapy treatment. The
psychological advantage was great and seemed to contribute to a more
independent adolescence and a better quality of life for these patients. The economical benefits for individuals and for society were
impressive.

PHYSICAL EXERCISE AND CYSTIC FIBROSIS

D. M. Geddes

Brompton and London Chest Hospitals

Physical exercise is an important part of normal life both for
health and pleasure.  Recently interest in the subject has been
growing very rapidly and exercise is often promoted as the panacea
for all man's ills whether physical, mental or social (32,39).
However, the amount of scientific proof that exercise is good
medicine is very limited and in trying to define its value in
cystic fibrosis we must see evidence of benefit before we impose
another time consuming procedure on our patients.

So far there is relatively little experience of the role of
exercise in the management of CF.  Some centres have studied
exercise physiology and some have evaluated short term programmes
of exercise with measures which are inevitably quite crude.  In
contrast there is a considerable experience of exercise in
assessment and therapy of both childhood asthma (36) and adult
chronic obstructive lung disease (18).  Much of this experience is
directly relevant to cystic fibrosis.  The cardio-pulmonary
dysfunction is similar and the psychosocial consequences of chronic
pulmonary disability and the vicious cycles of immobility and
dependence that it sets up are undoubtedly similar to the situation
in CF.  Although the experience gained from the studies of exercise
in these conditions is somewhat varied all reports suggest a
benefit and none have demonstrated any harm.  In CF, no claim has
yet been made that exercise has any particular place in long term
management and given the paucity of data no such claim could be
made.  Nevertheless there are many theoretical reasons to suggest
that exercise may be good for the lungs in CF as well as compelling
arguments that it may benefit psychosocial adaptation to the
condition.  It is certainly important that the role of exercise in
the management of CF should be evaluated further.

## EXERCISE IN CF - PATHOPHYSIOLOGY

Physical activity results in profound physiological adaptations in
many organ systems and these have been well reviewed (2).  The
normal changes of particular relevance to CF include:

## 1. <u>Ventilation</u>

### A. Normal (2)

Respiratory rate and frequency increase resulting in a rise in total ventilation from 5 l/min at rest to a maximum of about 150 l/min. This closely matches the increase in $O_2$ consumption and $CO_2$ production with the result that arterial blood gas tensions remain unchanged until very high work loads are reached. The respiratory muscles work harder as the ventilation rises and so the oxygen cost of breathing is increased.

### B. CF

While there have been relatively few studies of exercise responses in CF the changes reported are similar to those found in other forms of chronic airflow obstruction. Cropp et al (13) and Cerney et al (8) assessed 20 patients, mean age 15 years, and compared them with 17 age matched normal controls. Patients were grouped according to the severity of CF lung disease as assessed by a pulmonary function score which correlated well with Taussig scores. Patients with mild (FEV1 80%, FVC 90% predicted) or moderate (FEV1 55%, FVC 79% predicted) lung function abnormality had normal peak work capacity (Fig I). Those with severe lung disease (FEV1 32%, FVC 57% predicted) had a limited peak work capacity (51% expected) with reduced maximum ventilation (39% predicted). Ventilation for a given work load ($\dot{V}_E/\dot{V}O_2$) tended to be high in most CF patients suggesting an increase in dead space ventilation (Fig II). These findings are similar to those of Godfrey & Mearns (20) who suggested that exercise dead space ventilation may be one of the most sensitive indications of pulmonary dysfunction in CF.

The severely affected patients also showed arterial blood gas changes at peak work load: $SaO_2$ fell by a mean of 7.3% and $PaCO_2$ rose by 5 mmHg (Fig III). These changes in blood gas tensions were attributed to both deteriorating ventilation perfusion ratios and also alveolar hypoventilation. The arterial oxygen desaturation in severely affected patients confirmed the findings of Goldring et al (21) and German et al (19). These changes could be dangerous and emphasise the need for caution and initial supervision in any exercise programme. Conversely the relatively normal performance of those with mild/moderate disease and their normal $SaO_2$ levels are reassuring and suggest that high work loads in these patients are safe.

In cystic fibrosis the combination of the increased $\dot{V}_E/\dot{V}O_2$ and airflow obstruction increases the oxygen cost of breathing . In patients with COPD up to 40% of total oxygen consumption may be needed for breathing alone (29) (normal < 5%) and this may be an important factor in limiting exercise tolerance. Supplementary oxygen during exercise reduces ventilation and also increases the $SaO_2$. While oxygen on exercise has been shown to be beneficial in chronic lung disease (18) there is only limited information on its use on CF during exercise (see below). Undoubtedly oxygen reduces exercise ventilation (about 12% in CF) and limits the risk of exercise hypoxaemia in patients with severe pulmonary dysfunction.

Exercise oxygen therapy merits further study in relation to CF.

The role of respiratory muscle fatigue and training in chronic lung disease is controversial. Some measures of respiratory muscle function are abnormal and it has been suggested that muscle fatigue may contribute to both acute and chronic respiratory failure as well as to breathlessness and disability (22). Furthermore Leith and Bradley (28) were able to demonstrate changes in respiratory muscle function after regular ventilatory training and Belman and Mittman (5) claimed that ventilatory muscle training improved exercise capacity in patients with chronic obstructive pulmonary disease. Although the relevance of some respiratory muscle function tests to real life is uncertain and the importance of specific ventilatory training rather than a general exercise programme is not established these studies are clearly relevant to CF. Keens et al (27) compared 55 CF patients with 30 controls and showed a reduction in maximum sustained ventilatory capacity during normocapnic breathing. However when this ventilatory capcity was corrected for the lung function abnormality the patients appeared to perform better than the controls suggesting that chronic lung dysfunction had actually strengthened ventilatory muscles. The same workers went on to compare the effects of a ventilatory muscle training programme with a general physical activity programme (swimming, canoeing, etc) and showed definite increases in sustained ventilatory capacity (27). The improvements were greater in CF than controls and the general physical activities were at least as good as specific ventilatory muscle training. Orenstein et al (34) showed a similar increase in respiratory muscle endurance following a three month running programme. While these results were encouraging they are somewhat dampened by the findings of Asher et al (1) who showed an improvement in inspiratory mouth pressures in 11 patients with CF as a result of inspiratory muscle training but no change in exercise test results. The present evidence then suggests that respiratory muscles function well in most patients with CF and regular exercise is as good as any specific muscle training.

## 2. Circulation

### A. Normal (2)

Heart rate and stroke volume increase and the resulting rise in cardiac output from 5 l/min at rest to a maximum of about 30 l/min provides increased $O_2$ delivery to the tissues. $O_2$ delivery matches consumption until high work loads when a part of muscle metabolism becomes anaerobic with the result that lactic acid spills over into the circulation and produces a lactic acidosis. The increase in cardiac output is reflected in an increased blood flow to the lungs where ventilation and perfusion are matched at the alveolar level.

### B. CF

The heart is not involved primarily by cystic fibrosis but may fail due to a combination of hypoxia and pulmonary hypertension. Golding et al (21) showed normal pulmonary arterial pressures in patients with mild disease but significant elevation (20-30 mmHg) in those with the worst lung function. These same patients usually showed a fall in $SaO_2$ on exercise. Administration of 100% oxygen at rest and exercise reduced the pulmonary artery pressure in all patients but this reduction was slight and the pressure usually remained abnoraml. The studies of Cropp (13) & Cerney (8) referred to above showed normal heart rate responses to exercise in mild and moderately affected patients. Those with severe lung disease had a higher heart rate at rest and at each level of exercise (Fig IV). However, the rate of rise was similar to that of the groups with milder lung disease ie: the resting difference was maintained throughout exercise. Orenstein et al (34) found somewhat low maximum heart rates on peak exercise, probably a reflection of the slightly reduced peak work load achieved. The heart rate for a submaximal work load fell following training. These and other studies indicate an appropriate circulatory response to exercise in all except the most severely affected patients when a raised pulmonary artery pressure and arterial oxygen desaturation become important. It is therefore not suprising that a controlled trial of the effect of digoxin on exercise performance in CF (10) showed no benefit in terms of maximum work load or heart rate. There was a slight fall in stroke volume with the drug which may have contributed to a lower exercise $PaO_2$. It is reasonable to conclude therefore that cardiac function does not limit exercise capacity in most patients with CF.

## 3. Heat, Water and Electrolytes

A. Normal (2)
Exercising muscles produce heat as well as mechanical energy and so the body core temperature tends to rise. This rise is limited by heat loss from the skin (convection, radiation and evaporation), and respiratory tract (evaporation). Evaporation dominates at temperatures of over $20^{\circ}C$. Heat losses of over 100 KJ/min occur commonly during exercise of which about 20% is via the respiratory tract. Many litres of water can be lost by evaporation from skin and respiratory tract in a few hours with associated cooling and drying of the airways and loss of sodium and chloride via sweat. Clearly these losses depend highly on climate and clothing. In comparison to these changes the renal losses of water and electrolytes are relatively trivial.

B. CF
Since the sweat sodium and chloride are high in cystic fibrosis the effect of exercise on the overall loss of water and electrolytes and their resulting changes in different body compartments may be very important. Similarly the effect of exercise on body core temperature may be unpredictable. Sweat volume and secretion rates are normal in CF at rest and during exercise or heat stress (35) while sodium and chloride levels are around three times higher than normal. This three fold increase in NaCl loss appears to be well tolerated, presumably because the overall losses during moderate exercise are relatively small compared with body reserves. Nevertheless there have been well documented reports of salt and water depletion during very hot weather in CF. Prolonged heavy

exercise in temperate conditions seems to be safe as shown by the
successful completion of the Oslo Marathon in 3 hr 51 min by a 16
year old male with cystic fibrosis (43). He lost 0.9 Kg during
this time in spite of a fluid intake of 1L. Since he took no added
salt total salt losses must have been about 180 mequiv and there
was no change in serum sodium or chloride.

Although renal handling of salt and water is relatively normal in
CF. Some abnormalities have been reported. Interestingly
Orenstein et al (35) found that patients with CF had higher urinary
sodium and chloride losses than normals during 90 mins heat and
exercise stress. Also patients with CF do not show the expected
rise in urine potassium. These differences have not been explained
but are small in absolute terms and would not lead to salt
depletion. The risks of exercise are therefore slight under normal
temperature conditions and no special precautions need to be
recommended. Similarly CF changes in core temperature due to
exercise are normal.

The effect of evaporation from the respiratory tract in CF has not
attracted much attention. There are two potential problems:
exercise incuded asthma which has been investigated and adverse
effects on mucociliary clearance which has not.

### Exercise Induced Asthma (36)

Airway narrowing occurs during or following exercise if heat
losses from the airways are great enough. The important
variables are therefore ambient temperature and humidity,
the total ventilation and the degree of bronchial
reactivity. Thus if the ventilation is high when
temperature and humidity are low then almost all asthmatics
will develop an attack and this is true whether the
hyperventilation is due to exercise or eucapnic
voluntary overbreathing in a laboratory. Other factors
must be involved as swimming provokes less asthma than
running even when respiratory heat loss is idential (33).

Prevention of EIA is relatively simple. Respiratory heat
losses can be minimised by nose breathing (nasal airflow
resistance falls sharply on exercise (17)) but this is only
possible for moderate work loads. There is also some
evidence to suggest that repeated short sprints can be used
to induce a refractory period so that subsequent exercise
will not result in asthma (25). Exercise induced asthma  can
be prevented always by a beta adrenergic stimulant inhaler,
often by disodium cromoglycate and sometimes by methylxanthines. β stimulant inhalers are also effective at
reversing the attack.

The frequency of EIA in CF is not certain because
studies have not always controlled the temperature and
humidity precisely. Zambie et al (48) reported that 10
of 36 patients with CF (28%) had post exercise falls in

peak flow of > 15% (range 16-38%). Resting lung function or skin prick tests failed to predict which individual would wheeze. However, other studies have reported frequencies as high as 65% (14) or as low as 2% (42). Since the frequency is bound to vary with exercise load and climatic conditions it must be prudent to warn all patients with CF of the possibility of EIA and perhaps to suggest prophylactic $\beta$ stimulant inhalers in every case. The individual who has no risk of EIA will still benefit from a bronchodilator during exercise.

## Mucociliary Clearance

Some CF secretions are relatively deficient in water and while this has not been convincingly demonstrated in CF sputum, dry respiratory secretions may well play a part in altering mucociliary function and predisposing to lung infection. In theory exercise induced airway water loss might therefore worsen any mucociliary dysfunction. On the other hand most runners notice that running promotes sputum production and detailed studies by Woolf et al (45) have convincingly demonstrated increased clearance of radiolabelled aerosolised particles from all zones of the lung as a result of exercise on a bicycle ergometer. This increase was not due to increased ventilation alone as eucapnic voluntary overbreathing improved clearance is due to better mucociliary function or to increased secretion of mucous or both. Mucociliary clearance on exercise in CF has not been systematically studied and it is important that this should be done. If it can be shown that exercise is good physiotherapy and that airway drying is irrelevant then this will be a powerful reason to encourage exercise in patients. Furthermore it may be possible to discontinue regular physiotherapy and replace it with regular exercise which would be popular with patients and might well improve compliance. Compliance with physiotherapy is often poor especially among adolescents. The reports of training programmes in CF (see below) are encouraging in this respect.

## 4. Hormones

A. Normal (2)
The secretion and clearance of a wide range of circulating hormones are altered during exercise. In particular catecholamines, cortisol, growth hormone and endorphins have been shown to rise. These rises become less marked as a result of physical training.

B. CF
The hormonal response to exercise in CF has not been studied in any detail. There is some evidence of abnormal endocrine status at rest and on exercise in other forms of chronic lung disease (40) and so information about CF would be of some interest. In

particular the normal rise in catecholamines on exercise may be blunted or even absent in exercise induced asthmatics (4) and may also be abnormal in adults with chronic obstructive pulmonary disease. Since catecholamines stimulate mucous production, speed ciliary beat frequency, and may enhance mucociliary clearance these observations are clearly relevant to CF.

## 5. Nutrition

A. Normal (2)

The energy for exercise comes from the oxidation of food. Fat is the richest fuel with an energy density of 39 KJ/g compared with 17 KJ/g for carbohydrates. Furthermore fat can be stored as pure droplets while carbohydrate is stored in association with water which reduces the energy density to about 4 KJ/g and is therefore much less efficient as a portable fuel store. Normally fat stores are 50 x greater than carbohydrates. Protein is not used as a fuel while fat or carbohydrate are available. Fat requires 10% more oxygen than carbohydrate for the same energy yeild and anaerobic metabolism is only 5% as efficient as aerobic and can only use carbohydrate as fuel. At rest fat and carbohydrate are used in equal proportions but as work increases in severity or duration plasma free fatty acid levels rise and more and more energy comes from fat. Nevertheless prolonged exercise may be limited by hypoglycaemia when glycogen stores become depleted. The balance of fat and carbohydrate metabolism depends on many factors including the hormonal changes referred to above. Also carbohydrate food taken shortly before exercise increases the proportion of carbohydrate used as fuel.

Exercise tends to stimulate appetite approximately by the amount required to compensate for increased energy consumption (jogging uses about 400 Kcal/hour of extra energy.)

B. CF

Under nutrition has a profound affect on exercise capacity (3). While this is clearly important in CF and has been widely studied there is little data relevant to exercise. Coates et al (9) examined the relative importance of lung function, clinical status, body build and serum lipids on maximum exercise capacity. Lung function correlated with work load achieved (r = 0.68) and the variance in exercise capacity could be accounted for predominantly by a combination of airflow obstruction and body mass percentile (Wt/Ht$^2$). These in turn correlated well with Schwachman score. In other words fit patients are well from every point of view and patients with poor clinical scores are also those with poor weight, poor lung function and impaired exercise ability. Serum lipids were abnormal but the abnormalities did not go with chemical or functional status. In the absence of more data the following questions need to be answered: are nutritional factors important in sustained exercise (as opposed to short maximal exercise tests); does regular exercise lead to an improvement in appetite and nutrition or deplete essential stores; should any special dietary advice be given to patients with CF who exercise either long term or in relation to a bout of activity.

## Exercise and the Mind

The links between body and mind in health are many.  The number and complexity of these interactions naturally increase with disease and are notoriously difficult to study.  It is therefore not surprising that there are many more unsupported statements about the effect exercise has on the mind than there are hard facts. However reliable data is accumulating and the subject has been fully reviewed recently (39,41).  The influence of the mind on the body is on the whole easier to document than the other way round.

Exercise appears to influence mood and sleep, at least in the short term.  Immediately after exercise normal subjects record less anxiety, depression and hostility, and subjective pleasantness increases (30).  Exhaustive exercise profoundly alters the pattern of sleep (7) and may improve insomnia.  These short term effects are likely to be related at least in part to exercise induced hormonal changes.  Longer term studies have also shown improvements in anxiety and depression both in cardiac patients (16) and chronic obstructive pulmonary disease (11).  However not all studies are positive and in particular exercise may be less helpful in the mentally ill:  only 2 of 7 clinically depressed subjects improved as a result of an exercise programme (23).

The effect of play and sports on education, development and social integration are often stated but seldom studied.  Obviously such studies are almost impossible to conduct because of the time involved and because of the range of confounding variables. Intuitively sports may appear healthy but such intuition is based very much on culture and upbringing.  The Anglo-Saxon enthusiasm for exhaustion is seldom shared by Mediterranean races and this together with learned parental attitudes may make the difference between success and failure of an exercise programme.

The links between body and mood have been quite well studied in chronic pulmonary disability.  Anxiety and depression are prevelant and are probably caused by the disability (18).  Conversely breathlessness and exercise tolerance are definitely influenced by mood.  Depression, and the patients attitudes and beliefs about their lung disease are more important in limiting walking distance than any measure of pulmonary function (31).  It is therefore easy to see how vicious cycles of disadvantage can become established.

In CF mood and psycho-social adaptation to disease are remarkably normal and so the effects of exercise on mental health may not be very impressive.  However as mental factors in relation to exercise tolerance and their modification by training have not been formally studied in CF, and it would certainly be interesting to include some simple measures in the assessment of an exercise programme. Whatever the results it is important to remember that exercise and sports should be fun in themselves and so make a direct contribution to good quality of life and happiness.  Such a contribution might well be missed by a psychologist's questionnaire.

### Exercise Programmes

Doctors have prescribed exercise for their patients for centuries, usually in an unstructured way and almost always without any attempt to measure the benefits. The history of such advice has been concisely reviewed by Fitch (15) starting from the Archbishop of St. Andrews in 1551 whose asthma appeared to benefit from regular horse riding, although the relative contributions of exercise and hyposensitisation are opaque, through the private gymnasium with attendant doctor of Theodore Roosevelt in 1880 which led inexorably to the Presidency and a Nobel Prize, up to modern times when the UK Asthma Research Council recommended remedial breathing exercises only. Subsequently doctors have become more interested in measurement and a few controlled trials of exercise programmes in chronic lung disease, asthma and cystic fibrosis have been reported:

### Chronic Lung Disease (18)

Patients with smoking related airflow obstruction have usually been studied although Keens has reviewed the subject from the pediatric point of view (26). In a recent UK study (12) swimming, cycling and rowing resulted in a significant improvement in twelve minute walking distance as compared with controls and this was reflected in an increased maximum oxygen uptake measured on a treadmill test. The improvements were still present seven months later. The changes although small, were similar to those found in previous controlled studies when reduction in ventilation and heart rate at given work loads were also often found. Interestingly the control group, who attended the rehabilitation centre but did not exercise, also improved although more slowly. Both the exercise and the control group showed an improvement in psychological scores for anxiety, depression, anger and fatigue (11) together with an increase in vigour although these changes were not analysed statistically. There was no association between the psychological changes and the increase in walking distance. Lung function did not change. In summary, exercise produces independent benefits in exercise tolerance and psychological scores without change in lung function and these can be maintained after the formal programme ends. The benefits for the chronically disabled appear worthwhile.

### Asthma

Exercise programmes in asthma aim not only to improve exercise tolerance and psychological factors but also to improve the disease itself. A number of studies (24,44) have demonstrated a training effect with improved atheletic ability and maximum oxygen uptake. This improvement does not always happen and naturally the changes will be greatest when very unfit subjects enter the study and when the programmes are long and the work is hard. Exercise induced asthma seems to improve but only because of fitness. As an asthmatic trains so he can do the same amount of exercise more easily with less ventilation, respiratory heat loss is therefore less. If the work load is increased to offset the training effect then EIA is unaltered. This is well illustrated by a fit asthmatic marathon runner who developed EIA after four hours running when the effect of his pre-race bronchodilator inhaler had worn off (36).

Peterson & McElhenney (38) in an uncontrolled study reported improved exercise tolerance and vital capacity following an 8 month physical fitness programme in asthmatic boys. The most striking benefits were in school attendance with aggregate days lost falling from 185 to 69. Parents, teachers and personality questionnaires administered to the boys all recorded imporvement. This study is important in the range of measurements made and it is unfortunate that so many studies have assessed physical variables only. However the lack of a control group and the tendency of childhood asthma to improve with time are major drawbacks. Most people involved with asthmatic training programmes claim great psychological benefits and it is essential that more are measured in future controlled trials.

A recent controlled study of short term physical training in adult asthmatics is particularly encouraging (6). The training group improved their maximal oxygen consumption, marginally improved their pre-exercise peak flow (an effort dependent measurement) and significantly reduced their bronchodilator usage. Whether the changes were due to improved asthma or to improved fitness (doing daily tasks at a lower proportion of $VO_2$ max) is unclear but whatever the mechanism the results are desirable.

In summary, asthmatics can train safely and while no disadvantages have been reported, there are definite benefits in fitness with associated psychological and schooling advantages. Exercise may also reduce the frequency and severity of the asthma so that less treatment is needed.

## Cystic Fibrosis

There are additional considerations in exercise programmes for cystic fibrosis as well as the effect on chronic pulmonary disability, EIA, and the psyche. The effect on sputum production and pulmonary infection are probably the most important. The relatively poor nutritional state and muscle development of many patients, which may well be improved by physical activity, nevertheless make exercise more difficult and unpleasant for the individual and exercise programmes must be designed with this in mind. At present there is only limited published data although many of those caring for CF have considerable experience in practice.

Orenstein et al (34) compared 21 patients (FEV1 61%, FVC 82% predicted) who underwent a three month running programme with 10 well matched controls. The exercise consisted of three sessions per week lasting one hour each and comprising one initial warm up followed by 10-30 minutes of jogging/ walking and then games after a rest period. There was a significant improvement in $\overset{\bullet}{V}O_2$, the heart rate response to exercise, and respiratory muscle endurance. Since there was no change in RQ or peak heart rate it was unlikely that the improvements were due to increased effort alone. There was no assessment of sputum production but the FEV1 remained stable in the exercise group while falling slightly in the controls.

Zach et al (47) in an uncontrolled study assessed the effect of swimming on forced expiration and sputum clearance. Ten patients (clinical score 73, range 43-90) each had 17 sessions of one hour over a seven and a half week period. Forced expiratory volumes and flows were higher after the programme but none of these changes were sustained ten weeks later. Perhaps the most interesting finding was a 16% increase in sputum volume following swimming. The improvements were attributed to either the effects of exercise itself or to more subtle changes of submersion on the pressure volume relationships of the lungs. The same workers (46) reported the effect of a 17 day exercise programme of swimming, hiking and other physical activities in 12 children with CF median age 10.5 years Schwachman score 37-86. Again there were improvements in spirometric volumes which had returned to pre-exercise levels 8 weeks later. An important part of this study was that all the patients stopped their physiotherapy during the exercise period, eleven suffered no disadvantage while one child with difficulty in clearing secretions had to restart physiotherapy.

These studies show that exercise is safe and that short programmes can produce changes which seem to be beneficial. The effect on secretions has not been assessed adequately but there is nothing to suggest deterioration in lung clearance and some indications that it might be improved. The patients who took part were relatively well so these findings cannot be extended to those with severely deranged lung function whose exercise capacity is poor (see above). There is no data on nutrition or muscle mass and no psychological measurements have been made; these measures should probably be included in future studies.

### Practical Considerations

The experience above all suggests that exercise can be useful in chronic lung disease in general and cystic fibrosis in particular. However, if exercise is to have any routine place in the management of CF a number of practical questions need to be asked. What exercise? Which work load? How long and how often? What precautions should be taken?

The activities chosen must be enjoyable otherwise will not be done and ideally should be varied to avoid monotony. Group activities are more enjoyable and have psycho-social advantages but are much more difficult to organise, need special premises and involve travelling. Some activities which have been evaluated, such as cross-country skiing or mountain walking, have very limited application and are in any case unsuitable for the severely disabled. Jogging is simple but tedious while dancing has much to recommended it as different dances can be learned in groups and continued alone at home. There are a few references to jazz dancing and classical ballet in the literature (36) but no detailed information and clearly some practical experience of dancing in cystic fibrosis would be worthwhile. Otherwise swimming is probably the best activity so far assessed. Even the most disabled can take part, group and solo activities are possible, there is a documented benefit in sputum production and swimming pools are quite widely available. Swimming is less likely than other sports to cause EIA (33) and although there has been concern that chlorine may irritate the airways this has not been born out in practice. However suitable swimming may be, there will be limits to the number of times that patients will be prepared to go and so some form of home exercises would also be essential if exercise were to replace physiotherapy. Whatever solo exercise is done regular attendances at a group centre should also be continued to get the group benefits, to keep up enthusiasm and to vary the programme.

The intensity and duration of exercise used to be tailored to the individual. A work rate of around 70% predicted maximum is probably ideal since this is not unpleasant and can be sustained for some time. There is no reason to try to exceed this, but lower work loads have less effect in terms of training. Oseid has recommended the following valuable guidelines (37).

1. An initial assessment of exercise ability by a doctor or group leader. This assessment need not be a formal physiologists progressive exercise test unless this is a requirement of an experimental protocol.
2. Premedication with drugs against EIA. This is a sensible precaution in all CF patients even in the absence of EIA since the bronchodilator and possibly mucociliary clearance effects will be valuable.
3. Low intensity warm up lasting 10-15 minutes in which the individual sets the work rate according to comfort.
4. Interval training with work periods of a few minutes alternating with periods of reduced activity but not necessarily rest. Ball games and relay races are good structured examples.
5. Training with submaximal work load aiming at heart rates of 160-170 /min.

These guidelines are specifically aimed at training for the child with EIA. The principles are however suitable for any training programme and can be used for swimming or dancing. This programme lasts about an hour but could be shortened to two period of half an hour to be done twice a day. Most patients with CF give up at least this amount of time for daily physiotherapy.

Although there are virtually no reports of adverse effects of exercise programmes a number of possible dangers exist especially in CF. The worst patients may have pulmonary hypertension and a low $PaO_2$ with worsening on exercise. Whether such patients would benefit in any case is unknown but clearly they should only be included under close supervision to begin with and formal monitoring of transcutaneous blood gas changes on exercise would be a sensible precaution. Similarly patients with an infective exacerbation could be harmed both by unpredictable changes in exercise physiology and also by the debilitating effect of exercise at a time when resources are needed to combat infection. Exercise induced asthma and airway drying have been discussed above. The psychological benefits of exercise have been discussed but patients may also feel inadequate and depressed when faced with their inability to do physical work and be reluctant to display this inadequacy to the group. While such problems can usually be overcome by a sympathetic and experienced group leader, inevitably some patients will not adjust and they must be allowed to stay away if they wish - ideally they should not have been included in the first place.

Finally the aim of any exercise group or programme should be to start a good habit which will then continue independently. The patients should continue at home or join a local club so that exercise becomes a part of his life which he enjoys and does willingly. The medical aspects may continue to be important but should not be the chief reason for exercising.

### Conclusions

Although there is a great deal of information about exercise in chronic lung disease and much of this is directly relevant to CF there are still relatively few certainties. It may therefore be useful to list what we know and what we do not know.

We know.
1. Exercise is very safe.
2. Training improves peak performance and makes submaximal exercise easier.
3. In CF: (a) Cardiopulmonary responses are normal except in those with severe lung damage.
         (b) Cardiac function is seldom a limiting factor.
4. Exercise induced asthma is common but easily prevented.
5. Exercise affects the mind and the mind affects exercise capacity. Within this interrelationship is one aspect of the quality of life.
6. Many of the claimed benefits of exercise are unproven.

We do not know.
1. In CF, the effects of exercise long or short term on:
         (a) Nutrition
         (b) Hormone response
         (c) The psyche
         (d) Mucociliary clearance
         (e) Immune defenses.
2. The long term effects of exercise, beneficial or harmful.
3. The relative values of exercise and physiotherapy in practice.

4. Which form of exercise in CF is the most valuable and the most acceptable.

Since physical activity is so essential a part of normal life for development, pleasure and work and may also be actively beneficial for CF lung disease it is important that we try to answer these questions. As the outlook in CF continues to improve so the condition will change from a hospital based disease to a community based disability. Any measures which can help this transition and any form of therapy which emphasises normality rather than illness must merit a high priority in CF research.

## References

1. Asher, M.I., Pardy, R.L., Coates et al. 1982. The effects of inspiratory muscle training in patients with CF. American Review of Respiratory Disease, 126, 855-9.

2. Astrand, P.O., Rodahl, K., 1977. Textbook of Work Physiology New York, McGraw Hill.

3. Barac-Nieto, M., Spurr, G.B., Macksend, M.G., Zotero, H. 1978. Aerobic work capacity in chronically undernourished adult males. Journal of Applied Physiology, 44, 209-15.

4. Barnes, P.J., Brown, M.J., Silverman, M, Dollery, C.T. 1981. Circulating catecholamines in exercise and hyperventilation induced asthma. Thorax, 36, 435-40.

5. Belman, M.J., Mittman, C., 1980. Ventilatory muscle training improves exercise capacity in chronic obstructive pulmonary disease. American Review of Respiratory Disease, 121, 273-80.

6. Bundgaard, A., Ingerman-Hansen, T., Halkjaer-Kristewen, J., Schmidt, A., Bloch, I., Andesen, P.K., 1983. Short term physical training in bronchial asthma. British Journal of Diseases of the Chest, 77, 147-52.

7. Bunnell, D.G., Bevier, W., Horvath, S.M., 1983. Effects of exhaustive exercise on sleep of men and women. Psychophysiology, 20, 50-58.

8. Cerney, F.J., Pullano, T.P., Cropp, G.J.A., 1982. Cardiorespiratory adapations to exercise in CF. American Review of Respiratory Disease, 126, 217.

9. Coates, A.L., Boyce, P., Muller, D., Mearns, M., Godfrey, S., 1980. The role of nutritional status, airway obstruction, hypoxia and abnormalities in serum lipid composition in limiting exercise tolerance in children with CF. Acta Paed. Scand,69,353-8.

10. Coates, A.L., Desmond, K., Asher, M.I., 1982. The effect of Digoxin on exercise capacity and exercising cardiac function in CF. Chest, 82, 543-5.

11. Cockcroft, A., Berry, G., Brown, E.B., Exall, C., 1982. Psychological changes during a controlled trial of rehabilitation in chronic respiratory disability. Thorax 37,413-416.

12. Cockcroft, A.E., Saunders, M.J., Berry, G., 1981. Randomised controlled trial of rehabilitation in chronic respiratory disability. Thorax, 36, 200-203.

13. Cropp, G.J., Pullano, T.P., Cerney, F.J., Nathanson, I.T., 1982 Exercise tolerance and cardiorespiratory adjustments at peak work capacity in CF. American Review of Respiratory Disease, 126, 211.

14. Day, G., Mearns, M.B., 1973. Bronchial lability in cystic fibrosis. Arch. Dis. Child., 48, 355-9.

15. Fitch, K.D., 1983. Sport, physical activity and the asthmatic. The asthmatic child in sport and play. London, Pitman Press, 246-258.

16. Folkins, C.H., 1976. Effects of physical training on mood. Clinical Psychology, 32, 385-8.

17. Forsyth, R.D., Cole, P., Shephard, R.J., 1983. Exercise and nasal patency. Journal of Applied Physiology, 55, 860-5.
18. Geddes, D.M., 1984. Chronic airflow obstruction. Postgraduate Medical Journal, 60.
19. Germann, K., Orenstein, D., Horowitz, J., 1980. Changes in oxygenation during exercise in cystic fibrosis. Med. Sci. Sports Exercise, 121, 127.
20. Godfrey, S., Mearns, M., 1971. Pulmonary function and response to exercise in cystic fibrosis. Arch. Dis. Child., 46, 144-51.
21. Goldring, R.M., Fishman, A.P., Turino, G.M., Cohen, H.I., Denning, C.R., Anderson, D.H., 1964. Pulmonary hypertension and cor pulmonale in CF of the pancreas. J. Pediatr., 65, 501-24.
22. Green, M. and Moxham, J., 1983. Recent Advances in Respiratory Medicine. Ed. D. C. Flenley. 3, 1-20.
23. Hartz, G.W., Wallace, W.L., Coyton, T.G., 1982. Effect of aerobic conditioning upon mood in clinically depressed men and women. Percept. Mot. Skills, 55, 1217-20.
24. Henriksen, J.M., Nielson, T.T., 1983. Effect of physical training on exercise induced bronchoconstriction. Acta. Paed. Scand., 72, 31-6.
25. Henriksen, J.M. Dahl, R, Lundgrist, G.R., 1983. Influence of different degress of bronchoconstriction on refractoriness in EIA. The asthmatic child in sport and play. London, Pitman Press, p.85-91.
26. Keens, T.G., 1979. Exercise training programs for pediatric patients with chronic lung disease. Paed. Clin. N.America, 26, 517-24.
27. Keens, T.G., Krastius, R.B., Wannamaker, E.M., Levison, H., Crozier, D.N., Bryan, A.C., 1977. Ventilatory muscle endurance training in normal subjects and patients with cystic fibrosis. American Review of Respiratory Disease, 116, 853-60.
28. Leith, D.E., Bradley, M., 1976. Ventilatory muscle strength and endurance training. Journal of Applied Physiology, 41, 508-16.
29. Levison, H., Cherniak, R., 1968. Ventilatory cost of exercise in chronic obstructive pulmonary disease. Journal of Applied Physiology, 25, 21-7.
30. Lightman, S., Posner, E.G., 1983. The Effects of exercise on mood and cognitive functioning. J Psychosomat Res, 27, 43-52.
31. Morgan, A.D., Peek, D.F., Buchanan, D.R., McHardy, G.J.R., 1983 Effect of attitude and beliefs on exercise tolerance in chronic bronchitis. British Medical Jouranl, 286, 171-3.
32. Morris, J.N., 1983. Exercise , health and medicine. British Medical Journal, 286, 1597-8.
33. Newman, I., 1982. The effect of breathing dry or humid air on EIA caused by running or seimming. The asthmatic child in sport and play, London, Pitman Press, p 74-79.
34. Orenstein, D.M., Franklin, B.A., Doershuk, C.F. et al., 1981. Exercise conditioning and cardiopulmonary fitness in CF. Chest, 80, 392-398.

35. Orenstein, D.M., Henke, K.G., Costill, D.L., et al., 1983. Exercise and heat stress in CF patients. Pediatr. Res. 17, 267-269.
36. Oseid, S., Edwards, A.M., 1983. The asthmatic child in sport and play. London, Pitman Press.
37. Oseid, S., Edwards, A.M., 1983. The asthmatic child in sport and play. London, Pitman Press, p.237-245.
38. Peterson, K.H., McElhenney, T.R., 1965. Effects of a physical program upon asthmatic boys. Pediatrics, 35, 295-9.
39. Physical activity and health: a documentation. Scand. J. Soc. Med., 1982, Suppl. 29, 5-269.
40. Semple, P.D.A., Watson, W.S., Beastall, G.H., Betnel, M.I.F., Grant, J.K., Hume, R., 1979. Diet, absorption and hormone studies in relation to body weight in obstructive airways disease. Thorax, 34, 783-8.
41. Shepherd, R.J., 1983. Physical Activity and the Healthy Mind. Can Med Assoc J, 128, 525-8.
42. Skorecki, K., Levison, H., Crozier, D.N., 1976. Bronchial lability in cystic fibrosis. Acta Paed Scand, 65, 39-42.
43. Stanghelle, J.K., Skyberg, D., 1983. The successful completion of the Oslo Marathon by a patient with CF. Acta Paed Scand 72, 935-8.
44. Svenonius, E., Kantto, R., Arborelius, M., 1983. Improvement after training of children with exercise-induced asthma. Acta Paed Scand, 72, 23-30.
45. Wolff, R.K., Dolovich, M.B., Obuinski, G., Newhouce, M.T., 1977 Effects of exercise and eucapnic hyperventilation on bronchial clearance in man. Journal of Applied Physiology, 43, 46-50.
46. Zach, M.S., Oberwaldner, B., Hausler, F., 1982. CF: physical exercise versus chest physiotherapy. Arch Dis Child, 57, 587-90.
47. Zach, M.S., Purrer, B., Oberwaldner, B., 1981. The effect of swimming on forced expiration and sputum clearance in CF. Lancet, (2), 1201-3.
48. Zambie, M.F., Gupta, S., Lewen, R.J., Hilman, B., Waring, W.W., Sly, R.M., 1979. Relationship between response to exercise and allergy in patients with CF. Ann Allergy, 42, 290-4.

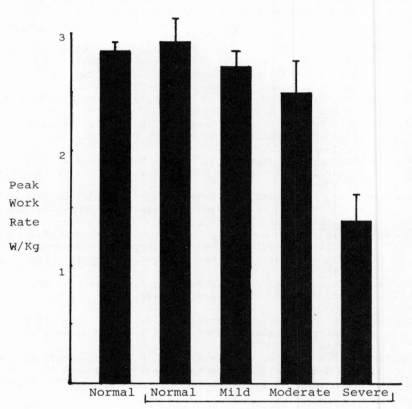

FIG I    PEAK WORK CAPACITY IN CF

(Cropp et al ARRD 1982 126 211)

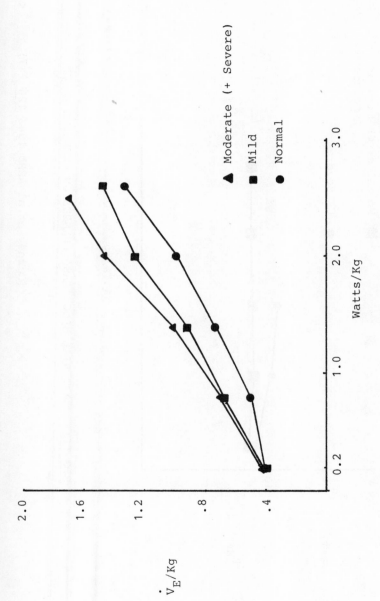

FIG II    VENTILATORY RESPONSE TO EXERCISE IN CF

(Cerney et al ARRD 1982 126 217)

136

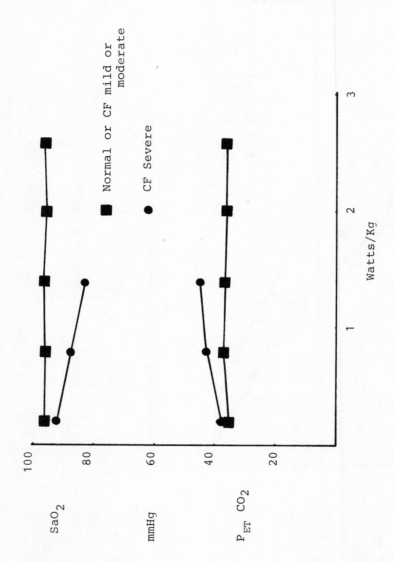

FIG III 'ARTERIAL BLOOD GAS' CHANGES ON EXERCISE IN CF

(Cerney et al ARRD 1982 126 217)

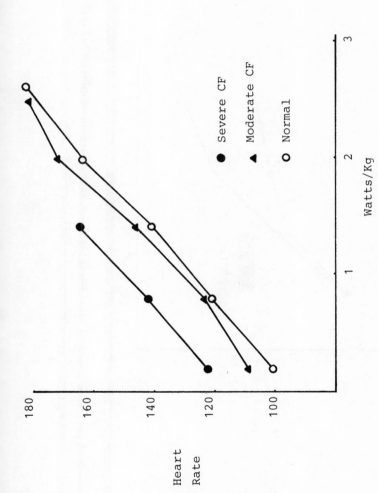

Heart
Rate

Watts/Kg

● Severe CF

▲ Moderate CF

○ Normal

FIG IV   CARDIAC RESPONSE TO EXERCISE IN CF

(Cerney et al ARRD 1982 126 217)

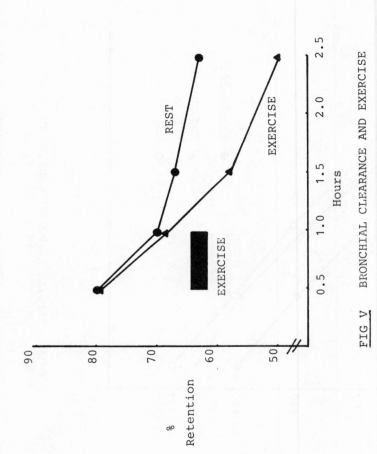

FIG V   BRONCHIAL CLEARANCE AND EXERCISE

(Redrawn from Wolff et al JAP 1977 43 46)

GENE CLONING - A TOOL TO FIND THE BASIC
DEFECT IN CYSTIC FIBROSIS?

R. Williamson, C. Gilliam, M. Blaxter,
P. Scambler, T. Robbins and K.E. Davies


Cystic Fibrosis Genetics Research Group,
Department of Biochemistry,
St. Mary's Hospital Medical School,
University of London,
London W2 1PG, England

In spite of a great many careful chemical pathology
studies of fluids and tissues from CF patients, the
basic biochemical defect remains a total enigma
(Williamson et al, 1983). The chromosomal location of
the mutated gene is not known, and there are no positive
linkage data. No selective advantage to account for the
high frequency of this disorder has been proven. In
spite of the clinical heterogeneity of the disease, the
genetic evidence is consistent with cystic fibrosis
being due to a mutation or mutations at a single DNA
locus (Romeo, 1983).

Defining a strategy aiming at either prevention by fetal
diagnosis, or a rational approach to treatment, would be
greatly simplified by a knowledge of the basic defect.
The lack of such knowledge is a most serious handicap to
CF research. However, the detection of the abnormal
gene must go hand in hand with advances in the study of
the physiology and biochemistry of the disease in order
to translate findings at the DNA level into improved
management of the patients.

There are many levels at which a mutation at a single
gene can cause pathology, and these have been best
defined for the haemoglobinopathies (Weatherall, 1982;
Weatherall and Clegg, 1982). Among these are:

(1) gene deletion, as for South-East Asian
$\alpha^{o}$-thalassaemia, where an entire coding gene, with
surrounding and intervening sequences, is lost from the
genome of affected individuals (Ottolenghi et al.,
1974). Some cases of pituitary dwarfism (Phillips et

al., 1982) and Christmas disease (Giannelli et al, 1983) are also due to deletions of portions of the genes coding for human growth hormone and clotting factor IX respectively.

(2) A mutation in a control region 5' to the structural gene, where RNA polymerase binds to the DNA and transcription of messenger RNA commences, as in some cases of $\beta^+$-thalassaemia (Orkin et al, 1982a).

(3) Transcription of a nuclear RNA containing the coding region specifying the protein, but with a mutation that causes a complete failure of processing to cytoplasmic mRNA. Such mutations may occur, for instance, at the boundaries of intervening sequences, so that splicing cannot occur, as in some Italian $\beta^b$-thalassaemias (Orkin et al, 1982a).

(4) Transcription with misprocessing due to a base change which introduces a new and inappropriate splicing site, which gives a messenger RNA containing either more or fewer nucleotides, often out of phase. Since splicing occurs at the correct site in a proportion of cases, this class of mutations is "leaky" and leads to inherited conditions such as Cypriot $\beta^+$-thalassaemia (Busslinger et al, 1981; Westaway and Williamson, 1981).

(5) Premature termination of translation due to a mutation where a coding base triplet is altered to give a stop codon, as in the Chinese variety of $\beta^o$-thalassaemia (Chang and Kan, 1979).

(6) Change of a single base pair, causing synthesis of an altered protein with different enzymatic or structural properties. Sickle cell anaemia is paradigmatic, but there are many examples (apolipoprotein E in hypercholesterolaemia (Rall et al, 1982; Wallis et al, 1983); $\propto$-1 antitrypsin deficiency in emphysema (Rogers et al., 1983). A single base change in a coding sequence can also generate a new splice site, as in the case of Haemoglobin E, where a single mutation gives a mixed molecular pathology.

Approximately twenty human inherited diseases have now been studied at the DNA sequence level (Williamson et al., 1983). It is early to generalise about classes of mutation, other than to state that structural gene deletions, splicing mutations and single base changes in coding sequences appear to be common relative to control mutations. This may reflect the small sequence complexity of control regions of the genome.

To define a strategy to identify the basic defect in CF, we must first surmise whether or not the mutated

sequence is transcribed.  There are many autosomal
recessive disorders known, and in every case the mutated
gene causes pathology through the absence or alteration
of a protein product.  (It should be noted that this may
not be true for X-linked or autosomal dominant
disorders.)  We are assuming that CF is caused by a
mutation in a structural gene coding for a protein.
There is no way of surmising whether the CF defect
causes the absence or instability of a protein, or the
synthesis of a stable variant which is non-functional
due to an amino acid substitution.  Examples of both
types of defect are known where the carriers are
symptomless.

## GENE ANALYSIS IN CYSTIC FIBROSIS

It is a relatively simple matter to make gene libraries,
consisting of bacterial colonies containing a set of
representative DNA sequences, from a patient with CF and
from normal controls.  Libraries may be complete
("genomic libraries"), and contain every DNA sequence
found in nuclear DNA; such libraries are complex and
difficult to analyse since the total human haploid
genome contains $3 \times 10^9$ base pairs.  Libraries can also
be prepared from DNA from a single human chromosome
(Davies et al., 1981) or from the genes expressed (as
messenger RNA) in a single tissue (Woods et al., 1980;
Crampton et al., 1980).  These libraries are each
specific to the tissue, chromosome and person from whom
they have been isolated, and can be compared with one
another.

If cystic fibrosis is due to a gene deletion, this can
in principle be identified directly as a missing DNA
sequence in a genomic library; also, by definition, if a
coding sequence is deleted, it cannot be transcribed,
and thus will be missing from a cDNA library prepared
from a tissue in which it is usually expressed.  The
problem, of course, is one of complexity; since a
genomic library contains very many sequences, it is
difficult to identify with certainty a single clone that
is absent; the signal is too weak against a high
background.  Also, DNA sequences are present at various
copy numbers (multiplicities) in the human genome, and
therefore those that are present only once (including
most of the coding sequences for proteins) are lost in a
high intensity signal from those present many thousands
of times.  Because of this, there have been no
comparisons of total human DNA between patients and
normal controls.

The general technique for analysis of human genomic DNA
is to cleave the DNA with specific enzymes known as
restriction endonucleases.  For a particular gene, the

fragment boundaries are fixed by the restriction enzyme
selected, and the restriction fragment obtained is of a
unique size. The DNA fragments can then be subjected to
electrophoresis and transferred to a nitrocellulose
membrane ("Southern blotting"). The DNA bound to the
membrane is then "probed" with a radioactively labelled
cloned gene (a DNA probe, or gene probe). Each probe
gives a characteristic pattern of bands on an
autoradiograph. However, as human DNA contains many
repeated sequences, single copy genes have to be used;
otherwise, a smear is obtained which is impossible to
interpret. Since single copy sequences are present at
levels of one part per million, the probe must be
labelled to a high specific activity.

When a defect is known, a cloned gene sequence that is
mutated in patients as compared to normal controls can
be used as a disease-specific probe. It may recognise
the mutation by the absence or alteration of
hybridisation (as for a deletion; Kan and Dozy, 1975) or
by instability of the double strand caused by mis-match
(as for single base changes: Conner et al., 1983).
Sometimes a restriction site is altered, and this can be
detected as a change in fragment size (Flavell et al.,
1978; Orkin et al., 1982b). For CF, the challenge is to
find a gene-specific probe which is also disease-
specific. One approach we have followed is to look for
potential disease-specific probes, starting with cloned
genes for proteins where it has been suggested that the
protein is the basic defect, however good or bad the
evidence!

Recently, we have had the opportunity to study one such
protein, complement C3, a component of the blood
coagulation pathway. It had been suggested that C3 is
mutated and this is the underlying defect in CF, based
on altered levels of C3 in CF patients and on the
inhibitory effect on ciliary movement seen when a
solution of C3, and its natural peptide fragments, are
placed on living oyster gill or rabbit trachea
preparations (Hann et al., 1974; Conover et al.,
1973,1974). We were fortunate to obtain a DNA clone
containing a portion of the structural gene for human C3
which we found recognised a restriction fragment length
polymorphism that is common in the population (Davies et
al., 1983). DNA from several families in which there
are three children with CF was tested using this probe,
and in some cases the parents were of different
genotypes, so the inheritance of different C3 alleles to
each child could be followed. If the basic defect were
a mutated gene for C3, each child with CF must inherit
the same pair of C3 alleles from father and mother,
while unaffected sibs must inherit at least one
different allele. Although each child had CF, they

inherited different alleles; this demonstrates conclusively that C3 cannot carry the mutation causing the basic defect in CF (Davies et al., 1983).

There have been many proposed candidates for the mutated protein causing CF, including ATPases, proteolytic enzymes, superoxide dismutase, and the various cystic fibrosis factors found in serum and with specific physiological or antigenic properties. As clones for these sequences become available, it will be possible to determine immediately whether they are the site of the mutation causing the basic defect, by using exactly the same technique as we have applied to complement C3.

A possible alternative method to select candidate genes involves comparison of cDNA libraries from normal and affected individuals, to seek differences between expressed sequences (Woods et al., 1980; Crampton et al., 1980). Sequences in cDNA libraries are made by transcribing mRNAs, and therefore contain only coding genes. Since the cDNA libraries are much less complex than genomic libraries, and contain only 8,000 or so different clones per tissue, this approach is feasible. We have compared libraries made from mRNAs from normal and CF lymphocytes, and to date have found no qualitative differences between sequences expressed at an intermediate to high level in the cells. These would include the more abundant structural proteins, and some of the enzymes present in high concentrations.

We have isolated several sequences which show decreased expression in CF compared to normal lymphocytes in a majority of patients. However, a double-blind study has revealed that these clones are not invariably decreased in CF, and therefore are likely to be secondary rather than primary to the disease. Other cloned sequences are expressed at higher levels in CF cells as compared to the level of expression in normal cells. We have looked at the sizes of the mRNAs corresponding to these genes in CFs and controls, and have found no differences. It is still necessary to determine the levels of expression of these apparently normal mRNAs, as it is possible that a splicing defect or point mutation can lead to a decrease in the number of normal gene transcripts.

## LINKAGE STUDIES

Genetic linkage exists when two genes are close to each other on a chromosome and are co-inherited at greater than random frequency. Conventional protein polymorphisms are found on several chromosomes, but only relatively small regions of the genome are sufficiently well covered with informative markers so that linkage studies with a disease are straightforward. In the case

of an autosomal recessive disease such as cystic
fibrosis, the absence of a carrier detection test causes
further problems, as it is not possible to follow a CF
haplotype with certainty in an extended family - only
affected persons, and their parents, have a known
genotype.  Attempts that have been made to link CF to
known highly polymorphic protein markers, such as blood
groups and histocompatibility antigens, have given
negative results (Goodchild et al., 1976).

Since the first demonstration of the use of a DNA
polymorphism unrelated to a disease for patient
diagnosis by Kan and Dozy (1978) for sickle cell
anaemia, it has been recognised that a relatively small
number of random cloned human DNA sequences exhibiting
polymorphisms would be sufficient to provide a
comprehensive human linkage map (Solomon and Bodmer,
1979).  Single base changes causing restriction fragment
length polymorphisms are particularly useful as family
markers, since it is relatively simple to determine
haplotype in a large pedigree (Little, 1981; Davies,
1981).  If a linkage is found, it identifies the
chromosomal location of the defect with sufficient
accuracy to allow a focussing of effort upon that
region.

Linkage to a phenotype which may be several hundred
thousand base pairs away may occur.  Whether linkage is
observed depends on the probability of crossing-over,
which occurs at a rate of only 2-3 per chromosome per
generation.  This type of analysis can always be applied
within families, but not always to populations (Davies
et al., 1982).  If there is selection for carriers of a
mutation, or a strong founder effect, linkage
disequilibrium may be found, in which case one haplotype
is preferentially associated with a mutant allele.

One advantage of the linkage technique is that it
is applicable to genomic DNA from any nucleated cell,
and does not depend on the availability of a particular
tissue where the disease is expressed.  About 40% of
single base pair changes generate a change in
restriction endonuclease sites which can in principle be
used as linked markers to identify the inheritance of
the mutation, although the enzymes are not always
available commercially.  These single base changes in
genomic DNA are quite common and usually appear to have
no phenotypic effect; Jeffreys has estimated single base
changes to occur approximately once in every 100-200
base pairs in the region of the human $\beta$-globin gene
family (Jeffreys, 1979).  Many of the mutations are to
intervening sequences, or DNA between genes, since
changes in coding sequences would be more likely to be
disadvantageous to the organism.  The mutations can be

followed through a family when each of the pair of chromosomes in one person give different restriction fragments for the same probe.

We have recently used linkage to locate the mutation causing the X-linked disease Duchenne muscular dystrophy (DMD) more accurately. First, a human X-chromosome library was made in bacteriophage, using the cytofluorimeter to estimate the DNA content of each stained chromosome (Davies et al., 1981). Single copy sequences were selected and located on the chromosome, and one clone was shown to co-inherit with DMD 85% of the time (Murray et al., 1982). A second clone was obtained from a colleague in Leiden, which also is linked to the disease, but on the opposite side of the mutation (Davies et al., 1983). Linked probes can be used to advise women who might carry the DMD mutation whether they have inherited the sequence that is more or less likely to be linked to the disease, by comparison with the chromosomes of their brothers (Harper et al., 1983; Pembrey et al., 1984). However, the markers are not close enough to DMD to allow fetal diagnosis; the error rate of 15% due to cross-over is, in our view, too high. Using these probes, Kingston et al. (1983) have shown that DMD is very close to, and perhaps allelic with, the mutation causing the milder Becker muscular dystrophy; this result is very interesting as Becker MD had previously been thought to be due to a mutation at the opposite end of the X-chromosome.

For cystic fibrosis, we do not have the advantage of knowing the chromosomal localisation of the gene defect. Because the CF heterozygote cannot be identified, we must rely completely upon families in which there are several affected children. However, if a linkage is obtained, then it will be possible to predict carrier status for unaffected sibs with a certainty depending only upon the closeness of the marker to the CF mutation. Such studies will also allow an analysis of heterogeneity for CF, and provide data which will indicate whether there is linkage disequilibrium, a pointer to selective heterozygote advantage.

### CHROMOSOMES 4 AND 19 - A START

To find the mutant gene in CF amongst all of the other autosomal DNA sequences is indeed a daunting task. However, the search will be cumulative in the sense that regions of chromosomes can gradually be excluded by a process of elimination. Each probe permits us to test for linkage over a region of about 1/250 of the human genome. Clearly, several hundred equally spaced probes would be sufficient, but since clones selected from a genomic library are random rather than evenly spaced, it

would take almost a thousand to analyse most of the
genome (Skolnick, 1982).

Fortunately, chances can be improved by isolating probes
from a single chromosome, as we have done for the
X chromosome for Duchenne muscular dystrophy.  Using
this technique, only 500 probes must be studied.  By
linking probe to probe, a network of linked DNA
sequences can be constructed to trawl the entire genetic
length of a chromosome for the CF mutation.  Should no
linkage to CF be found in the families, that chromosome
can be "discarded" and a new one considered.  This
approach has already been used with protein markers to
assign the MNS blood group locus to a region of
chromosome 4 with a high degree of probability (Cook et
al., 1980).

For no particular reason, we have started by considering
one large and one small chromosome, 4 and 19.
Chromosome-specific bacteriophage libraries were
prepared, and clones selected at random.  Testing for
the presence of these sequences in rodent/human hybrid
cell lines with known, partial human chromosome
complements confirmed the chromosomal location of these
probes in many cases.  Those DNA sequences that also
detect RFLPs are now being used for linkage analysis in
our CF families, as are probes for coding genes known to
be on chromosomes 4 and 19.

Seven such probes on chromosome 4, and four on 19, are
presently under study.  Whilst on chromosome 19 we have
almost completed the probe-probe linkage analysis our
linkage data for the much larger chromosome 4 is in its
early stages.  At the moment we cannot exclude the CF
mutation with sufficient certainty from either of these
chromosomes.

We have received encouragement by recent results from
the laboratory of Jim Gusella, in Boston, who has found
a clone linked to the autosomal dominant disorder,
Huntington's disease.  This condition, which begins in
middle years after childbearing age and causes severe
neurological and mental handicap, is equally baffling at
the biochemical level as CF.  After studying only 12
probes, Gusella and his colleagues found one which is
closely linked to Huntington's disease.  The existence
of a very large Venezuelan pedigree, and the ease of
following alleles causing a dominant disease, certainly
helped this group, and there was also an undoubted
element of luck.  However, once the probe is found (as
for HD), the entire research perspective for this
disease is changed, with new opportunities for both
fetal diagnosis and carrier detection.

Candidate genes selected from a cDNA library can also be studied as family linkage markers, but for a different reason. As for complement C3, once a sequence is thought to be the site of the mutation, it must always track with one allele of the gene in a pedigree. Therefore, linkage is the simplest method of confirming or excluding the identity of a candidate for the basic defect. We have shown that a 1% chance of recombination in a generation corresponds to a DNA distance between two loci of about one million base pairs (Davies et al., 1983); therefore recombination is unlikely to occur within a locus, as most genes are much smaller than this.

Once a linkage has been found, it is still essential to move along the chromosome to the basic defect. Genetic techniques should permit the location of the defect within a stretch of several million base pairs of DNA, and it will then be necessary to "walk" the genome using large overlapping fragments of genomic DNA (Hadfield, 1983). Each step in the walk can be as large as approximately half the size of the fragment that is cloned. With 50 kb fragments cloned in cosmids one can "walk" in 25 kb steps, identifying coding genes in each fragment by studying messenger RNAs in tissues which are affected in CF. It is often easier to use bacteriophage, for although the inserts of human DNA are only half the length, the clones are much easier to handle, and tricks exist where the gene walk is carried out biologically by a bacterium (Seed, 1983). Ultimately, a combination of linkage and mRNA analysis should allow the basic defect to be identified.

FETAL DIAGNOSIS

Fetal diagnosis followed by termination of affected pregnancies represents an acceptable method for prevention of a severe genetic disease for many families. The diagnosis of an inherited disease usually involves the measurement of the structure or function of the protein which is mutated, as for Tay-Sachs or Lesch-Nyhan Syndromes. In general, the availability of fetal diagnosis decreases the frequency of abortion, as in the absence of diagnosis many families chose to terminate all pregnancies at risk.

There are several promising approaches to fetal diagnosis for CF (see Brock, this volume), but none of them have yet been proven in several centres, and do not appear to measure the basic defect in any case. If the gene defect can be determined, antenatal analysis can be carried out on genomic DNA from any fetal tissue. This was first done using amniocytes (Kan et al, 1976). However, the late stage of pregnancy (18-19 weeks) at

which diagnosis is possible using present technology
raises difficult psychological and social problems for
many families. We have demonstrated the  usefulness of
obtaining chorionic villi for diagnosis at a much
earlier time in pregnancy (Williamson et al., 1981;
Elles et al., 1983).  This is now in use for fetal
diagnosis of sickle cell disease and thalassaemia using
gene probes, and for chromosome analysis where there is
a risk of Down's syndrome (Old et al., 1982; Brambati et
al, 1983).  However, before this technique can be
applied more widely, it will be necessary to prove an
acceptably low level of fetal morbidity and mortality.

One implication of the molecular biological approach to
the CF gene is that it may be possible to offer
heterozygote detection and fetal diagnosis prior to
understanding the pathophysiology of the disease.
Population linkage disequilibrium will indicate a
heterozygote advantage.  However, the delineation of the
gene defect will not in itself necessarily lead to
advances in therapy; this will require further research
to identify and characterise the gene product in a
series of families.

## ACKNOWLEDGEMENTS

Our research is supported by generous grants from the
Cystic Fibrosis Research Trust and the Medical Research
Council.

## REFERENCES

Brambati, B. and Simoni, G., 1983.  Diagnosis of fetal
    trisomy 21 in first trimester.  Lancet, I, 586.

Busslinger, M., Moschnas, N. and Flavell, R.A., 1981.
    $\beta^+$-thalassemia: abberant splicing results from a
    single point mutation in an intron.  Cell, 27,
    289-298.

Chang, J.C. and Kan, Y.W., 1979.  $\beta^o$-thalassemia; a
    nonsense mutation in man.  Proc. Natl. Acad. Sci.
    U.S.A., 76, 2886-2889.

Conner, B.J., Reyes, A.A., Morin, C., Itakura, K.,
    Teplitz, R.L. and Wallace, R.B., 1983.  Detection of
    Sickle Cell  $\beta$ -Globin Allele by Hybridization with
    Synthetic Oligonucleotides. Proc. Natl. Acad. Sci.
    U.S.A., 80, 278-282.

Conover, J.H., Conod, E.J. and Hirschhorn, K., 1973. Complement components in cystic fibrosis. Lancet, II, 1501-1502.

Conover, J.H., Conod, E.J. and Hirschhorn, K., 1974. Studies on ciliary dyskinesia factor in cystic fibrosis: IV, its possible identification as anaphylatoxin (C3a)-IgG complex. Life Sci., 14, 253-256.

Cook, P.J.L., Noades, J.E., Lomas, C.G., Buckton, K.E. and Robson, E.B., 1980. Exclusion Mapping illustrated by the MNS Blood Group. Ann. Hum. Genet., 44, 61-73.

Crampton, J.M., Humphries, S., Woods, D. and Williamson, R., 1980. The isolation of cloned cDNA sequences which are differentially expressed in human lymphocytes and fibroblasts. Nucl. Acids Res., 8, 6007-6017.

Davies, K.E., 1981. The application of DNA recombinant technology to the analysis of the human genome and genetic disease. Hum. Genet., 28, 1-7.

Davies, K.E., Gilliam, C. and Williamson, R., 1983. Cystic Fibrosis is Not Caused by a Defect in the Gene Coding for Human Complement C3. Mol. Biol. Med, 1, 185-190.

Davies, K.E., Hartley, D.A., Murray, J.M., Harper, P.S., Hill, M.E., Casey, G., Taylor, P. and Williamson,R., 1982. The characterisation of sequences from a human X chromosome library for the study of X-linked diseases. Banbury Report, (Cold Spring Harbour Laboratory), 14, 279-290.

Davies, K.E., Jackson, J., Williamson, R., Harper, P.S., Ball, S., Sarfarazi, M., Meredith, L. and Fey, G., 1983. Linkage analysis of myotonic dystrophy and sequences on chromosome 19 using a cloned complement 3 gene probe. Journal of Medical Genetics 20, 259-263.

Davies, K.E., Pearson, P.L., Harper, P.S., Murray, J.M., O'Brien, T., Sarfarazi, M. and Williamson, R., 1983. Linkage Analysis of Two Cloned DNA Sequences Flanking the Duchenne Muscular Dystrophy Locus on the Short Arm of the Human X-Chromosome. Nucl. Acids Res. 11, 2303-2312.

Davies, K.E., Young, B.D., Elles, R.G., Hill, M.E. and Williamson, R., 1981. Cloning of a representative genomic library of the human X chromosome after sorting by flow cytometry. Nature, 293, 374-376.

Elles, R.G., Williamson, R., Niazi, M., Coleman, D.V. and Horwell, D., 1983. Absence of Maternal Contamination of Chorionic Villi Used for Fetal Gene Analysis. New Engl. J. Med., 308, 1433-1435.

Flavell, R.A., Kooter, J.M., De Boer, E., Little, P.F.R. and Williamson, R., 1978. Analysis of the β-, δ-Globin Gene Loci in Normal and Hb Lepore DNA. Cell, 15, 25-41.

Giannelli, F., Choo, K.H., Rees, D.J.G., Boyd, Y., Rizza, C.R. and Brownlee, G.G., 1983. Gene deletions in patients with haemohilia B and anti-factor IX antibodies. Nature, 303, 181-183.

Goodchild, M.C., Edwards, J.H., Glenn, K.P., Grindey, C., Harris, H., Mackintosh, P. and Wentzel, J., 1976. A search for linkage in cystic fibrosis. Journal of Medical Genetics 13, 417-419.

Gusella, J.F., Wexler, N.S., Conneally, P.M., Naylor, S.L., Anderson, M.A., Tanzi, R.E., Watkins, P.C., Ottina, K., Wallace, M.R., Sakaguchi, A.Y., Young, A.B., Shoulson, I., Bonilla, E. and Martin, J.B., 1983. A polymorphic DNA marker genetically linked to Huntingdon's disease. Nature, 306, 234-238.

Hadfield, C., 1983. Chromosome Walking, in Focus, 5:4, pp 1-5. Bethesda Research Laboratories Inc., Maryland, U.S.A.

Hann, S., Holsclaw, D.S. and Shin, H.S., 1974. Complement components in cystic fibrosis. Lancet, II, 520-521.

Harper, P.S., O'Brien, T., Murray, J.M., Davies, K.E., Pearson, P. and Williamson, R., 1983. The use of linked DNA polymorphisms for genotype prediction in families with Duchenne Muscular Dystrophy. Journal of Medical Genetics, 20, 252-254.

Jeffries, A.J., 1979. DNA Sequence Variants in the $^G\gamma$-, $^A\gamma$-, δ- and β-Globin Genes of Man. Cell, 18, 1-10.

Kan, Y.W. and Dozy, A.M., 1978. Polymorphisms of DNA Sequence Adjacent to the Human β-Globin Structural Gene: Relation of Sickle Mutation. Proc.Natl.Acad. Sci. U.S.A., 75, 5631-5635.

Kan, Y.W., Globus, M.S. and Dozy, A.M., 1976. Prenatal diagnosis of α-thalassemia: Clinical application of molecular hybridization. New Eng. J. Med., 295, 1165.

Kingston, H.M., Thomas, N.S.T., Pearson, P.L., Sarfarazi, M. and Harper, P.S., 1983. Genetic linkage between Becker Muscular Dystrophy and a polymorphic DNA sequence on the short arm of the X chromosome. Journal of Medical Genetics, 20, 255-258.

Little,P.F.R., 1981. DNA Analysis and the Antenatal Diagnosis of Haemoglobinopathies, in Genetic Engineering Vol 1, (ed. R. Williamson), pp 61-102. Academic Press, London.

Murray, J.M., Davies, K.E., Harper, P.S., Meredith, L., Muller, C.R., Goodfellow, P.N. and Williamson, R., 1982. Linkage relationship of a cloned DNA sequence on the short arm of the X chromosome to Duchenne muscular dystrophy. Nature, 300, 69-71.

Old, J.M., Ward, R.H.T., Karagozlu ,F., Petrou, M., Modell, B. and Weatherall, D.J., 1982. First-Trimester Fetal Diagnosis for Haemoglobinopathies: Three Cases. Lancet, II, 1413-1416.

Orkin, S.H., Kazazian, H.H., Antonarakis, S.E., Goff, S.C., Boehm, C.D., Sexton, J.P., Waber, P.G. and Giardina, P.J.V., 1982a. Linkage of $\beta$-thalassemia mutations and $\beta$-globin gene polymorphisms with DNA polymorphisms in the human $\beta$-globin gene cluster. Nature, 296, 627-631.

Orkin, S.H., Little, P.F.R., Kazazian, H.H. and Boehm, C., 1982b. Improved Detection of the Sickle Mutation by DNA Analysis. New Engl.J.Med, 307, 32-36.

Ottolenghi, S., Lanyon, W.G., Paul, J., Williamson, R., Weatherall, D.J., Clegg, J.B., Pritchard, J., Pootrakul, S. and Boon, W.H., 1974. Gene Deletion as the Cause of $\alpha^o$-thalassaemia. Nature, 251, 389-392.

Pembrey, M.E., Davies, K.E., Winter, R.M., Elles, R.G., Williamson, R., Sazzoni, T.A. and Walker, C., 1984. The clinical use of DNA markers linked to the gene for Duchenne muscular disease. Arch. Dis. Childhood, in press.

Phillips, J.A., Hjelle, B.L., Seeburg, P.H. and Zachmann, M., 1981. Molecular Basis for Familial Isolated Growth Hormone Deficiency. Proc.Natl.Acad. Sci.U.S.A., 78, 6372-6376.

Rall, S.C., Weisgraber, K.H., Innerarity, T.L. and
    Mahley, R.W. 1982. Structural basis for receptor
    binding heterogeneity of apolipoprotein E from type
    III hyperlipoproteinaemic subjects. Proc. Natl. Acad.
    Sci. U.S.A., 79, 4696-4700.

Romeo, G., Menozzi, P., Mastella, G., Giulta, A., Lodi,
    G., Constantini, D., Micalizzi, C., Gargani, G.,
    Romano, C., Bappispini, A., Grzincich, G.L.,
    Antonelli, M., Quattrucci, S., Follo, B., Marianelli,
    A. and Ansaldi, N., 1982. Genetic and epidemiologic
    study on cystic fibrosis in Italy. Italian Journal
    of Pediatrics, 7, 201-209.

Rogers, J., Kalsheker, N., Wallis, S., Speer, A.,
    Coutelle, C., Woods, D. and Humphries, S.E., 1983.
    The Isolation of a Clone for Human $\alpha$1-Antitrypsin
    and the Detection of $\alpha$1-Antitrypsin in mRNA from
    Liver and Leukocytes. Biochem.Biophys.Res.Comm,
    116, 375-382.

Seed, B., 1983. Purification of Genomic Sequences from
    Bacteriophage Libraries by Recombination and
    Selection in vivo. Nucl. Acids Res., 11, 2427-2445.

Skolnick, M., 1982. Use of chromosome specific DNA
    libraries for mapping and modeling genetic diseases.
    First European Congress on Cell Biology. Paris 1982
    p349.
Solomon, E. and Bodmer, W.F., 1979. Evolution of sickle
    variant gene. Lancet, I, 923.

Wallis, S.C., Rogne, S., Gill, L., Markham, A., Edge.
    M., Woods, D.L., Williamson, R. and Humphries, S.,
    1983. The isolation of cDNA clones for human
    apolipoprotein E and the detection of apo E RNA in
    hepatic and extra-hepatic tissues. The EMBO Journal,
    2, 2369-2373.

Watson, J.D., Tooze, J. and Kurtz, D.T., 1983.
    Recombinant DNA: A Short Course. W.H. Freeman,
    New York.

Weatherall, D.J., 1982. The New Genetics and Clinical
    Practice., Nuffield Provincial Hospitals Trust,
    London.

Weatherall, D.J. and Clegg, J.B., 1983. Thalassemia
    Revisited. Cell, 29, 7-9.

Westaway, D. and Williamson, R., 1981. An Intron
    Nucleotide Sequence Variant in a Cloned
    $\beta^{+}$-Thalassaemia Globin Gene. Nucl.Acids Res., 9,
    1777-1788.

Williamson, R., Casey, G., Humphries, S. and Davies, K., 1983.  Molecular Genetics - Basic Principles and Techniques,  in Advanced Medicine 19 (ed. K.B. Saunders), pp 196-201. Pitman, London.

Williamson, R., Eskdale, J., Coleman, D.V., Niazi, M., Loeffler, F.E. and Modell, B.M., 1981.  Direct Gene Analysis of Chorionic Villi: a Possible Technique for First-Trimester Antenatal Diagnosis of Haemoglobinopathies.  Lancet, II, 1125-1127.

Williamson, R., Crampton, J.M. and Clarke, B.E.,  1982. Research perspectives:  the basic defect in Cystic Fibrosis, in Cystic Fibrosis (Ed. Hodson, M.E., Norman, A.P. and Batten, J.C.), pp 260-272  Baillere Tindall, London.

Woods, D., Crampton, J.M., Clarke, B.E. and Williamson, R., 1980.  The construction of a recombinant cDNA library representative of the poly(A)+ RNA population from normal human lymphocytes. Nucl.Acids.Res , 8, 5157-5168.

Woo, S.L.C., Lidsky, A.S., Guttler, F., Chandra, T. and Robson, K.J.H., 1983.  Cloned human phenylalanine hydroxylase gene allows prenatal diagnosis and carrier detection of classical phenylketonuria. Nature, 306, 151-155.

# CYSTIC FIBROSIS: A SINGLE LOCUS DISEASE

Giovanni Romeo

Laboratory of Genetics, Institute of Neurology
University of Bologna Medical School
Via U.Foscolo 7, 40123 Bologna (Italy)

## ABSTRACT

The analysis of segregation for CF in a  sample of 624 Italian
families shows a segregation ratio of 0.252 in close agreement with
the value expected for autosomal recessive transmission. In two
successive studies carried out on 401 and 624 CF couples a definite
increase of the frequency of consanguineous marriages has been
observed with respect to that of the general population, which had
been accurately determined in the past taking advantage of the
existence in Italy of an Archive of consanguineous marriages. The
number of first-cousin marriages among CF parents closely matches
that expected from the hypothesis of a single locus disorder and is
in contrast with the model of mutations at two or more loci.
Finally the estimate of birth incidence of CF in Italy (1/2000)
obtained from consanguinity studies agrees with the most recent
incidence estimates deriving from neonatal screening, confirming
the reliability of the methodology used.

## INTRODUCTION

The question of genetic heterogeneity has been raised several times
in the past and recently published data on the incidence of Cystic
Fibrosis (CF) amongst first cousins of affected have been interpreted as favouring the hypothesis of mutations at more than one locus
which would cause clinically similar phenotypes (Danks et al., 1983).
This type of heterogeneity is defined in the present paper as
intergenic heterogeneity in order to keep it distinct from intrage-
nic  heterogeneity, or heterogeneity of mutations which belong
to the same locus. The latter type of heterogeneity represents the
rule rather than the exception when appropriate tools of analysis
at the molecular level become available as in the case of the different mutations of the ß-globin gene which cause the ß-thalassemia
phenotype (Treisman et al., 1983). On the contrary intergenic heterogeneity has serious implications on the search of the primary
genetic defect of a disorder like CF, because the molecular abnor-

155

mality might be different among families, thus hampering the comparison of data obtained from different populations.

Some of the classica. approaches used in human genetics may help in discriminating whether one or more loci are involved in the etiology of CF. To this end we have applied segregation analysis and analysis of consanguineous marriages to a sample of 624 Italian CF families (Romeo et al. 1984). The predictive value of segregation analysis in human genetics consists in its capability of establishing a simple mendelian mode of inheritance, thus taking away support from more complicated, and often proposed, modes of transmission, such as that advanced for CF some years ago (Schaap and Cohen, 1976). The main interest of the present paper is focused, however, on the problem of genetic (intergenic) heterogeneity in CF, as it can be analyzed through consanguinity. Our approach has taken advantage of an unique opportunity existing in Italy represented by the Archive of consanguineous marriages based on about 500,000 dispensations given by the Catholic Church for such marriages from 1910 through 1964 (Moroni, 1964) and for some regions even later (Moroni,1977). The Archive has made it possible to carefully establish the frequency of consanguineous marriages, up to second-cousin degree, in the general population for each of the 95 Italian provinces and for five-year periods (Zei,G. and Moroni,A., unpublished results). It has therefore been possible to compare the frequency of consanguineous marriages observed among CF parents with the frequency of consanguineous marriages of the same degree celebrated in the different Italian provinces during the same years. Since consanguinity varies enormously in space and time, such a fine subdivision of data from the general population allows to match an adequate control population with the sample of parents of patients instead of using frequencies of consanguineous marriages obtained from large populations and for long periods of time, as it is usually done with this type of studies. Such approach has already been shown valuable for estimating the incidence in Italy of different autosomal recessive disorders, like Friedreich ataxia (Romeo et al.1983a) and PKU (Romeo et al. 1983b). The rationale behind these estimates of incidence is represented: 1) by the possibility of measuring quite accurately the increase of consanguineous marriages in a sample of parents of patients with respect to a properly matched control population; 2) by the mathematical relationship, quantitatively determined by Dahlberg (1947) and subsequently by Barrai (1965), linking this increase of consanguineous marriages to the gene frequency of the same disorders. In descriptive terms this relationship can be summarized saying that the greater the proportion of consanguineous marriages observed among parents of patients, the rarer is the disorder.

The incidence of CF in Italy has been estimated in the past using

consanguinity data from 401 families (Romeo et al., 1981) belonging
to the larger sample of 624 families more recently analyzed (Romeo
et al., 1984). In addition to the segregation analysis of CF, this
paper will therefore present an updating of the incidence estimate
on the total sample of 624 CF families together with a discussion
of the test for genetic heterogeneity based on consanguineous marriages.

## PATIENTS AND METHODS

Patients had been diagnosed by 11 CF Centers following criteria
previously described (Romeo et al.,1981). Only those patients with
at least two consecutive positive sweat tests were considered as
affected and information regarding their family history for CF and
consanguinity of their parents was collected by each Center on
questionnaires through direct interview of at least one of the parents.
On the same questionnaires information regarding a possible history
of CF and sweat tests performed was collected for each sib of the
proband, and segregation tables were prepared and analyzed with
the aid of a computer program described elsewhere (Bianco ,1983).
An accurate pedigree was reconstructed for those families whose parents were consanguineous so that all degrees of consanguinity up to
second cousins could be clearly detected.

The weighted average of the frequencies of marriages among first
cousins ($C_1$) and among second cousins ($C_2$) in the general Italian
population was calculated as previously reported (Romeo et al.,1981,
1983a) using the consanguinity rates known for each of the 95 Italian provinces and for each 5 year period (Zei,G. and Moroni,A.,
unpublished results). Marriages among parents of CF patients celebrated according to the Catholic rite were checked in the Archive
and the answers concerning consanguinity, given through interviews,
always corresponded to the information contained in the same Archive.
The equation of Dahlberg (1947) which has been used in the present
study to test the genetic (intergenic) heterogeneity of CF is the
following: $C'_1 = C_1 (1 - 15q)/(C_1 + 16q - C_1 q)$ where $C'_1$ is the
frequency of first-cousin marriages in the sample of parents of
patients, $C_1$ is the weighted average of the frequencies for the same
type of marriages in the general population calculated as just defined, and q is the gene frequency. From the above equation the gene
frequency (q) can also be derived as already shown (Romeo et al.,
1981): $q = C_1 (1 - C'_1 )/ C_1 (1 - C'_1 ) + 16 (C'_1 - C_1)$.
A more general equation formulated by Barrai (1965) which takes into
account all types of consanguineous marriages (in our case both
first and second cousins), has also been used to calculate gene and
disease frequencies.

RESULTS

Segregation analysis of CF.The data necessary for segregation analysis, collected by the different Centers for 624 sibships as described under Methods, are summarized in table 1. The results, presented
in greater details elsewhere (Romeo et al., 1984), are summarized
in table 2.

TABLE 1. Segregation table of 624 CF sibships according
to their size (s) and number of affected sibs (r).

| r | 1 | 2 | 3 | 4 | TOT. |
|---|---|---|---|---|------|
| s |   |   |   |   |      |
| 1 | 172 | 0 | 0 | 0 | 172 |
| 2 | 205 | 36 | 0 | 0 | 241 |
| 3 | 87 | 38 | 2 | 0 | 127 |
| 4 | 29 | 13 | 6 | 0 | 48 |
| 5 | 13 | 4 | 3 | 2 | 22 |
| 6 | 5 | 3 | 0 | 0 | 8 |
| 7 | 0 | 0 | 0 | 1 | 1 |
| 8 | 0 | 2 | 1 | 0 | 3 |
| 9 | 0 | 0 | 0 | 0 | 0 |
| 10 | 0 | 0 | 0 | 0 | 0 |
| 11 | 1 | 0 | 1 | 0 | 2 |
| tot. | 512 | 96 | 13 | 3 | 624 |

TABLE 2. Results of segregation analysis from the data of
table 1, under single, truncate and multiple selection (Bianco,1983)

| | Single selection | Truncate selection | Multiple selection |
|---|---|---|---|
| Estimate of p | 0.161 | 0.263 | 0.252 |
| $\chi^2_1$ df | 34.44 | 0.511 | --- |
| $\sigma(p)$ | 0.0152 | 0.0178 | --- |
| 95% intervals | $0.131<p<0.191$ | $0.227<p<0.298$ | --- |
| Estimate of $\pi$ (probability of ascertainment) | ---- | ---- | 0.925 |
| Estimate of x (sporadic cases) | ---- | ---- | 0.000 |

The segregation ratio observed under multiple selection is in accordance with that expected for an autosomal recessive disorder (p =
0.25) and with a model of ascertainment close to truncate selection
(which would have a probability of ascertainment $\pi$= 1).
Consanguineous marriages and birth incidence of CF. The two essential
requirements of epidemiological studies based on consanguinity, namely sample size and availability of an adequate control population,
have been met in this study thanks to the number of families studied
and to the existence in Italy of the Archive of consanguinity described in the Introduction.
The results summarized in table 3 present two estimates of consanguinity rates calculated at two different stages of this study. The
first estimate, calculated on a partial sample of 401 couples of CF
patients (Romeo et al. 1981) is quite similar to the more recent
estimate calculated from the whole sample of 624 couples (Romeo et
al. 1984).
The increase of first-cousin marriages varies from 3.2 fold in the
first study to 3.4 fold in the more recent one. The incidence of
the disease ($q^2$) calculated only from first-cousin marriages, using
the equation reported under Methods, varies from 1/1351 to 1/1635
in the two studies, while the incidence calculated from all consanguineous marriages, according to Barrai's equation (1965), remains
stable. The stability of the latter estimate is the result of variations, having opposite sign, of the $C'_1/C_1$ and $C'_2/C_2$ ratios,
which balance each other in the calculation of q when the equation
of Barrai is used. If the two estimates of $q^2$ obtained from the
sample of 624 couples are considered, namely 1/1635 and 1/2367, an
intermediate value of 1/2000 seems the most likely value of incidence of CF in Italy. The very nature of the procedure used indicates
that this is an estimate of incidence at birth.
Consanguinity and genetic heterogeneity of CF. Consanguinity data
can also be used to test the occurrence of genetic heterogeneity in
CF, in particular of that type of heterogeneity defined as intergenic in the Introduction, which hypothesizes mutations at more than
one locus. The rationale behind this test is based on the consideration that if CF were made of two (or more) separate genetic entities, the number of consanguineous marriages expected among CF
parents would be greater than that expected for a disorder due to
mutations of a single gene. In table 4 the two hypotheses just
mentioned are compared by solving Dahlberg's equation (see Methods)
for first-cousin marriages. In both cases the unknown value is $C'_1$
(or the proportion of first-cousin marriages expected among parents
of patients) and the equation can be easily solved if $C_1$ and q are
known. Under both hypotheses $C_1$ is the value obtained as the weighted average of first-cousin marriages in the general population,

TABLE 3. Rates of consanguinity and incidence of CF calculated from a partial sample of 401 CF couples of parents (Romeo et al., 1981) and from the present sample of 624 couples (Romeo et al.,1984).

| N. of couples (a) | Marriages among cousins 1st (b) | 2nd (c) | $C'_1$ % | $C_1$ % | $\dfrac{C'_1}{C_1}$ | Dahlberg * q | $q^2$ | $C'_2$ % | $C_2$ % | $\dfrac{C'_2}{C_2}$ | Barrai ** q | $q^2$ |
|---|---|---|---|---|---|---|---|---|---|---|---|---|
| 401 | 8 | 10 | 1.995 | 0.626 | 3.19 | 0.0272 | 1/1351 | 2.49 | 0.434 | 5.74 | 0.02059 | 1/2358 |
| 624 | 15 | 16 | 2.404 | 0.706 | 3.41 | 0.0247 | 1/1635 | 2.56 | 0.618 | 4.15 | 0.02055 | 1/2367 |

* q has been calculated from the frequencies of first-cousin marriages only, among parents of patients ($C'_1$) and in the general population ($C_1$) accordingto the equation reported under Methods derived from that of Dahlberg (1947). $C'_1$ represents the ratio b/a and $C_1$ is the weighted average calculated as described under Methods.

** q calculated from the frequencies of first-cousin marriages (see above) as well as of second-cousin marriages ($C'_2$ and $C_2$) according to the equation of Barrai (1965). $C'_2$ represents the ratio c/a and $C_2$ is the weighted average calculated as described under Methods.

TABLE 4. Test for genetic heterogeneity of CF from first-cousin marriages.

a) Incidence calculated from screening
   (1/3000 x 10/8)                                      0.000416

b) Gene frequency calculated from a)                    0.020412

c) Weighted average for first-cousin marriages
   in the general Italian population ($C_1$ for
   624 couples from table 3)                             0.00706

d) Observed frequency of first-cousin marriages
   ($C'_1$ from table 3) among 624 CF couples of
   parents                                              0.02404
   Total N. observed among 624 = 15

===================================================================
Hypothesis 1: mutations at only one locus

- Expected frequency of first-cousin marriages
  ($C'_1$) among CF parents (from Dahlberg's
  equation,using b and c)                               0.02764
  Total N. expected among 624 couples = 17.25
  ($\chi^2_{1\ df}$ = 0.29)

===================================================================
Hypothesis 2: mutations equally distributed between two loci($\alpha$ and $\beta$)

A) Incidence for each of the 2 genetic disorders
   deduced from screening (½ x 1/3000 x 10/8)           0.0002083

B) Frequency of each of the 2 genes ($\alpha$ or $\beta$)   0.014433

- Expected frequency of first-cousin marriages
  ($C'_1$)among CF parents (from Dahlberg's equation
  using B and c) for each genetic disorder
  ( $\alpha\alpha$  or $\beta\beta$)                               0.036102

- Total expected frequency of $C'_1$ for the 2
  genetic disorders                                     0.072203
  Total N. expected among 624 = 45
  ($\chi^2_{1df}$ = 20)

whereas q can be deduced, at least as a threshold value, from the
data available from neonatal screening. Several neonatal screening
programs for CF have been carried out in Italy in recent years and
the most recent data from the Veneto region indicate that screening
can detect 1 CF child among 3000 newborns (Pederzini et al., 1983).
This value can therefore be considered, after correction for false
negative results, as the lowest possible estimate of birth incidence.
Under the conditions used in this screening (Pederzini et al.,1983)
false negatives cause a loss of about 20% of the patients.
The estimated incidence of the disease from screening is therefore,
after correction, equal to 1/2400, which yelds a gene frequency of
0.020412 (Table 4). The latter estimate is true if the disease is
due to mutations affecting a single gene (hypothesis 1). If, on the
contrary, CF is made of two distinct genetic disorders having similar frequencies (hypothesis 2) as recently proposed (Danks et al.,
1983), the overall incidence has to divided by 2 and the gene frequency for each disorder is consequently lower. Since the observed
$C_1$ value remains identical under both hypotheses, the expected
value of $C'_1$ is greater under hypothesis 2, which predicts 45 first-
cousin marriages among the 624 couples of CF parents instead of the
15 observed (with a $\chi^2_{1df}$ = 20). On the contrary the number of first
cousin marriages expected under hypothesis 1 closely matches the
observed one, making this the more likely alternative ($\chi^2_{1df}$ = 0.29).

## DISCUSSION

The results of segregation analysis are      in close agreement
with the expected segregation ratio of 0.25 and confirm the autosomal recessive mode of inheritance of this disorder in spite of
the recurring proposals of alternative models of transmission
(Schaap and Cohen,1976) partly motivated by a supposedly higher
segregation ratio. However segregation analysis cannot discriminate
whether CF is a single genetic entity or is heterogeneously made of
two or more autosomal recessive disorders, all causing the same
clinical manifestations. The hypothesis of two distinct genetic disorders in CF recently proposed (Danks et al.,1983) is based on the
argument that the gene frequency for the disease (q = 0.0266) calculated from the proportion of affected first cousins of the probands
in Victoria, Australia, would be higher than the gene frequency
calculated by direct counting of cases (q = 0.0198). The agreement
between these two estimates is, according to the conclusions of the
Authors, poor but not poor enough to dismiss the one locus model
(Danks et al., 1983).

   In summary the analysis of consanguineous marriages among parents
of CF patients carried out in Italy during the last few years confirms the autosomal recessive transmission of the disorder and fully

supports the hypothesis of mutations at a single locus (Table 4).
At the same time the incidence of the disease calculated by the same
approach is in accordance with the most recent estimate deriving
from neonatal screening in Italy (Pederzini et al.,1983). This
concordance, together with the stability of our estimate at two
different moments in the course of this study (Table 3), is somewhat reassuring about the soundness of the methodology used.

## REFERENCES

Barrai,I., Mi,M.P., Morton,N.E., Yasuda,N., 1965. Estimation of
prevalence under incomplete selection. Am.J.Hum.Genet., 17, 221-
236.

Bianco,M., 1983. Metodo di studio statistico, epidemiologico e genetico applicato ad una malattia ereditaria: la fibrosi cistica
del pancreas. Tesi di laurea. Dipartimento di Scienze Statistiche
Università di Bologna.

Dahlberg,G., 1947. Mathematical methods for population genetics.
Basel, Switzerland, Karger, pp 61-67.

Danks,D.M., Allan,J., Phelan,P.D., Chapman,C., 1983. Mutations at
more than one locus may be involved in CF. Evidence based on
first-cousin data and direct counting of cases. Am.J.Hum.Genet.,
35, 838-844.

Moroni,A., 1964. Evoluzione della frequenza dei matrimoni consan-
guinei in Italia negli ultimi cinquant'anni. Atti A G I, 9, 220.

Moroni,A., 1977. Human ecology studies in Sardinia, with special
reference to human consanguinity, in Human Adaptability (Eds.
Collins and Weiner), pp 153-155. London, Taylor and Francis.

Pederzini,F., Armani,P., Barbato,A., Borgo,G. et al., 1983.
Newborn screening for cystic fibrosis. Two methods compared on
229,626 newborns tested in 8 years in the Veneto region. Ital.
J.Pediat., November,

Romeo,G., Menozzi,G., Mastella,A., Giunta,G. et al., 1981. Studio
genetico ed epidemiologico della fibrosi cistica in Italia. Ri-
sultati di un'indagine policentrica del gruppo di lavoro per la
fibrosi cistica della Società Italiana di Pediatria. Riv.It.Ped.
7, 201-209.

Romeo,G., Menozzi,P., Ferlini,A., Fadda,S. et al., 1983a. Incidence
of Friedreich ataxia in Italy estimated from consanguineous
marriages. Am.J.Hum.Genet., 35, 523-529.

Romeo,G., Menozzi,P., Ferlini,A., Prosperi,L. et al., 1983b. Incidence of classic PKU in Italy estimated from consanguineous
marriages and from neonatal screening. Clin.Genet., 24, 339-345.

Romeo,G., Bianco,M., Menozzi,P., Mastella,G. et al., 1984. Segregation analysis and analysis of consanguinity on 624 Italian
families with Cystic Fibrosis  (Submitted for publication).

Schaap,T. and Cohen,M.M., 1976. A proposed model for the inheritance
   of CF. In CF: projection into the future. (Eds. Mangos and Talamo)
   pp 291-303. Stratton Int.Co.
Treisman,R., Orkin,S.H., Mainatis,T., 1983. Specific transcription
   and RNA splicing defects in 5 cloned ß-thalassemia genes. Nature
   302, 591-596.

# POPULATION AND MOLECULAR GENETIC ANALYSES OF CF IN THE OHIO AMISH

Katherine Wood Klinger    Dept. of Mol. Biol. and Microbiol. and the Cystic Fibrosis Center, Case Western Reserve Univ. Sch. of Med., Cleveland, Ohio   USA 44118

CF  is an inherited disease of unknown etiology: however, no chromosomal location or linkage to classical genetic markers have been discovered. Advances in molecular genetics have made it theoretically possible to identify gene sequences specifically related to the basic defect responsible for CF. These DNA sequences could represent the CF gene, but are more likely to be DNA sequences closely linked to the CF locus. The probability of success of these studies can be improved by using population genetics to support the molecular genetic techniques. For this reason, and because the success of linkage studies is generally a function of the quality of the families chosen for study, I have characterized the inheritance of CF in an inbred population, the Ohio Amish.

There are two major Amish populations in Ohio, one in southern Ohio and one in eastern Ohio. The results of this study indicated a difference in the incidence of CF between the two populations. The incidence in the southern community was 1/569 live births, nearly four times the national incidence in the United States. No cases of CF occurred in the eastern population. Founder effect was responsible for the difference in CF gene frequency between the two populations. Thus the eastern population is essentially free of the CF allele, and an excellent source of normal donors for controls for the DNA analyses. Nineteen cases of CF were identified in children born in the southern Ohio Amish community between 1950 and 1982. These cases were distributed among 6 sibships that form one large extended family. Because of inbreeding, distribution of affected children within the kinship, and the quality of genealogic records, this population is maximally informative for linkage analysis.

Inherited sequence differences in the DNA prepared from peripheral white blood cells isolated from the Amish CF families were used as genetic markers. These differences (restriction fragment length polymorphisms) are detected by southern blot analysis using cloned gene probes. The probes used in this study are concentrated on chromosomal regions 6p and 11p, so that an exclusion map can ultimately be generated for these regions. To date we have seen no linkage of CF to an HLA A-locus specific probe, an HLA B-locus specific probe, or a random chromosome 6 probe.

USE OF DNA RESTRICTION FRAGMENT LENGTH POLYMORPHISM FOR LINKAGE
STUDIES IN CYSTIC FIBROSIS

Lap-Chee Tsui, Natasa Plasvic, Dara Kennedy, Martha Zsiga and Manuel
Buchwald. Genetics Department, The Hospital for Sick Children,
Toronto, Ontario, Canada M5G 1X8.

We have recently taken a new approach to the Cystic Fibrosis (CF)
problem by searching for a DNA marker for the disease. The method
relies on the DNA sequence heterogeneity prevalent among different
individuals and on the fact that these sequence variations are
genetically inherited. These polymorphic sequences sometimes occur
within restriction endonuclease recognition sequences and may therefore be detected as restriction fragment length polymorphisms (RFLPs).
By correlating the inheritance pattern of the RFLPs and that of the
disease trait in affected families, it is possible to identify DNA
fragments which are closely linked to the CF gene. This RFLP approach
has been proven successful in the study of Huntington disease.

Due to the recessive nature of CF, only two-generation families
with two or more affected children are likely to provide significant
statistical information in the linkage analysis. With the assistance
of several CF clinics in Canada,we have identified over 100 such
families and collected blood samples from 28 of them, 7 of which have
at least 3 affected children. We have already established lymphoblast
lines for all the participating individuals and begun screening their
DNAs with RFLP probes identified in our own laboratory and some of
those made available to us by other investigators.

Mapping the CF gene will require the use of markers distributed
over most of the human genome,since it has not yet been unequivocably
assigned to any chromosome (although it is clearly not X-linked).
Theoretically, only 150 evenly spaced markers are needed to cover all
possible chromosomal locations so that at least one of the markers is
within 10 centimorgans (10% recombination) of the disease locus.
Although this approach is time consuming,a systematic search should
eventually lead to the CF gene. Once close linkage of a RFLP marker
to the CF gene is established, we will have the opportunity to provide
a reliable method for carrier detection and prenatal diagnosis. Most
importantly,the marker will be a foundation for identification of the
basic defect of this disease.

To date we have excluded the possibility of close linkage of the
CF gene to 10 markers. The data and their analysis will be presented
and discussed in the context of the clinical characteristics of the
patients in each family.
(Supported by the Canadian Cystic Fibrosis Foundation and the Sellers
Foundation).

On a Unified Theory of Cystic Fibrosis
Lung Disease

Richard C. Boucher, Michael R. Knowles,
C. Cotton, M. Jackson Stutts,
James R. Yankaskas and John T. Gatzy

University of North Carolina
Chapel Hill, North Carolina, USA

## I. INTRODUCTION

Recent studies have identified specific functional abnormalities
in epithelia of the sweat duct (Quinton and Bijman, 1983) and
several airway regions (Knowles, Gatzy and Boucher, 1981). However, neither the normal physiology nor the dysfunction in CF of
these and other target epithelia are sufficiently well characterized to assign the abnormality to a single gene defect. Our
report will use data from one relatively well-studied epithelium,
proximal airway epithelia, to illustrate the dilemma. Specifically, we will focus on (1) the epithelial ion transport functions
which may play a major role in the maintenance of the volume and
composition of surface liquid in normal and CF subjects; (2) two
hypotheses that may account for the origin of the CF syndrome in
this region; and (3) gaps in our knowledge that make the formulation of a unified theory premature.

## II. NORMAL FUNCTION

A. Organ Level Physiology

The epithelia that line pulmonary surfaces appear to participate
in the production and control of the volume and composition of
surface liquids. These functions are divided between the two
major anatomic units of the airway mucosa: (1) the surface epithelium, which, depending on region and need, can either absorb
sodium (salt and water) or secrete chloride (salt and water); and
(2) glands, which appear to be confined to more proximal airways
and are solely secretory.

The functions of the pulmonary epithelia are determined by the
stage of development. The work of Olver, Strang (Olver and
Strang, 1974) has demonstrated that the fetal sheep lung produces
a relatively large volume of liquid that flows from the lung
through the glottis and oropharynx into the amniotic fluid. The

primary driving force for liquid secretion is active chloride
transport by the pulmonary epithelium. Liquid secretion creates a
slightly positive pressure in the lung that reflects the flow of
lung liquid through the resistive elements of the glottis. The
positive pressure generated appears to be an important stimulus
for normal lung growth (Fewell et al., 1983).

A rapid change in epithelial function occurs at birth when the
lung is converted from a liquid-filled to a gas-filled organ.
Several processes contribute to the rapid clearance of liquid from
the pulmonary air spaces. For example, upon delivery, the first
breaths are accompanied by large negative interstitial pressure
that favors liquid absorption. Inflation also increases the
radius of "pores" in the epithelial barrier that provide paths for
liquid movement from lumen to the interstitial compartment.
Active ion transport systems may also contribute to the clearance
of liquid from the lung. Brown and associates have shown that
isoproterenol infusions into the near-term sheep fetus can slow
secretion of lung liquid or even induce volume absorption (Brown
et al., 1983). Because the effect induced by isoproterenol is inhibited by amiloride, a relatively selective antagonist of sodium
absorption, these investigators have speculated that circulating
catecholamines, which increase in concentration near term, stimulate the active absorption of $Na^+$ by an action on beta receptors.
Cotton and co-workers have recently shown chloride secretion by
the trachea of fetal sheep in vitro (Cotton et al., 1983). However, isoproterenol only increased chloride secretion and did not
induce sodium absorption. Consequently, the isoproterenol actions
observed by Brown and co-workers must be attributed to regions
distal to the trachea.

The pattern of ion translocation in mature proximal airways is
quite different than that of the fetus. Chloride secretion is not
detectable in tracheas excised from adult sheep and is replaced by
active $Na^+$ absorption (Cotton et al., 1983). Isoproterenol is ineffective. Similar patterns of ion translocation have been
described for proximal airways in many other adult animal species,
including both the nasal and bronchial epithelium of man. The capacity to absorb sodium and a counter ion (chloride) and water
reflects the need to modulate the depth of liquid on proximal
airway surfaces that are continually receiving a relatively large
volume of liquid that is swept by ciliary activity from distal
airways towards the mouth.

Mechanisms are available to modulate the volume and content of
proximal airway "secretions". For example in some circumstances,
e.g. during fever or exercise, water may evaporate from the airway
surface. Water can be conserved on proximal surfaces by slowing
the rate of $Na^+$ absorption. In addition, excised proximal airways
can, under appropriate conditions, generate a counter-flow (secretion) of $Cl^-$ that also may serve to add liquid to the surface.
Interestingly, the ability to secrete chloride is greatest when

the absorption of sodium has been slowed by inhibition of Na+
entry into cells (Boucher et al., 1983). These interrelationships
between sodium and chloride flows probably reflect the function of
superficial epithelial cells. Glands, that are located mainly in
proximal regions, can also secrete liquid onto airway surfaces
when stimulated. However, their main function may be to add mucin
glycoproteins onto airway surfaces in response to irritants.

Although the ion transport and permeability of airways in proximal
regions has been characterized, almost nothing is known about the
ion transport by distal lung units and the origin of the airway
surface liquid that moves up the airway surfaces. Recent evidence
from the primary cultures of alveolar Type II cells isolated from
adult animals suggests that these cells absorb sodium by an amiloride sensitive mechanism, and the rate of sodium absorption may be
stimulated by beta agonists (Goodman and Crandall, 1982; Mason et
al., 1982). If Na+ absorption is the dominant ion transport by
cells of this region in vivo, then liquid would tend to be driven
away from alveolar surfaces and net flow onto the surface would
have to reflect:    (1) passive hydrostatic forces; or (2) the
active secretory functions of cells other than Type II on the alveolar surfaces, i.e., Type I cells. Alternatively, liquid may
not be transferred from alveolar surfaces to airways and the primary site of distal "secretion" may be small airways.

B.  Respiratory Epithelial Ion Transport at a Cellular
    Level

A model for ion transport by a normal bronchial epithelial cell is
shown in Figure 1.  The mode of sodium translocation in this

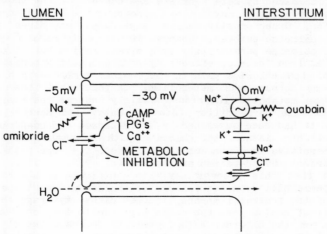

Fig. 1.    Ion transport and permeability of bronchial
epithelial cell.

tissue appears to be similar to that described for many other epithelia. Sodium crosses the apical or luminal membrane of the cell
through an electrically conductive path. Entry is favored by both
the chemical and electrical gradients. This entry step is amiloride sensitive. The $ED_{50}$ for amiloride of $10^{-6}M$ is in the range
reported for tight epithelia. Sodium is extruded from the cell
across the basolateral barrier by a process that involves a
sodium-potassium ATPase and is ouabain sensitive.

Surprisingly little is known about the factors that control the
rate of sodium absorption in the main airways in vivo. Like other
epithelia, the rate of sodium entry into the cell may be limiting
for net $Na^+$ transport in the basal state. For example, amphotericin B, a cation ionophore that increases the rate of $Na^+$ entry,
can increase the rate of sodium absorption by mammalian airways
two-fold. However, naturally occurring agents that might be expected to increase the number of sodium channels e.g., aldosterone
or antidiuretic hormone, do not affect mammalian airways.

Chloride flow across the epithelial barrier under basal conditions
is passive and follows sodium. Consequently, electroneutrality is
preserved under the conditions of NaCl absorption that prevail in
vivo. There are two major paths for chloride absorption: through
(transcellular) and around (paracellular) the cell. Chloride flow
across epithelial cells of most proximal airway regions appears to
be divided about evenly between the two paths. The permeability
of the individual barriers in the cell path has been characterized
in bronchial and tracheal epithelia (Widdicombe and Welsh, 1980;
Boucher and Gatzy, 1982). The permeability of the apical chloride
path is increased by beta agonists and certain of the prostaglandins, i.e., $PGE_1$, that may act by increasing the rate of cyclic AMP
generation. Other prostaglandins, e.g. $PGF_{2a}$, may directly stimulate the chloride pathway. Changes in cytosolic calcium may also
modulate chloride permeability by a direct action but it is difficult to exclude indirect effects by prostaglandin generation. In
addition, the chloride path in the luminal membrane is highly dependent on normal cell metabolism. Exposure of the cell to
hypoxia or metabolic inhibitors rapidly reduces the luminal membrane chloride permeability (Stutts, Gatzy and Boucher, 1983).
Finally, it has been suggested by Hviid-Larsen and co-workers that
like excitable tissues, the chloride path in amphibian epithelia
may be sensitive to transmembrane voltages, i.e. the path is voltage dependent (Hviid-Larsen and Rasmussen, 1982). There is some
evidence that this process may also contribute to the regulation
of $Cl^-$ permeability in respiratory epithelia because hyperpolarization of the luminal membrane, induced either by drugs that limit
the entry of sodium into the cells e.g., amiloride, or removal of
sodium from the external bath, appear to decrease the $Cl^-$ permeability of the apical barrier. In summary, considerably more is
known about modulation of apical $Cl-$ than $Na^+$ permeability.
However, the contribution of modulators to the regulation of
apical $Cl^-$ permeability in vivo has not been determined.

Cl⁻ moves across the basolateral barrier by a neutral, coupled, NaCl co-transport process. We have recently speculated that a conductive path for Cl⁻ also may be located in the basolateral barrier of canine bronchial but not resting tracheal epithelium. This difference may account for the absence of chloride secretion by unstimulated bronchial epithelium.

Finally, the paracellular or shunt path is a major route of passive ion permeation through the bronchial epithelium. Although the total surface area occupied by these paracellular pathways or pores is relatively small, the equivalent pore radius is large (~10nm). Several lines of evidence suggest that most if not all of the passive flow of sodium and about half of the passive Cl⁻ flow across bronchial epithelia occurs via this route.

### III. CYSTIC FIBROSIS

A. Organ Level Dysfunction

Mucus plugging, airflow obstruction, and infection with Staphylococcus aureus and Pseudomonas aeruginosa are common characteristics of CF lung disease. Pulmonary function and pathologic studies of newborn CF subjects suggest that the lung has developed a normal pattern of alveolarization and is of normal size at birth. These findings are compatible with normal secretion of lung liquid *in utero* and, hence, if chloride secretion participates in these secretory process in humans, as it does in sheep and dogs, then the chloride path may be normal in CF lungs at birth. There is no evidence for material that resembles meconium in the lung at birth. The earliest pathologic changes in the lung appear during the neonatal period and include obstruction of small airways by mucus and mucus gland obstruction in the proximal airways. Accordingly, it is reasonable to propose that the lung progressively develops the dysfunction associated with CF some time after birth.

Direct study of epithelial function in the lungs of CF subjects is difficult. However, two clues suggest that an abnormality(ies) of the epithelium that lines airway surfaces may be important in the pathophysiology of lung dysfunction. Two studies of airway surface liquid composition in CF show that the CF pulmonary liquids are characterized by a lower than normal water content and higher than normal potassium content. However, concurrent infection was present in the CF subjects so that these abnormalities may not be a primary epithelial dysfunction. More recently, the transepithelial electric potential difference, which reflects active transepithelial ion flows shunted by passive ion movement, was shown to be abnormally raised in the CF patients (Knowles, Gatzy and Boucher, 1981). This abnormality has been observed both in the nasal cavity and lower airways, and has been detected before infection occurs. Consequently, it appears likely that an abnormality of the surface epithelium characterizes the CF lung and that this abnormality may be reflected in the abnormal composition of "secretions".

## B.   Clues to the Nature of the CF Dysfunction at the Cellular Level

The origin of the raised transepithelial potential difference in CF proximal respiratory epithelia has been a subject of some controversy. Because the PD is related to transepithelial current flow (active ion transport) and barrier resistance to ion flow, abnormalities in one or both of these variables can result in an abnormal voltage. Our original interpretation of the raised PD suggested that the active flow of sodium in the absorptive direction (increased current) was raised. Subsequently we and others suggested that an abnormally low passive chloride permeability (which increases resistance) also contributes to the raised voltage. In vitro data accumulated over the past year suggest that dysfunctions in both the rate of active absorption of sodium and epithelial permeability to chloride combine to contribute to the abnormally raised transepithelial potential difference in CF airways .

For example, we have recently shown that the electrically measured short circuit current (Isc) of nasal polyps excised from CF subjects is an accurate reflection of sodium transport. This equivalency has been demonstrated both by radioisotopic measurements of $Na^+$ flow and the sensitivity of Isc to amiloride. Moreover, the Isc in the basal state of normal nasal epithelium and polyps excised from atopic individuals also is accounted for almost entirely by the active absorption of sodium. We compared the basal rate of sodium transport (Isc) in 54 polyp tissues obtained from 18 CF subjects with 38 normal turbinate tissues from 24 subjects and 23 atopic polyp tissues obtained from 12 subjects. The mean short circuit current of the CF tissues was almost twice ($146 \pm 11 uA \cdot cm^{-2}$) that observed in the normal turbinate tissue (mean = $77 \pm 5 uA \cdot cm^{-2}$). In addition, the mean current of CF tissue exceeded that of patients with atopic polyps ($94 \pm 11 uA \cdot cm^{-2}$). We also found that the absorption of sodium may be increased by exposure of CF but not normal tissue to beta agonists. Consequently, the response of CF nasal epithelium is qualitatively different from that of normal tissues or atopic polyps which are stimulated to secrete $Cl^-$ by beta agonists.

The genesis of the increased transport activity has not been elucidated. Amiloride's inhibition of transepithelial conductance (the reciprocal of resistance) can be taken as an index of the number of sodium entry sites that are blocked by this drug. Because the amiloride-induced reduction in conductance is, if anything, smaller in CF than normal tissues, the number of functioning apical sodium channels is probably not increased in CF tissues. However, because amiloride may also reduce apical membrane chloride permeability (conductance) of normal airway epithelia, (this permeability is smaller in CF than normal tissue, see below), a quantitative comparison of apical sodium channels is not possible. Other studies have demonstrated that the sensitivity of these channels in CF tissues to amiloride is not different than normal tissues. Little information is available about other possible sites of $Na^+$ transport dysfunction such as the number of $Na^+$-$K^+$ ATPase pumps or their activity.

There is considerable evidence that the chloride permeability of the CF respiratory epithelium is abnormally small. Absolute flows of $Cl^-$ across the barrier are reduced and this is reflected in a smaller transepithelial G (Knowles et al., 1983). Several observations suggest that the defect is in the cell path for $Cl^-$. For example, if mannitol is taken as a marker of paracellular flow, then the flow of $Cl^-$ through a non-restrictive paracellular path can be estimated. About 50% of total $Cl^-$ flow occurs through the paracellular path in normal tissues but approxmiately 75% of the transepithelial $Cl^-$ flow takes place through this path in CF tissues. Because total $Cl^-$ flow is also reduced in CF, the absolute magnitude of $Cl^-$ flow through the cell is clearly low. In addition, after amiloride treatment $Cl^-$ flow in the absorptive direction across normal tissues decreases, a phenomenon that may reflect the hyperpolarization of apical barrier. This phenomenon accounts, at least in part, for the persistence of a PD after amiloride treatment in normals because $Cl^-$ flow in the secretory direction persists and hence $Cl^-$ secretion is induced. Exposure of CF tissues to amiloride induces smaller changes in the flow of $Cl^-$ in the absorptive direction and a smaller residual current. This difference in amiloride effect can be explained by an apical membrane of CF tissue that is poorly permeable to $Cl^-$. The bi-ionic diffusion potential generated by superfusing the luminal membrane of CF cells _in vivo_ or _in vitro_ with a solution where all $Cl^-$ is replaced by a poorly permeant organic anion (gluconate) is reduced in CF compared to normal tissue (Knowles, Gatzy and Boucher, 1983a). This result suggests a defect in luminal membrane chloride permeability in CF subjects. This hypothesis was confirmed when Cotton and co-workers impaled airway epithelial cells with microelectrodes and established that the change in luminal membrane electrical potential generated by removal of chloride from the luminal compartment was blunted in CF.

Recent evidence also indicates that the apical chloride conductance of CF epithelia cannot be increased by treatment with agonists that increase $Cl^-$ conductance in normal respiratory epithelia. For example, _in vivo_ superfusion of nasal surfaces with beta agonists or prostaglandins ($PGE_1$, $PGF_{2a}$) increases the $Cl^-$ diffusion PD of normal but not CF subjects (Knowles, Gatzy and Boucher, 1983b). Further, chloride secretion can be induced _in vitro_ by beta agonists, prostaglandins, or a calcium ionophore (A23187) in normal but not in CF tissue. Consequently, it appears that the reduced chloride conductance of CF airway epithelia may not reflect an insufficient concentration of endogenous modulators _in_

vivo. Microelectrode experiments showed that the magnitude of the
apical membrane potential is not different in CF and normal subjects, so it is unlikely that the relative chloride impermeability
reflects the effects of a greater transapical membrane voltage and
a voltage-dependent mechanism.

Paracellular pathways have not been well characterized in CF tissues.    The   permeation   of  a  marker  of  paracellular  flow,  $^{14}C$
mannitol, has been measured and is not substantially different in
CF tissues.   Similarly,  the magnitude of the bi-ionic potentials
when, in the presence of amiloride, luminal sodium is replaced by
choline,  are  similar  in  magnitude  (~2 millivolts) in vivo or in
vitro.  These results suggest that the contribution of the selec-
tivity of the paracellular paths to the PD is about the same for
both groups.  However, estimates of equivalent pore radii with un-
charged,  polar  solutes  of different size will be needed to better
characterize this path.

### IV.  SPECULATION

There are at least two hypotheses that may account for the abnormalities noted in CF respiratory epithelial cells.   The first,
based on studies of the sweat ductal epithelium, would suggest
that  the  abnormality  in  the  chloride channel is the primary
defect.  This abnormality could reflect a structural absence of
the channel, or a change in the ability of the existing channel to
permit $Cl^-$ flow.   The other abnormalities in cellular function
would presumably be secondary to (1) the "absence" of a chloride
path, (e.g. by differences in electrical potentials); or (2) the
spillover of the action of intracellular mediators into other
pathways, e.g. sodium transport.  The second hypothesis would
state that there is a primary abnormality in paths that control
ion permeation through the cell.  The CF abnormality would then
reflect the inability of the cell to maintain the chloride pathway
in an "open" state and to appropriately regulate the rate of
sodium absorption.

Rigorous experiments that select between these hypotheses are difficult to design.   However,  there are bits of information that
help focus their relative merits.  For example, several lines of
evidence suggest that chloride channels in adult CF respiratory
epithelial cells are not completely absent.  For example, amiloride superfusion onto CF nasal surfaces in vivo does not reduce
the PD to zero, which suggests the induction of some $Cl^-$ secretion.   In addition, the response of the CF nasal epithelium in
vivo to superfusion with chloride free solutions (bi-ionic potentials) is ~17 or 18 millivolts. Although this response is smaller
than normal ( PD=35mV) it is larger than the response predicted
for a bi-ionic potential generated exclusively at a non-selective
paracellular path (~9mV).  Accordingly, some chloride permselec-
tivity may exist in the apical membrane of CF cells. In vitro,
the ratio of $P_{Cl^-}$ to $P_{mannitol}$ is lower in CF than in normal tis-

sues, but the ratio does not approach that which would be expected for exclusive Cl⁻ movement through a free solution paracellular pathway (4.1 vs. 2.9 respectively). These results are compatible with some Cl⁻ permeation through the cell. In addition, amiloride induces approximately a 90% inhibition of short circuit current in CF epithelia. Since net Na⁺ transport is abolished, it is possible that the residual 10% of current reflects the induction of a small chloride secretion. This contention is supported by the observation that pretreatment with indomethacin increases the efficacy of amiloride (98% inhibition of Isc). If indomethacin acts in CF tissues, as it does in other tissues to reduce chloride permeability by inhibition of prostaglandin synthesis, then this action is also consistent with the presence of chloride permeation through the apical membrane of the CF cell. In summary it appears that the respiratory epithelium probably is not completely devoid of cell Cl⁻ channels.

It also is clear that an abnormality in chloride channels is not generalized to all tissues. For example, gastric acid and chloride secretion appear to be normal or even supernormal in CF subjects. These results are consistent with a gastric epithelium with a normal chloride permeability. Similarly, other epithelia, e.g. esophagus, do not manifest an abnormality in chloride permeability. Chloride paths in nonepithelial structures have not been as rigorously studied. Recent experiments with circulating blood elements, e.g. lymphocytes and red blood cells, have not revealed abnormal chloride permeation in cells from CF patients.

Perhaps the most compelling evidence against the proposal that an abnormality in Cl⁻ permeability is the primary defect in CF respiratory epithelia is the observation that pharmacologic inhibition of chloride permeability does not, by itself, induce a substantial increase in sodium absorption by normal tissues. For example, if normal tissues are pretreated with indomethacin and bumetanide, both inhibitors of chloride permeability, sodium absorption either in model systems (canine trachea) or human nasal epithelium is not increased. Further, adrenergic agents do not stimulate Na⁺ transport by normal tissue after blockade of the Cl⁻ path.

We are left with the notion that CF lung disease is the consequence of an abnormality in the control of ion pathways. This general hypothesis could be framed in several different ways. In one, chloride secretion by the lung in utero and during the early neonatal period may be normal. However, the conversion to the mature or adult pattern of airway ion transport, that is accompanied by the development of sodium absorption and suppression of chloride secretion, "overshoots" in CF airways. Alternatively, regional differentiation of function of epithelial function may be faulty. For example, adult alveolar Type II cells are reported to absorb sodium in vitro, and this transport process is accelerated by adrenergic agonists. These characteristics are shared by proximal airway epithelial cells from CF but not normal subjects. Consequently, it is conceivable that the CF cells of proximal airways are regulated by the same processes that control ion permeation in more distal pulmonary epithelia. The relative Cl⁻ permeability of these distal cells is of major interest.

One observation that argues against the general concept of abnormal regulation in CF epithelia is the inability to increase Cl⁻ permeability with known modulators. This observation would fit the hypothesis only if regulatory signals are included that maintain the Cl⁻ channel in a closed state.

In conclusion, it is premature to establish a unified theory about the pathophysiology of CF, even for one region of a single structure that is affected by CF. It is obvious that better tools for the study of Cl⁻ channels are necessary to quantitate their number and characteristics. A more complete understanding of the control of sodium and chloride pathways in the adult epithelium, the signals that switch functions during maturation, and the specialization of the control of ion paths in distal from proximal cells, are also obviously required. Only when these studies have been performed and contrasted with parallel studies in other epithelia that are affected by CF, will a unified theory of the disease emerge.

Supported by HL 22924, HL 16674, HL 00787, and a CFF RRDP R002. Dr. Boucher is American Heart Established Investigator.

### REFERENCES

Boucher, R., and Gatzy, J., 1983. Relative ion permeability of apical and basolateral barrires of canine bronchial (CB) epithelium. Federation Proceedings, 42, 461.

Boucher, R., Knowles, M., Stutts, M., Fischer, N., and Gatzy, J., 1983. Induction of Cl⁻ secretion across excised human nasal epithelium. Clinical Research, 31, 856A.

Brown, M., Olver, R., Ramsden, C., Strang, L., and Walters, D., 1983. Effects of adrenaline and spontaneous labor on the secretion and absorption of lung liquid in the fetal lamb. Journal of Physiology, 344, 137-152.

Cotton, C., Lawson, E., Boucher, R., and Gatzy J., 1983. Bioelectric properties and ion transport of airways excised from adult and fetal sheep. Journal of Applied Physiology: Respiratory Environmental Exercise Physiology, 55, 1542-1549.

Fewell, G., Hislop, A., Kitterman, J., and Johnson, P.,1983. Effect of tracheostomy on lung development of fetal lambs. Journal of Applied Physiology: Respiratory Environmental Exercise Physiology, 55, 1103-1108.

Goodman, B., and Crandall, E., 1982. Dome formation in primary cultured monolayers of alveolar epithelial cells. American Journal of Physiology, 243, C96-100.

Hviid-Larsen, E., and Rasmussen, B., 1982.    Chloride channels in toad skin. <u>Phil. Trans. R. Soc. Cond. B.</u>, 299, 413-434.

Knowles, M., Gatzy, J., and Boucher, R., 1981.  Increased bioelectric potential difference across respiratory epithelia in cystic fibrosis. <u>New England Journal of Medicine</u>, 305, 1489-1495.

Knowles, M., Gatzy, J., and Boucher, R., 1983a.  Relative ion permeability of normal and cystic fibrosis nasal epithelium. <u>Journal of Clinical Investigation</u>, 71, 1410-1417.

Knowles, M., Stutts, M., Spock, A., Fischer, J., Gatzy, J., and Boucher, R., 1983.  Abnormal ion permeation through cystic fibrosis respiratory epithelium. <u>Science</u>, 221, 1067-1070.

Knowles, M., Gatzy, J., and Boucher, R., 1983b.  Modulation of nasal epithelial ion permeability in normal and cystic fibrosis subjects in vivo. <u>Clinical Research</u>, 31, 858A.

Mason, R., Williams, M., Widdicombe, J., Sanders, M., Misfeldt, D., and Berry, L., 1982.  Transepithelial transport by pulmonary alveolar type II cells in primary culture.  <u>Proceedings National Academic Science</u>, 79, 6033-6037.

Olver, R., and Strang, L., 1974.  Ion fluxes across the pulmonary epithelium and the secretion of lung liquid in the fetal lamb. <u>Journal of Physiology, London</u>, 241, 327-357.

Quinton, P., and Bijiman, J., 1983.  Higher bioelectric potentials due to decreased chloride absorption in sweat glands of patients with cystic fibrosis. <u>New England Journal of Medicine</u>, 308, 1189-1191.

Stutts, M., Gatzy, J., and Boucher, R., 1983.   Metabolic inhibition of bronchial ion transport. <u>Federation Proceedings</u>, In Press.

Widdicombe, J., and Welsh, M., 1980.   Ion transport by dog tracheal epithelium. <u>Federation Proceedings</u>, 39, 3062-3066.

178

# ADRENERGIC AND CHOLINERGIC STIMULATION OF CF SWEAT GLANDS

Sean Harper and Paul M. Quinton, Biomedical Sciences, University of California Riverside, Riverside, CA 92521, U.S.A.

Recent reports indicate that eccrine sweat glands of cystic fibrosis (CF) patients differ in their secretory response to certain pharmacological agents (1). We have studied the sweating response of cystic fibrosis patients, ill control (IC) patients without cystic fibrosis, and healthy control (HC) subjects to three classes of autonomic nervous system (ANS) agonists. IC patients were selected without regard to specific disease, but with regard to diseases associated with limited physical activity. After iontophoretically administering cholinergic (acetylcholine, Ach); $\alpha$-adrenergic (phenylephrine, Phe); or $\beta$-adrenergic (isoproterenol, Isp) agonists, the number of active sweat glands was counted in a standard circular area of 20 $mm^2$ on the forearm and the sweat rate for single sweat glands was determined as described previously (2). The sweat rate for each subject was taken from the mean of four randomly selected glands. All subjects responded to Ach and the total number of glands/$cm^2$ stimulated in 23 CF (210 $\pm$ 50)* was not significantly different from 11 HC (240 $\pm$ 115) or 7 IC (245 $\pm$ 90) subjects. All subjects except one CF patient responded to Phe stimulation and again the number of glands/$cm^2$ stimulated in CF (195 $\pm$ 90) patients, was not different from HC (235 $\pm$ 115) or IC (200 $\pm$ 90) subjects. The number of glands/$cm^2$ responding to Isp stimulation was significantly less in CF (85 $\pm$ 85) patients than in HC subjects (145 $\pm$ 75) but not different from IC (75 $\pm$ 70) patients. All HC subjects gave at least some response, but 2 of the 7 IC and 6 of the 23 CF patients failed to respond to Isp. Subsequent studies revealed that atropine prior to Isp blocked sweating in 11 of 17 HC subjects and all of 7 CF patients. The average maximum sweat rates (nl/min/gland) of CF patients closely matched for age and sex were less than, but not significantly different from, 8 HC subjects when stimulated by Ach (CF = 5.4 $\pm$ 1.3; HC = 7.2 $\pm$ 4.6)*, Phe (CF = 1.4 $\pm$ 0.6; HC = 2.9 $\pm$ 1.2), or Isp (CF = 0.9 $\pm$ 1.1; HC = 1.5 $\pm$ 0.9). In contrast, the average maximum sweat rate of CF patients was greater than, but not significantly different from, 7 closely matched IC patients when stimulated by Ach (CF = 4.0 $\pm$ 1.4; IC = 3.4 $\pm$ 2.5); Phe (CF = 1.8 $\pm$ 0.6; IC = 0.6 $\pm$ 0.6), or Isp (CF = 1.0 $\pm$ 0.9; IC = 0.4 $\pm$ 0.4). These results suggest that the influence of the $\beta$-adrenergic stimulation on sweat secretion may involve secondary factors such as exercise, heat stress, and general condition of health. Nonetheless, the uniform failure of the CF group to respond to B-adrenergic stimulation after muscarinic blockage may indicate some ANS abnormality. The finding that some control subjects also failed to respond to Isp may indicate that the characteristic is not unique to CF.

1.    Sato, K. and F. Sato. Clin. Res. 31: 253A, 1983.
2.    Quinton, P.M. and J. Bijman. N. Engl. J. Med. 308: 1185, 1983.
The generous cooperation of Dr. Chun-I Wang, Director, CF Clinic, Children's Hospital of Los Angeles and Dr. R.C. Dooley, Director, CF Clinic, San Bernardino County Medical Center is deeply appreciated.    * mean $\pm$ S.D.

**POSTER GROUP ONE No. 1.01**

CHROMOSOMAL LOCALISATION OF DNA SEQUENCES BY IN SITU
HYBRIDISATION

Gillian Bates, Tim P. Robbins, Dave Hartley and
Bob Williamson
Department of Biochemistry, St. Mary's Hospital
Medical School, University of London, W2 1PG, England.

As cloned DNA probes of interest are isolated, it
is important to be able to determine their precise
chromosomal location.  In recent years it has become
possible to map single copy DNA sequences by in situ
hybridisation (1).  This technique provides a direct
visualisation of the position of the probe on human
metaphase chromosomes.  Metaphase spreads are prepared,
and the chromosomes denatured, to allow the
radiolabelled probe to anneal to its complementary
sequence.  The site and extent of hybridisation is
detected by autoradiography after an exposure time of
approximately three weeks.  This is correlated to the
G-banding pattern, which can be produced either before
hybridisation by treatment with lipsol and Leishman's
stain, or after by staining with quinacrine mustard.

In situ hybridisation has now been used to map a
number of single copy gene sequences, for example, the
human myosin heavy chain gene to 17p (2) and insulin to
11p (3).  We have so far exploited this technique to
locate specific cloned sequences on the X-chromosome
and autosomes (4).

1.  Harper, M.E. and G.F. Saunders (1981) Chromosoma
    83:431-439.
2.  Rappold,G.A. and H.P. Vosburg (1983) Hum. Genet.
    43:195-197.
3.  Harper, M.E. et al., (1981) PNAS 78:4458.
4.  Hartley, D. et al. submitted.

**POSTER GROUP ONE No. 1.02**

LINKAGE MARKERS FOR CF ON CHROMOSOME 19

Peter Scambler', Gillian Bell', Kay Davies',
Patricia Tippett", Art Boylston^, Steve Humphries' and
Bob Williamson'.
'Departments of Biochemistry and ^Pathology, St.
Mary's Hospital Medical School, University of London W2
1PG England. "MRC Blood Group Unit, Wolfson House,
University College, London, NW1 2HE.

In the research for the genetic locus of the CF
defect we have chosen two chromosomes for study,
numbers 4 and 19. Our strategy with chromosome 19, as
for 4, is to establish a genetic map of the chromosome.
We then aim to exclude the CF locus from the length of
chromosome between two linked probes by following
segregation of the disease and marker pairs through
families. As this method takes some time each probe is
also used to generate linkage data in the conventional
way. One set of markers we have used is the polymorphic
blood group loci for which linkage data is presented.
In addition we have several recombinant DNA probes
including Apo-C-2, Complement factor 3, $\beta$HCG and TCGF.
Some of these probes have been shown to recognise RFLPs
and linkage data for CF is now available.

To complement this approach we have used a FACS
to prepare chromosome 19 DNA for a 19 specific library,
from which we hope to generate RFLP markers.
Preliminary data suggests a good enrichment for
chromosome 19 DNA. Further work utilizing probes for
structural genes and random RFLPs will result in a
genetic map of chromosome 19.

**POSTER GROUP ONE No. 1.03**

LINKAGE MARKERS FOR CF ON CHROMOSOME4

Tim P. Robbins, Peter J. Scambler, T. Conrad Gilliam,  Bob Williamson, Caroline A. Ingle, Kay E. Davies
Department of Biochemistry, St. Mary's Hospital Medical Scool, University of London, W2 1PG, England.

CF is most often considered to be an autosomal, single gene defect. As such, the study of CF can be approached by means of genetic linkage analysis in that the segregation of defined markers and the mutant CF gene can be compared in CF families, the degree of co-inheritance reflecting physical proximity. In the past this was often done using protein polymorphisms such as those of the blood group loci (1), but the new recombinant DNA technology enables a wealth of hitherto undetected DNA sequence variations to be tapped, such that almost any cloned sequence ("probe") can be applied to linkage studies.

Physical mapping of these probes to specific chromosomal locations enables one to conjecture, and later confirm by family studies, the genetic linkage relationships between probes. Once any two probes are linked, segregation analysis in CF families will give a definitive answer to the question, "Does the CF mutation lie between these marker loci?" By considering successive regions of the human genome we hope to eventually map the gene involved in CF.

Individual chromosomes present a convenient unit of the genome upon which to focus, thus we have concentrated on chromosomes 4 (this poster) and 19 (see poster, Scambler et al.). At the time of writing we have 7 cloned sequences mapped to chromosome 4 by somatic cell genetics or in-situ hybridisation (see poster, Bates et al.). Using a chromosome 4 enriched library of cloned sequences we hope to increase this number still further, such that through linkage analysis the exclusion/inclusion of the CF mutation from chromosome 4 may be achieved.

1.  Goodchild et al., (1976) Journal of Med. Gen. 13: 417.

182

**POSTER GROUP ONE No. 1.04**

IMMUNOREACTIVE PANCREATIC LIPASE (IRL) ASSAYED USING DRIED BLOOD SPOTS A NEW TEST FOR THE NEONATAL DETECTION OF C.F.

Keith B. Hammond, Christine G. Ask, Dianne C. Watts; Dept. of
Pediatrics, Univ. of Colorado, School of Medicine, Denver, CO 80262,
USA.

We have previously reported the adaptation of a commercial radio-immunoassay kit for serum pancreatic lipase (NuClin Diagnostics, Northbrook, IL 60062) to dried blood specimens, and demonstrated elevated IRL levels in neonates with C.F. (Lancet i, 42, 1984). Our preliminary data suggested that the dried blood spot IRL assay might be a more specific neonatal screening test for C.F. than the IRT assay, while retaining the sensitivity of the latter. This report describes a prospective comparison of this assay with the IRT test routinely used in the Colorado neonatal screening program.

Dried blood specimens obtained from 1046 newborn infants (2-3 days) were assayed for both IRL and IRT. The mean and 95% ranges (determined nonparametrically) for both analytes were 18 (10-40) ng/mL and 29 (10-87) ng/mL respectively (values expressed as ng/mL of serum and assuming an average hematocrit of 50%). Only 3 of the 1046 newborn specimens (0.29%) had levels that simultaneously exceeded the 97.5th percentile of "normal" for both analytes. In 2 of these the IRT value exceeded the 99.8th percentile used in this laboratory for screening purposes. Repeat specimens from both infants showed normal levels for IRT and IRL at 4 weeks of age.

In a separate study IRL values were measured only when the IRT values exceeded the 99.8th percentile "cut-off" Of the approximately 13,500 newborn specimens tested in October through December 1983, a total of 35 (0.25%) were re-assayed for IRL. Of these 35 "positives" only 17 (48.6%) had IRL levels in excess of the 97.5th percentile. To date (January 1984) we have received follow-up specimens on 21 of the 35 infants (60%). 4 of these had elevated IRT and IRL levels and sweat testing confirmed the diagnosis of C.F. in each case.

This study confirms our earlier suggestion that the IRL assay might be useful in reducing the number of "false positive" IRT tests. However, the increase in predictive value of a positive test result (in this case from 19% to 36%) is insufficient to justify elimination of the "two-tier" approach to screening, in which a second blood specimen is obtained at approximately 4-6 weeks of life and used to determine whether or not a confirmatory sweat test is indicated.

Further studies are required to establish the optimal "cut-off" value for IRL, both in the context of a secondary(confirmatory) screening test and as a possible substitute for the IRT assay as the primary screening method. In the latter case the predictive value of a positive IRL test, either alone or in combination with IRT, awaits completion of a larger prospective evaluation.

**POSTER GROUP ONE No. 1.05**

HUMAN LEUCOCYTE ANTIGENS (HLA) AND HAPLOTYPES IN CYSTIC FIBROSIS
PATIENTS: POSSIBLE INCREASE OF HLA-B8 IN THOSE WITH LIVER DISEASE.

Mario Mondelli, Peter T. Donaldson, Alex P. Mowat
Depts.of Child Health and Liver Unit, King's College Hospital,London.

A variety of immunological abnormalities has been described in
patients with cystic fibrosis (CF), including immune complexes in
serum and sputum, immediate hypersensitivity reactions to allergens,
antinuclear factors and lymphocyte sensitisation to pancreas and
lung derived antigens. Recent data would suggest that immune
responses to liver antigens may play a role in symptomatic liver
disease complicating cystic fibrosis.[1]

In this preliminary study we have examined, using a standard
lymphocyte microcytotoxicity assay, the frequencies of HLA antigens
and haplotypes in 38 children with cystic fibrosis of whom 14 had
clinical and biochemical evidence of liver disease, to determine
whether the development of liver disease in this condition may be
due to HLA-linked genetic susceptibility. HLA-B8 was more frequently
detected in patients with liver disease compared with subjects without liver disease (50% and 20.8% respectively: p = 0.054, HLA Workshop control figure 15.7%). Class II (DR) antigen type was obtained
in 26 of the patients and a similar trend was noted. The frequency
of HLA-B8-DR3 being 54.5% in patients with liver disease and 26.7%
in those without (HLA Workshop control figure 7%). Increased
frequencies of HLA-DR2 (50%) and HLA-DR3 alone (54.5%) were also
observed  in children with cystic fibrosis and liver disease (HLA
Workshop control figures 25.1 and 20.4% respectively), but similar
values were obtained in children without liver disease (35.7 and 40%
respectively).

Immune regulation has been shown to be defective in several of
the B8-DR3 associated diseases such as systemic lupus erythematosus,
thyrotoxicosis and autoimmune chronic active  hepatitis. These
preliminary results showing an increased percentage of HLA-B8 and
HLA-B8 B3 in cystic fibrosis subjects with overt liver disease,
should be extended to confirm whether an HLA-associated genetic
factor controlling immune responses to liver antigens may contribute
to the liver damage (overt or latent) found in cystic fibrosis.

REFERENCE:
1.   Arch.Dis.Childh. 55:696, 1980.

**POSTER GROUP ONE No. 1.06**

EXCLUSION MAPPING OF CANDIDATE STRUCTURAL GENES IN CF

Kay E. Davies, Bob Williamson, Conrad Gilliam,
Christine Leeson and Kevin Davies
Department of Biochemistry, St. Mary's Hospital
Medical School, University of London, W2 1PG, England

It is difficult to determine whether a single
cloned gene sequence, or other inherited polymorphic
marker, is linked to a genetic disease unless
(a) large families are available for study or
(b) the marker is very close to the mutation causing
the disease. For an autosomal recessive disease such
as CF, where there is no proven method of carrier
detection, the only informative members in most
families are affected children and their parents.
Therefore, the family resources are in general too
small for positive linkage analysis of the type that
has been so successful in finding a marker for
Huntington's disease (1).

However, even with small families, it is possible
to determine whether any candidate gene sequence
exhibiting a restriction fragment length polymorphism
is mutated to cause CF. This is because the mutation
must track with one or other of the polymorphic
alleles from each parent to each affected child. We
have used DNA from several families in which there
are three affected children to determine whether a
mutation of the serum protein, complement three, is
the basic defect causing CF, as proposed by Conover
et al (2). We were given a cloned gene probe for C3
by George Fey, Scripps Institute, San Diego, and
found a common RFLP which occurs in some of our
families (3). In two families, three affected
children each inherited different RFLPs for C3 from
the parents, demonstrating that C3 is not the basic
defect causing CF (4).

1. Williamson et al., plenary lecture, this Congress.
2. Conover et al., Lancet ii (1973) 1501.
3. Whitehead et al., ProcNatAcadSciUS 79 (1982) 5021.
4. Davies et al., MolBiolMed 1 (1983) 185.

**POSTER GROUP ONE No. 1.07**

MESSENGER RNA'S PRESENT AT HIGH LEVELS IN
LEUKOCYTES:DIFFERENCES ASSOCIATED WITH CYSTIC FIBROSIS.

Mark Blaxter, Julian Crampton, Kay E. Davies and
Bob Williamson
Department of Biochemistry, St. Mary's Hospital
Medical School, University of London, W2 1PG, England

Using recombinant cDNA clone banks we have
isolated cloned sequences, corresponding to messenger -
molecules present at high levels in blood leukocytes,
which show differences in level of expression between
cystic fibrosis (CF) patients and normal individuals.

Messenger RNA was isolated from leukocytes of CF
and normal individuals. From these mRNA samples,
complementary DNA was synthesised, double stranded and
cloned into pAT153 to give two cDNA clone banks of
several thousand different clones each (1). These
clone banks provide a stable and easily accessible copy
of all the messenger RNA species present in the cells.

The clone banks were then screened in duplicate
using either CF or normal leukocyte mRNA as a probe.
The mRNA was radiolabelled and then hybridised to
selections of the clones immobilised on nitrocellulose
sheets. This identifies clones which are highly
expressed or which contain repetitive sequences (2).
Clones which are differentially expressed between the
two probes can also be identified (3). None of the
clones examined showed a qualitative difference in
expression between normal and CF individuals. Several
clones were isolated which showed quantitative
differences, however, and several of these were studied
further. The difference in expression of one of the
sequences was characteristic of the phenotype in 80% of
a small sample of CF patients (4). Other sequences
show less concordance with the CF phenotype, and we
conclude that the differences we are studying are
probably secondary to the basic defect.

1.  Woods et al., (1980) Nucl. Acids Res. 8:5157-5168.
2.  Crampton et al., (1981) Nucl. Acids Res. 9:
    3821-3834.
3.  Crampton et al., (1980) Nucl. Acids Res. 8:
    6007-6017.
4.  Crampton et al., (1984) Biochim. Biophys. Acta.
    in press.

**POSTER GROUP ONE No. 1.08**

THE EFFECT OF SPUTUM SOL FROM CYSTIC FIBROSIS PATIENTS ON HUMAN AND
RABBIT RESPIRATORY TRACT CILIA.

Wayne Griffin, Jonathan Rutland[*] and Peter Cole.
Host Defence Unit, Department of Medicine, Cardiothoracic Institute,
Brompton Hospital, Fulham Road, London, SW3 6HP, England.
* Respiratory Unit, Concord Hospital, Sydney, Australia.

Ciliary dyskinesia factor(s) (CDF) has been demonstrated in serum,
sweat, saliva, sputum and in the supernatant medium from cultured
cells of CF patients (Danes BS. Tex Rep Biol Med. 1976;34:135).  We
have demonstrated no ciliostatic effect of serum from patients with
CF on human nasal and bronchial cilia but have confirmed its ciliostatic effect for rabbit tracheal cilia (Rutland J et al. Am Rev
Respir Dis. 1983;128:1030).  A ciliary dyskinesia factor in the serum
of asthmatic patients has been described by Wilson and Fudenberg
(Nature 1977;266:463) which has some similarity to that of cystic
fibrosis.  Subsequently Dulfano et al (Clin Sci. 1982;63:393) have
reported that some sputum sols obtained from asthmatic patients
induced ciliostasis when applied to the isolated frog palate.
We therefore studied the effect of sputum sols from 10 CF patients
on normal human nasal and rabbit tracheal cilia.  Sputum samples were
centrifuged at 30,000g for 90 mins at $4^{\circ}C$.  The supernatant sols were
removed and stored in liquid nitrogen.  They were added to human
nasal and rabbit tracheal ciliated epithelium, obtained by brushing,
and incubated in sealed microscope slide preparations at $37^{\circ}C$ for 3
hours.  Ciliary beat frequency (CBF) was quantitated during this
period by a photometric technique (Rutland J and Cole PJ.  Lancet
1980;2:564).  Ciliary motility in neat sol and in sol diluted 25%, 50%
and 75% with tissue culture medium 199 was compared with that of cilia
in medium alone.  Similarly, CBF in CF sol to which CF serum had been
added was compared with that in medium alone and CF serum alone.  No
sol-induced ciliostatic effect was observed in normal human and rabbit
respiratory tract cilia.  However, a CF sol:serum mixture in a ratio
of 1:3 caused immediate ciliostasis of rabbit cilia, a ratio of 1:1
caused late cilioinhibition and a ratio of 3:1 caused no ciliostasis.
It is unlikely that this response is due to a simple dilution effect
of CF sol on CF serum because our previous studies showed the cilioinhibition induced by neat CF serum to be unchanged when the serum
was diluted to 25% concentration in medium.
It is possible that CF sputum sols contain substances (eg enzymes)
able to inactivate the CDF(s) responsible for the slowing induced in
rabbit cilia by CF sera.

**POSTER GROUP ONE No. 1.09**

THIRTY-ONE CASES OF CYSTIC FIBROSIS IN AN AMISH-MENNONITE KINDRED: Robert H. Schwartz, M.D. and Richard A. Doherty, M.D., Department of Pediatrics, University of Rochester Medical Center, Rochester, New York, United States 14642.

In 1976 a search was undertaken to find relatives of a male proband with cystic fibrosis (CF) to enlist their participation in future genetic studies of CF. A linkage of any biological aberration to the basic defect in CF must be tested in families to prove its genetic nature.

An Amish-Mennonite family from Alsace-Lorraine, embarked from Le Havre, France and arrived in New York City on June 19, 1833. They were children (5/10) of Christian J.(1766-1828) and Anne F.(1771-1816). Although their final destination was to be "Ohio", this group settled mainly in Ontario, Canada (Waterloo Co.) and Upstate, New York (Lewis Co.) which are separated by more than 300 miles. Because of secularization, 7/19 ascertained families are now located in 5 other states. There are over 10,000 direct descendents of the founding couple. Thirty-one cases of CF (born between 1951 and 1983) in 19 families have been documented (52 non-affected siblings). Consanguinity has been documented in 6/19(32%) matings of parents of CF children. Seven other consanguineous matings are known to have occurred in previous generations. Despite common ancestry, recording of heritage, and CF within each family, several families were unknown to each other.

The recessive hypothesis of CF is supported by the similarity (P>0.7) of observed(31) vs expected(29.6) CF births (method of Apert). CF births have occurred at the rate of 1 per yr. since 1951 and deaths at the rate of 1 per 2 yrs. 13/20 CF males are living (mean age =17.2yrs.;range = 1.5 - 32yrs.). 7 males have died (mean age = 5.6yrs.;range = 1 day - 10.7yrs.). 4/11 CF females are living (mean age = 11.2yrs.; range = 4 mos. - 20.9yrs.). 7females have died (mean age = 5.1yrs.; range = 4mos. - 12yrs.). 5/31 (16%) had meconium ileus at birth(1/5 died). All others presented with failure to thrive due to maldigestion. 7/11 (64%) who lived to or beyond age 15 years have had nasal polyps.

Members of this kindred (113 plus 17 with CF) are participating in research to find a restriction fragment length polymorphism (RFLP) of DNA closely linked to the CF gene. Permanent lymphoblastoid cell lines as a source of genomic DNA have been established for each person. This phase of research is being conducted at Integrated Genetics, Inc., Framingham, Massachusetts.

188

COULD NORMOTENSION PROVIDE THE HETEROZYGOTE ADVANTAGE
IN CYSTIC FIBROSIS?

Authors:  M Super, N Mann, G Hambleton, D. MacGlashan
Cystic Fibrosis Clinic, Royal Manchester Childrens
Hospital, Pendlebury, Manchester M27 1HA.

There have been a number of theories which attempt to
explain the frequency of cystic fibrosis in
Caucasians.   Most of these invoke a heterozygote
advantage though no convincing mechanism of its action
has been discovered.  Reduced infections in earlier
generations in carriers have been invoked but were
this the mechanism one would expect a reducing
incidence of CF nowadays, with most infections under
control.  There is no evidence that the incidence of
CF is falling.
It is estimated that a heterozygote advantage of 2.2%
would explain a CF incidence of 1/2000.   Were the
healthy carriers of CF to suffer less from
hypertension, this could provide an advantage of that
order, with fitness over a longer period of time than
in those prone to hypertension.   Such an advantage
would be operative today and explain how the incidence
of CF remains in equilibrium.  While the incresed
sodium in the sweat of carriers might not be
sufficient to identify them accurately, nevertheless a
number of studies are agreed that such an increase
exists.  This could provide the mechanism for reduced
hypertension in carriers.  A small pilot study among
the parents of children who attend the CF clinic at
RMCH, revealed normal blood pressure in all 80 tested
and a history of high blood pressure in only one of
310 first degree relatives.  These bald figures give
the hope that the heterozygote advantage may work in
this way.   A large study, with comparison of
actuarial tables of blood pressure at various ages
could allow a definitive answer to this hypothesis.
Delegates will be invited to join us in such a study.

**POSTER GROUP ONE No. 1.11**

MOLECULAR POLYMORPHISM AND SERUM RATE OF TRANSFERRIN (Tf) AND VITA_
MIN D BINDING GLOBULINE (GC) IN CYSTIC FIBROSIS (CF).

Antonelli M., Pascali V.L., Bravo E., Stancati M., Bertasi S.
Dept. Pediatrics and Cistic Fibrosis Center. "La Sapienza" University
ROME. Dept. Pediatrics Civil Hospital AREZZO.  ITALY.

Studies dealing with the behaviour of glycoproteins in CF
pointed out differences in serum protein patterns among CF individuals (1), describing a "CF protein". More recent studies have been
devoted to the eletrophoretic pattern and quantitative rate of common plasma glycoproteins (2-3). The molecular polymorphism and serum rate of transferrin (Tf) and vitamin D binding globulin (Gc)
were ascertained in fibrocystic patients, heterozygotes and in a
control group in order to evaluate the extention of the protein
derangement, and search for a possible marker for the detection of
heterozigotes.
Quantitative rate of prealbumin, retinol binding globulin
(RBG) and alpha-glycoprotein were also investigated as a reference
for the evaluation of quantitative data. Neither different allele
distribution nor abnormal electrophoretic pattern was observed in
CF serum. Quantitative data indicated a lower serum rate of Tf,Gc,
prealbumin and RBC, likely due to malnutritional condition in CF.
A non homogeneous behavior was marked off among glycoproteins.

REFERENCES

1) Wilson G.B., Fudenberg H.H.. Pediatr. Res. 9:635  (1975).

2) Bowman B.H., Barnett D.R. and Coppenhaver D. Hum. Hered.
   31:248  (1981).

3) Coppenhaver D. et al.. Hum. Genet. 57:399  (1981).

**POSTER GROUP ONE No. 1.12**

THERMOINACTIVATION OF PLASMA HYDROLASES IN CYSTIC
FIBROSIS PATIENTS AND CARRIERS.

O.Guy-Crotte*,C.Figarella*; C.Galabert°,J.P.Chazalette°;
J.C.Mazière,L.Mora,*INSERM U31, 46 Bd.de la Gaye,13009,
Marseille, °Hop.R.Sabran, Giens, and CHU St.Antoine, 27
rue Chaligny, 75012, Paris, France.

In 1979, HOSLI and VOGT could successfully discriminate
between cystic fibrosis (CF) patients, obligate heterozygotes (parents) and normal controls by the heat inactivation of alpha-mannosidase and acid phosphatase in
plasma. In this test, these enzymes retained full activity (80-100%) in normals, only 40-60% in heterozygotes,
and lose almost all activity in homozygotes from CF (0
to 10%). A very recent double bind study performed on
45 samples of the three genotypes confirmed these findings. However, other authors were not able to reproduce this technique. We thus decided to investigate this
method in our own laboratories.
Plasma were carefully collected as described in the original method on the three genotypes, in Hopital Renée
Sabran (Giens), and CHU Saint-Antoine (Paris). In some
experiments, substrates and buffers were provided by
HOSLI and VOGT, and in others prepared with commercial
reagents (Sigma) and distillated water from our laboratories. In most of the experiments, we found that homozygotes were clearly distinguishable from normal by
thermal inactivation at 48°C during 2 to 4 hours. Heterozygotes were discriminated from normal and homozygotes
by slow inactivation at 43°C in some cases, but clearcut
differences were not obtained in all experiments.
Despite of the difficulties encountered, we think that
the phenomenon initially described by HOSLI and coll.
is undeniable, and that the technique could be possibly
used, with careful adaptations to each laboratory conditions, for reliable diagnosis of CF and carrier screening.

**POSTER GROUP ONE No. 1.13**

PROPOSAL OF A TEST FOR SCREENING CYSTIC FIBROSIS (C.F.)
HETEROZYGOTES

I. Cigui, A. Luchesi, M.A. Mangiarotti, D. Faraguna, A.G. Marchi
Istituto di Puericultura e Cattedra Genetica dell'Università -
Istituto per l'Infanzia di Trieste.

A reliable test for screening cystic fibrosis (C.F.) heterozygotes is still lacking. Previously(1) we demonstrated that lymphocyte $\beta$-glucuronidase response to in vitro phytohaemagglutinin (PHA)
stimulation was reduced by serum of both C.F. homo and heterozygotes.
The complexity of the test, however, limited the application to an
at risk population.
Recently we tried to simplify the test; this goal was achieved
by employing normal subject lymphocytes and a 2 ml sample of proband's serum.
To find out other possible markers, we studied four different
lymphocyte lysosome enzyme activities: $\beta$-glucuronidase, $\alpha$-mannosi-
dase, $\alpha$-glucosidase, $\beta$-glucosidase. In vitro cultures were performed in the presence of serum of 12 c.f. homozygotes or 12 c.f. heterozygotes or 12 controls. Result can be summarized as follows:

1 - lymphocyte $\beta$-glucuronidase and $\alpha$-glucosidase activities showed
significantly reduced response to PHA stimulation when serum of both
c.f. homo and heterozygotes was added to culture medium;

2 - no differences in lymphocyte $\alpha$-mannosidase or $\beta$-glucosidase
activity response were observed;

3 - in culture medium the same values of the four lysosome anzyme
activities, in the presence of c.f. or normal serum, were found.
Therefore an altered exocytosis of in vitro cultured normal lymphocytes can be excluded.

Reference

1 - Marchi A.G., Mangiarotti M.A., Cigui I., Perticarari S., Uxa F.,
    Nordio S. - Beta glucuronidase activity in c.f. 8th Annual
    Meeting EWGCF, Badgastein, 1978

This work was supported by grant: Progetto Finalizzato Inge-
gneria Genetica e Basi Molecolari Malattie Ereditarie obiettivo 15
- Consiglio Nazionale delle Ricerche, 1983

**POSTER GROUP ONE No. 1.14**

INVESTIGATION OF SERUM PROTEINS IN CYSTIC FIBROSIS USING
ISOELECTRIC FOCUSING AND IMMUNOAFFINITY CHROMATOGRAPHY.

Jamieson, A.; Aitken, D.A.; Cooke, A.C.; Yaquoob, M.;
McKinley, Eliz. ; Ferguson-Smith, M.A.
Duncan Guthrie Institute of Medical Genetics,
Yorkhill, Glasgow.
Patients and most carriers of the Cystic Fibrosis allele
have been shown to possess a serum protein rarely detected
in the normal population (Wilson et al,Clin.Chim.Acta. 49,
79). This 'cystic fibrosis protein' (CFP) is identifiable
as extra banding patterns on isoelectric focusing (IEF)
run under stringent conditions. Using the LKB Multiphor
apparatus and pH2.5-10 gel gradients we have consistently
observed a number of different banding patterns in serum
from different affected and heterozygote individuals in
the pH8-9 region of the gel. These range from a single
band to mutiple bands and are in accord with the results
of Hallinan et al (Clin.Chim.Acta.117,103,1981). With
this criterion of positivity we have obtained positive
results in 93% of affected homozygotes (n=29), 66% of
obligate carriers (n=71), and 16% of controls (n=31). Thus
in this form the IEF method cannot be used as a reliable
carrier detection test. The higher than expected frequency of positivity in the control group suggests that CFP
may be a normally occuring serum protein which is present
in increased concentration in carriers and homozygotes of
the CF gene (Hallinan et al,1981). Preliminary results
from our laboratory using·more sensitive gel-staining
techniques following IEF of normal serum samples and γ-
globulin enriched fractions supports this hypothesis. In
addition, using various sample pretreatments prior to IEF
we have found the banding pattern to be relatively stable.
Attempts to develop a quantitative immunoassay (e.g. Bullock et al,Clin.Gen.21,336,1982) have shown the potential
of an anti-CFP antibody in a carrier detection test. However there are severe practical difficulties in maintaining a supply of such antisera. Preparation of monoclonal
antibodies to CFP would surmount many of these difficultie
s. This is the aim of our work. The preparation of a
purified antigen would increase the probability of success
in obtaining such antibodies. Our recent attempts at purification of CFP based on immunoaffinity chromatography
have resulted in enrichment of CFP as demonstrated on IEF.

ISOELECTRIC FOCUSING OF SERUM IN GENETIC COUNSELLING OF
FAMILIES WITH  CYSTIC FIBROSIS.

Authors: Maurice Super, Christine Swindlehurst, Michael
Super    Cystic   Fibrosis   Clinic,   Royal   Manchester
Childrens Hospital Pendlebury M27 1HA England.

The development of a good carrier detection test for
cystic fibrosis (CF) awaits discovery.    Siblings of
children with CF or of their parents frequently seek
genetic advice.    A risk figure based on the carrier
frequency as estimated from the incidence of the disease
is generally given.

We have confirmed the findings of others of a band at
pI 8.5 on isoelectric focusing of the serum of most
subjects with CF and most of their obligate heterozygote
parents. The band is seldom seen in healthy controls.
    Taking account of the prior probability of being a
carrier, based on the disease incidence or its presence
in the family, we combine the isoelectric focusing
results of the family members and their spouses in
providing a risk figure.  The high incidence of carriers
in the child-bearing Caucasian population, 1/22, allows
this less than perfect test to be applied in this way as
a (hopefully) temporary measure, until a definitive test
is discovered.  We have been able to counsell siblings
of CF subjects and their spouses with no CF family
history a risk of having affected children 1/12, 1/55,
1/625 or 1/2777 depending on their test reaction.   With
no test one would have to counsell all such couples a
figure of 1/132.
The Bayesian mathematics is given on the poster and
examples of the gels will be shown.

REFERENCE:   Brock D, Heywood C, Super M.   Controlled
trail of serum isoelectric focusing in the detection of
the cystic fibrosis gene.  Hum.Genet. 1982;60:30-31

**POSTER GROUP ONE No. 1.16**

PROBLEMS ENCOUNTERED IN RAISING MONOCLONAL ANTIBODIES TO CYSTIC
  FIBROSIS ANTIGEN

Veronica van Heyningen, Caroline Hayward*and David Brock*,
MRC Clinical & Population Cytogenetics Unit, and *Human Genetics,
Unit, Edinburgh.

Cystic fibrosis antigen (CFA) is a serum protein recognized by a
guineapig antiserum raised against the material at pI 8.4 when
appropriately collected serum from CF patients is run on urea-IEF
gels.  When the antiserum is used in a rocket immunoelectrophoresis
system, sera from cystics,heterozygotes and normals give high,
intermediate and absent peaks respectively.  Using this rocket
system to track the antigen, several methods of antigen purification
have been tried, including the use of antiserum as an affinity
reagent.

Partial purification of the antigen has been achieved.  Material
obtained in this way has been used to immunize mice which were then
used to produce large numbers of hybridomas in several fusions.
Devising suitable screening systems to detect all likely positive
clones and rejecting those which bind to irrelevant antigens has
been a major problem.  Success is dependent on having some idea of
the nature of the antigen molecule and of how it may relate to the
basic defect in cystic fibrosis.  We trace the evolution of our
ideas to our current position.

**POSTER GROUP ONE No. 1.17**

RESULTS OF SWEAT TESTS IN CHILDREN WITH DECREASED
ACTIVITY OF GAMMA-GLUTAMYL-TRANSPEPTIDASE ( GMT )
IN AMNIOTIC FLUID

H. Tomášová, M. Macek, V. Vávrová, I. Hrycejová, J Bur-
janková, V. Fuchs, Z. Hájek, E. Čech and J. Král

Research Institute for Child Development, Faculty of
Pediatrics, V úvalu 84, 150 06 Prague 5-Motol, Czecho-
slovakia.

Carbans et al ( 1983 ) indicated possible relationship between decreased activity of GMT in amniotic fluid
and the development of the foetus affected by cystic
fibrosis. Therefore we have performed sweat tests and
we report their results in all children delivered after
amniocentesis from the genetic indications where the
decreased values of GMT were discovered in the second
trimester of the pregnancy. The samples under investigation cover only pregnancies with normal results of prenatal genetic examinations, with normal development of
the pregnancy, birth weight higher than 2 000g and without risk to be carriers of hemophilia A, B, Duchenne
myopathy or metabolic diseases investigated prenatally.

The decreased values were selected on the basis of
normal variation of GMT in amniotic fluid in the range
of 16 - 24 weeks of pregnancy. That was ascertained by
our investigation of 455 samples of amniotic fluids from
pregnancies where the normal prenatal genetic findings,
normal development of the pregnancy were confirmed by
the delivery of a normal baby without any clinically
detectable anomaly.

196

MORPHOLOGICAL AND PHYSIOLOGICAL STUDIES OF THE HUMAN FETAL EXOCRINE PANCREAS AT MID-GESTATION

R.C. Pocknee[1], S.W.B. Ewen[2], D.R. Abramovich[3], H.D.A. Gray[2] and F. Fullerton[1].

Departments of Chemical Pathology[1], Pathology[2] and Obstetrics and Gynaecology[3], Foresterhill, Aberdeen, Scotland.

Following our original observation that amniotic-fluid obtained during mid-gestation contains significant concentrations of immuno-reactive trypsin (IRT), we have undertaken a study to investigate both the ultrastructure and the physiological behaviour in vitro of the human fetal exocrine pancreas in order to ascertain the functional capabilities of this organ in early and mid-gestation. Pancreases were dissected from normal fetuses within ten minutes of delivery (induced by extra amniotic prostaglandins). For histological examin-ation fragments of the pancreas were fixed in 10% neutral buffered formalin and embedded in wax. Sections were examined by light micro-scopy using an indirect immunoperoxidase technique utilising a primary antiserum raised in rabbits against purified human cationic trypsin. For studies in vitro, whole pancreases were placed immediately into cold buffer, but into small segments and transferred to an incubation cell pumped continuously with buffer at 37°C at 1 ml/min. Pancreatic function was assessed by monitoring continuously the amylase activity of the cell effluent by an automated fluorimetric method. The con-centration of IRT was also measured in 3 ml aliquots by radioimmuno-assay using the antiserum described earlier. Positive staining for IRT was present in all 17 pancreases investigated from 12 weeks gest-ation, but an 8 week old embryo pancreas was negative. At 12 weeks IRT is faintly detectable in the epithelial cells of the proliferating duct system, and by 14 weeks small clumps of acinar cells are present at the distal ends of the tubules, most of which stain strongly for IRT to a varying intensity. Acini of older·specimens all contain cells staining for IRT to a varying intensity. Studies on 4 fetuses (15-18 weeks) utilising acetylcholine and CCK as pancreatic stimu-lants failed to demonstrate any amylase production by the fetal pan-creas, although adult mouse pancreas showed typical increased enzyme production. However, a significant increase in the concentration of IRT over basal levels was observed in response to both acetylcholine and CCK in those fetuses studied to date. Further investigations are continuing utilising other secretagogues and inhibitors of pancreatic function. These observations are further evidence that the exocrine pancreas of the human fetus at mid-gestation is funct-ional in utero. At what stage therefore is fetal pancreatic function affected in CF and could the measurement of IRT in blood be used to diagnose CF in the fetus as in the neonate?

**POSTER GROUP ONE No. 1.19**

INHIBITION OF RABBIT TRACHEAL CILIARY MOTILITY BY HUMAN SERUM.   A
POSSIBLE METHOD FOR DETECTING CYSTIC FIBROSIS CARRIERS.

Wayne Griffin, Jonathan Rutland* and Peter Cole.
Host Defence Unit, Department of Medicine, Cardiothoracic Institute,
Brompton Hospital, Fulham Road, London, SW3 6HP, England.
* Respiratory Unit, Concord Hospital, Sydney, Australia.

In 1967 Spock et al (Pediatr Res. 1967;1:173) showed that the serum
of cystic fibrosis (CF) patients and their parents (CF heterozygote
carriers, CFHC) contained a ciliary dyskinesia factor (CDF) which
resulted in disco-ordination and slowing of ciliary motility in rabbit
tracheal explants.  Cystic fibrosis serum-induced disturbances of
ciliary function have since been demonstrated in a variety of animal
species.  In previous studies we found no effect of CF sera on human
nasal and tracheal ciliated epithelium in vitro (Rutland et al. Amer
Rev Respir Dis. 1983;128:1030) but we confirmed Spock's observations
in the rabbit by using a quantitative photometric method for measurement of ciliary beat frequency (CBF).  More recently, we have found no
effect of CFHC serum on human nasal and tracheal cilia.
   We have now studied the in vitro effect at $37^{\circ}$C of sera from CF,
CFHC, apparently healthy and disease controls on fresh rabbit tracheal
cilia obtained using a brushing technique (Rutland J and Cole PJ.
Lancet 1980;2:564).  In a blind study, conducted using coded and randomised sera, the mean CBF, expressed as a % of control beat frequency,
of rabbit tracheal cilia was slower when incubated for 60 mins with
41 CF (14±5%) and 51 known CFHC (42±6%) sera than with 129 normal
control sera (92±1%) (p<0.001).  All CF and CFHC sera were ciliostatic.  Mean time to ciliostasis was less in homozygote (48±6 min SEM)
than heterozygote (98±10 min SEM) sera (p<0.001).  However, ciliostasis was also induced by sera from 8/8 patients with sarcoidosis and
6/6 with acute severe asthma.  Sera from 2/20 bronchiectatics (one
with chronic Pseudomonas carriage, the other with panhypogammaglobu-
linaemia) and 9/129 apparently healthy subjects were ciliostatic.  No
sera from chronic bronchitics (20), chronic asthmatics (13) and patients with recurrent respiratory infections (11) were ciliostatic.
   The ciliostatic property of sera from patients with sarcoidosis and
acute asthma is being further investigated but it is possible that the
9 sera from apparently healthy controls which caused ciliostasis were
from CFHC.  These 9 ciliostatic sera in a population of 129 apparently
healthy controls would give a gene carrier frequency of 1:14 compared
to the estimated frequency in the normal population of 1:20 (Wood et
al, Amer Rev Respir Dis. 1976;113:833).
   The usefulness of this method as a screening test for cystic
fibrosis carriers will depend on the results of a larger blind study
in progress using sera from a larger normal population and from a
larger variety of gastrointestinal and respiratory disease controls.

**POSTER GROUP ONE No. 1.20**

AMNIOTIC FLUID MICROVILLAR ENZYME ANALYSIS AND THE
PRENATAL DIAGNOSIS OF CYSTIC FIBROSIS

D.A. AITKEN, M. YAQOOB AND M.A. FERGUSON-SMITH
DUNCAN GUTHRIE INSTITUTE OF MEDICAL GENETICS, YORKHILL,
GLASGOW G3 8SJ

Carbarns & colleagues (Lancet I,p329,1983) first reported
reduced activity of two microvillar enzymes ɣ glutamyl
transpeptidase (GGT) and amniopeptidase M(APM) in amniotic
fluid(AF) from pregnancies with cystic fibrosis(CF). These
findings have been confirmed (Baker & Dann,Lancet I,p
716,1983) and similar results obtained for a group of disaccharidases (Van Diggelen et.al.Lancet I,p817,1983) suggesting that the secretion of the fetal component of these
enzymes into the AF is somehow affected in pregnancies
with CF. Brock has further proposed (Lancet 2,p941,1983)
that the analysis of alkaline phosphatase (ALP) isoenzymes
may offer a more sensitive and specific prenatal diagnostic test, since the intestinal component of AF ALP activity
is almost exclusively fetal in origin. We have attempted
to confirm these findings by measuring GGT and ALP in a
series of AF samples from pregnancies with a I in 4 risk
of CF. GGT activity was assayed kinetically at 30°c in
20 µl aliquots of AF using a commercial spectrophotometric
assay kit (Sigma). ALP isoenzyme activities were determined in 2 µl aliquots of AF using a fluorescence assay with
4-methylumbelliferyl phosphate as substrate and L-homoarginine and L-phenylalanine as differential inhibitors of
ALP isoenzyme activity. 19 pregnancies were investigated
retrospectively. 11 resulted in the birth of an unaffected child and gave normal AF enzyme results. 7 pregnancies
resulted in the birth of a child with CF. AF from two of
these pregnancies had normal enzyme activities and five
had clearly abnormal enzyme results. The diagnosis in one
other case with normal enzyme results remains uncertain.
To date 12 pregnancies have been monitored prospectively.
One pregnancy which had low GGT but normal ALP activities
was found to have trisomy 18 on termination. One other
pregnancy gave abnormal ALP isoenzyme ratios but normal
GGT activity. This pregnancy and the remaining 10 (all
with normal enzyme results) are continuing. The outcome
of these pregnancies will be presented and the prospects
for reliable prenatal diagnosis of CF discussed.

**POSTER GROUP ONE No. 1.21**

---

ACTIVITY LEVELS AND THERMOLABILITIES OF LYSOSOMAL HYDROLYTIC ENZYMES ARE NOT ABNORMAL IN PLASMA AND SUBMANDIBULAR SALIVA OF CYSTIC FIBROSIS PATIENTS. L. Oglesbee, T.W. Seale, J.S. Mayes, S. Young, M. Flux, and O.M. Rennert. Departments of Biochemistry and Pediatrics, University of Oklahoma Health Sciences Center, P.O. Box 26901, Oklahoma City, OK, U.S.A. 73190.

The biochemical basis of cystic fibrosis (CF) is unknown. Currently no well accepted chemical markers are available for prenatal diagnosis or heterozygote detection. Hosli, et al. have proposed that CF arises from a subtle form of lysosomal storage disease in which lysosomal enzymes are qualitatively altered and improperly compartmentalized in lysosomes. A post-translational processing defect in the glycosylation of these enzymes is proposed to result in increased thermolability of these glycoprotein enzymes in CF compared to normal. Hosli, et al. have advocated the use of thermostability determinations of plasma acid phosphatase and α-mannosidase as reliable markers for detection of CF individuals and for the discrimination of heterozygous carriers from homozygous normal individuals. However, this assertion has remained controversial because conflicting results have been reported by several investigators. The goal of the research we present here was to investigate further the value of glycolytic enzymes as useful markers for CF detection. We determined total and specific activity levels and thermostability properties of α-mannosidase and acid phosphatase in plasma samples from 25 CF patients (with a variety of clinical scores) and compared these to 25 age and sex-matched normal controls. The mean total activity of α-mannosidase was $3.2 \pm 1.0$ mU/ml in CF plasma with a corresponding control value in normal plasma of $2.8 \pm 0.7$ mU/ml; acid phosphatase was $6.5 \pm 2.7$ mU/ml in CF plasma with a control value of $7.6 \pm 3.4$ mU/ml. The % total activity remaining after 4 hrs. of heat inactivation was $78.5 \pm 10.9$ for CF plasma with a control value of $80.3 \pm 8.8$; acid phosphatase was $61.0 \pm 18.5$ for CF plasma with a control value of $65.0 \pm 12.5$. There was no significant statistical difference between the values for CF and normal controls for either enzyme. We also investigated the activity level of these and four other lysosomal enzymes in saliva isolated from the submandibular gland, an exocrine gland affected in CF. The total enzyme activity for CF vs normal controls reported in mU/ml were: α-galactosidase ($0.51 \pm 0.3$ vs $0.50 \pm 0.5$), β-galactosidase ($0.05 \pm 0.2$ vs $0.11 \pm 0.2$), α-glucosidase ($0.16 \pm 0.1$ vs $0.09 \pm 0.02$), α-L-fucosidase ($1.29 \pm 0.9$ vs $0.87 \pm 0.6$), α-mannosidase ($0.20 \pm 0.1$ vs $0.19 \pm 0.2$), and acid phosphatase ($4.36 \pm 2.1$ vs $3.32 \pm 1.2$). No differences in activity per ml or specific activity were observed for five of the above enzymes and no significant differences in thermostability were observed for α-mannosidase and acid phosphatase in saliva from CF patients and normal controls. The activity per ml for α-glucosidase was increased twofold in CF plasma; however, the specific activity was not different from controls. We conclude that there is no significant increase which occurs in either lysosomal hydrolytic enzyme activities or altered thermostabilities which characterize CF and that these enzymes are not useful as diagnostic markers for this disease.

**POSTER GROUP ONE No. 1.22**

ULTRASTRUCTURAL AND BIOCHEMICAL ANALYSIS OF DISACCHARIDASES
IN CYSTIC FIBROSIS AND CONTROL ILEUM

H. Sips, J.M. van Dongen, A.T. Hoogeveen, A. Claass, M.
Sinaasappel[*], H.-P. Hauri[**] and H. Galjaard

Department of Cell Biology, Erasmus University Rotterdam,
P.O. Box 1738, 3000 DR Rotterdam, the Netherlands
[*] Department of Pediatrics, Subdivision Gastroenterology,
Erasmus University and University Hospital Rotterdam/
Sophia Children's Hospital, the Netherlands
[**] Department of Pharmacology, Biocentre University Basel,
Klingelbergstrasse 70, CH-4056 Basel, Switzerland

Recently it has been demonstrated in our laboratory
that the activities of four intestinal disaccharidases are
markedly decreased in the amniotic fluid from pregnancies
resulting in children affected with cystic fibrosis.
An explanation for this observation could be an abnormality in the ultrastructural localization affecting the
activities of these enzymes in cystic fibrosis. In order
to test this hypothesis we investigated the localization
and activity of sucrase in both cystic fibrosis and control
ileum.
Ultrathin cryosections of ileum were first incubated
with monoclonal antibodies against human sucrase-iso-
maltase, subsequently with a Protein A-colloidal gold
complex and analyzed by electron microscopy. In cystic
fibrosis and control ileum a similar localization in the
brush border membrane was observed; no significant differences in the amount of immunoreactive material was detectable.
Biochemical analysis of the sucrase activity in cystic
fibrosis and control ileum shows a similarity with respect
to the $K_m$-values (10 mM), pH-optimum (5.9) and heat-
stability. Moreover, the enzyme from cystic fibrosis and
control ileum precipitated in the same way with monoclonal
antibodies.
We conclude that the decreased disaccharidase activities in the amniotic fluid from pregnancies with cystic
fibrosis fetuses cannot be explained by an abnormal sub-
cellular localization of these enzymes.

**POSTER GROUP ONE No. 1.23**

Prenatal diagnosis of cystic fibrosis based on the values of intestinal enzymes in the amniotic fluid.    A follow-up study.

Muller F., Cezard J.P., Gasser B., Berg S., Frot J.C., Boué J.,
Philippe E., Boué A.

Unité de Recherches de Biologie Prénatale INSERM U.73, Château de Longchamp, 75016 Paris; Laboratoire de Biochimie, Hôpital Ambroise Paré, 92100 Boulogne; Service de Gastro-entérologie Pédiatrique (Pr. Navarro), Hôpital Bretonneau, 75018 Paris; Institut d'Anatomo-Pathologie, 67006 Strasbourg.

An approach to the prenatal diagnosis of cystic fibrosis has been proposed by assays of intestinal enzymes in the amniotic fluid in order to detect abnormality in microvillar membrane surfaces ( D. Brock; Van Diggelen et al.)

In this study we selected several enzymes : gamma-glutamyl transpeptidase, alkaline phosphatase isoenzymes, sucrase, maltase and leucine amino peptidase.

The technique for determination of alkaline phosphatase isoenzymes has been improved and the dispersion of the normal values of alkaline phosphatase residual activities has been reduced thus allowing a better separation of abnormal values.

The normal values of these enzymes, their kinetics in relation to gestational age, their correlations have been determined on several hundred amniotic fluids from pregnancies with a normal outcome after prenatal diagnosis for maternal age indications.

Some stored amniotic fluids from pregnancies at risk of cystic fibrosis in which the outcome was known were tested first.

Then, these assays have been used prospectively in at risk pregnancies. 18 prenatal diagnosis have been performed (January 25). A trisomy 13 was detected in one fetus. Four CF affected fetuses were diagnosed. Among these pregnancies two are in progress. The parents elected for the termination of the pregnancy in´ two cases, and the diagnosis of cystic fibrosis was confirmed on abortus material.

The follow-up study of these pregnancies and the pathological findings will be presented.

202

AFFINITY CHROMATOGRAPHY ON CON A-SEPHAROSE OF PEPTIDASE ENZYMES IN
AMNIOTIC FLUID AND SERUM: IMPLICATION FOR THE PRENATAL DIAGNOSIS OF
CYSTIC FIBROSIS.

J.R. Green, M.J. Lentze & D. Sidiropoulos*

Kinderklinik-Inselspital & Frauenklinik*, Universität Bern,
CH-3010 Bern, Switzerland.

It has recently been suggested that peptidase activity in amniotic
fluid might be decreased in pregnancies affected by cystic fibrosis
(CF) and could thus offer an opportunity for the prenatal diagnosis
of this disease (1). As preliminary results indicated an overlap in
the range of activities exhibited by affected and non-affected pregnancies, it was proposed that discrimination might be improved by
assaying specific isoenzymes.

In order to obtain information on the number and origin of the peptidase isoenzymes present in amniotic fluid, we have fractionated
samples of amniotic fluid, maternal serum, infant's serum and normal adult serum by affinity chromatography on a column of Con A-Sepharose eluted with 0.2 M methyl-a-D-mannopyranoside. One sample
of amniotic fluid came from a confirmed CF pregnancy. The column
eluates were assayed fluorimetrically for 4 known peptidase enzymes:
gamma-glutamyltranspeptidase (GGT), microsomal aminopeptidase (AMP),
aspartate aminopeptidase (APM) and dipeptidyl peptidase IV (DAP IV).

Overall, it was possible to detect 3 peaks of mixed peptidase activity; a major peak (I) of unretarded activity eluted in the column
void volume, a minor peak (II) of weakly bound activity appeared as
soon as the eluting mannopyranoside buffer was applied, and finally
a large peak (III) of strongly bound peptidase activity came off
after a further 2 column volumes of this buffer. In serum samples
from normal adults and pregnant mothers at term, peaks I and II were
very low relative to a large peak III. A similar pattern was observed with a serum sample from a premature infant. By contrast, in amniotic fluid at mid-term or during the last trimester, peak I predo-
minated and peaks II and III were smaller. There was no obvious
qualitative difference between the peptidase elution profile of the
CF amniotic fluid and that of a normal fluid of comparable gestational age. These results suggest that the large peak of unbound peptidase activity in amniotic fluid is not of maternal origin and thus
it could be relevant for the prenatal diagnosis of CF and other congenital disorders.

Ref. 1: Carbarns NJB, Gosden C & Brock DJH (1983) Lancet 329-331.

**POSTER GROUP ONE No. 1.25**

INTERPRETATION OF THE SWEAT TEST IN THE DIAGNOSIS OF
CYSTIC FIBROSIS

Harry Shwachman, M. D. and Abbas Mahmoodian, PhD.

Children's Hospital Medical Center
300 Longwood Avenue, Boston, Ma. 02215, USA

This study concerns the evaluation of patients
referred to our CF clinic for diagnosis, specifically for
the sweat test, performed in 30,000 patients over the
past 30 years. The sweat test is the most reliable
diagnostic test today. In our laboratory the quantitative
pilocarpine iontophoresis sweat test has a sensitivity of
98%, a specificity of 83%, and a predictive value of 99.5%.
The age of patients ranged from newborns to adults.
The diagnosis of CF is a clinical one, based on signs and
symptoms, family history, chest X-ray findings, and PFT's
confirmed by a positive sweat test, performed by the
standard QPIT method of Gibson and Cooke. The sweat test
is positive if either or both of the Na and Cl concentrations is above 70 m.e./l, negative if the values are below
45 m.e./l, and borderline if between 45 and 70. The
accuracy of the sweat test is critical to this study.
We have no difficulty with patients who have either a
positive or a negative sweat test, if this result is
consistent with the clinical situation. We have difficulty
in making a decision when the results are in the borderline zone.
This report deals with 100 patients with borderline
results from a series of 30,000 referred to our clinic to
determine whether they had CF. In addition to sweat tests
these patients were studied clinically. Repeat tests were
usually performed in duplicate by the same person on
subsequent visits. On follow-up, 75 patients did not have
CF. Many had allergies or asthma, or miscellaneous conditions including growth failure, the cilia dyskinesia
syndrome, neonatal intestinal obstruction, and azospermia
in adult males. Seventeen patients were diagnosed as
having CF, and are still under treatment. Eight have
succumbed. Six patients were lost to follow-up.
Less than 2% of patients with CF have borderline
sweat tests when first seen. Repeat tests and follow-up
studies are essential. This study points to the need of
a specific test for CF.

**POSTER GROUP ONE No. 1.26**

A NEW SIMPLIFIED METHOD OF SWEAT COLLECTION FOR DIAGNOSIS OF CYSTIC FIBROSIS

Wayne K. Barlow, H. Lewis Webster, Ph.D.
Wescor, Inc, 459 South Main Street, Logan, UT 84321 USA

The sweat test for laboratory diagnosis of cystic fibrosis involves three consecutive procedures: (1) sweat stimulation, (2) sweat collection, and (3) sweat analysis. The test has been requested and performed with ever increasing frequency during the past twenty-five years, but has been accompanied by a high and clinically unacceptable frequency of false results, particularly false-positive, within hospital laboratories generally. Until recently, only central referral laboratories possessing the skills born of specialization and experience were likely to turn out consistently accurate sweat test results. Virtually all of these employ the pad absorption method of Gibson and Cooke as first reported in 1959. Laboratories that infrequently perform the test have difficulty with the method because it is tedious and involves many steps at which human error can intervene.

Several innovative methods, including some that were based upon cup collection, were introduced during the 1960's and early 70's. These were intended to simplify the procedures of the sweat test so that it could be reliably performed with less demand upon the technical skill of the operator. However, in practice all of the "simplified" methods exacerbated rather than mitigated the problem of false results. The scientific literature of recent years has been rife with pungent criticism of such methods and the lengthy method of Gibson and Cooke is still regarded by many clinical and laboratory professionals as the only procedure worthy of their official endorsement.

In the latter 1970's, scientific investigation supported by clinical studies identified and quantified the major intrinsic error that had confounded the cup collection methods. This led to the development of the first simplified sweat collection system capable of delivering a truly error-free sample of sweat. It used a heated metal collection cup to abolish condensate error. This system was demanding of operator skill and experience at only one critical point where the collected sweat was to be "harvested" for analysis.

The system for sweat collection that is described here, like the heated cup system, delivers an error-free sample for analysis, but all of the procedural steps have been greatly simplified so that no special skill or experience is required of the operator. The principal innovation in this system is a small disposable collection device that automatically "harvests" the sweat into a flexible plastic microbore tube. It is the first collection system to provide visual quantification of the collected sweat volume during the entire collection period.

**POSTER GROUP ONE No. 1.27**

A NEW RELIABLE SWEAT TEST

Hans Kollberg and Kristoffer Hellsing
Department of Pediatrics, University of Kuwait, Kuwait
and Department of Clinical Chemistry, University
Hospital Uppsala, Sweden.

A clinical study has been performed to compare a new
sweat test device (Medtronic Model 10098 sweat
stimulation system and 10133 chloride concentration
test patch) with the classical Gibson-Cooke sweat test.
The stimulation system consists of a miniature
iontophoretic generator preformulated positive
(pilocarpine) and negative (potassium sulfate) polymer
electrodes. The test patch, which is attached directly
to the site of pilocarpine iontophoresis, consists of a
central part with chloride-absorbing material, a
peripheral ring with silver chromate and a capillary
tab to indicate when about 50 mg of sweat has been
collected. According to the manufacturer no break in
the perimeter boundary between the central (white)
region and the peripheral (brown) ring indicates
$[Cl^-]<40$ meq/l; a partial break $[Cl^-]$ 40-60 meq/l; and
a complete break of the boundary $[Cl^-]$.60 meq/l.

We have studied the device in 30 individuals (17 CF
patients and 13 controls) and found it highly reliable
and accurate. All CF patients had completely broken
perimeters; no controls have touched the perimeter.
The area which indicates chloride absorbtion has mostly
been three times larger (always at least twice as
large) in CF patients as in controls. The correlation
between the absorbtion area (Medtronic) and the
chloride concentration (Gibson-Cooke) is very good. In
three subjects sweat collection·had to be repeated due
to insufficient amounts of sweat. The Medtronic method
gives a slight erythema but no oedema or burns; it was
preferred over the Gibson-Cooke method by most of our
subjects.

We intend to investigate 50 subjects (25 CF and 25
controls). The poster will present the method in
detail and give hints on how to avoid pitfalls when
using the device. The device is easy to handle and can
be used for screening in doctor's offices or small
clinics.

**POSTER GROUP ONE No. 1.28**

## SWEAT TESTING OF INFANTS AND YOUNG CHILDREN
## USING A 30 MICROLITER PAPER PATCH

Warren J. Warwick, University of Minnesota, Minneapolis, MN,
Nancy N. Huang, Temple University, Philadelphia, PA, William W.
Waring, Tulane University, New Orleans, LA, Rita M. Hirsch, Gary
A. Lattin, Paul D. Sorenson, Medtronic, Inc., Minneapolis, MN USA

Previous studies[1,2] of the CF Indicator™ sweat test–CFIS* (a
simple, rapid, laboratory-independent sweat test, which uses a
miniature sweat stimulator and an in-situ sweat collection and
chloride analysis patch) demonstrated that the CFIS could
discriminate CF from non-CF subjects as efficiently as the
Gibson-Cooke Sweat Test (GCST). However, a relatively high
incidence (25%) of failure to collect enough sweat occurred in
children under 6 years of age. This report deals with the
substantial decrease of insufficient sweat collection in children
of that age group. The decrease was achieved by reducing the
volume of sweat needed for analysis from 50 to 30 microliters and
by improving CFIS quality control. Despite the smaller amount of
sweat collected, the CFIS results continue to compare favorably
with the GCST. One hundred twenty-eight sweat tests were done on
101 subjects with the 30 microliter patch. One hundred one of
the 103 tests done on children 3 months to 6 years of age and 18
of 25 tests done on children age 3 days to 3 months yielded
sufficient sweat. When comparing results, the CFIS showed
complete agreement with the analogous GCST, i.e., Level 0 = $\leq$40
mm/l; Level 1 = >40 to 60 mm/l; Level 2 = >60 mm/l. Two CFIS
tests gave positive readings with GCST results of 44 and 49 mm/l.
The distributions for the 101 subjects were:

|           | NORMAL | 40-60 | CF | QTY INSUFFICIENT |
|-----------|--------|-------|----|------------------|
| Diagnosis | 77     | 2     | 22 |                  |
| CFIS      | 72     | 1     | 22 | 6                |
| GCST      | 76     | 2     | 21 | 2                |

This further work with the CFIS suggests that the experimental 30
microliter patch will yield 98% sufficient sweat quantities in
subjects 12 weeks of age and older, 72% sufficient sweat
quantities in younger subjects and CFIS chloride analyses will be
as reliable as the GCST results.

[1]Warwick, W.J., Yeung, W., Huang, N., DuHon, G., Waring, W.,
Cherian, A.G., Strominger, D., Evaluation of a New CF Sweat Test
Screening System; A Cooperative Study. 12th Annual Meeting of
the European Working Group for Cystic Fibrosis (EWGCF)
[2]Warwick, W.J., Brown, I., Lattin, G., Hirsch, R. and Spevak, R.
Ambulatory Sweat Stimulation Device. Europ. J. Pediatrics 1981,
137:116.
*Medtronic, Inc., Minneapolis, MN USA

**POSTER GROUP ONE No. 1.29a**

AGE RELATED IRT BLOOD LEVELS AND INCIDENCE OF TRYPSIN BINDING
IgG IN CF AND NORMAL CHILDREN.

G. TRAVERT, D. LAROCHE, J.F. DUHAMEL, C. BLANDIN.
C.H.U. de CAEN - 14040 CAEN - FRANCE.

Two tier screening for CF using IRT assay is now becoming a widespread procedure, the daily practice of which needs an accurate knowledge of the time related evolution in IRT blood levels, in CF and non
CF children with neonatal transient hypertrypsinemia (NHT)
    In addition, trypsin binding immunoglobulins (TBIgG) are found
with a high incidence in sera from patients with CF, and are likely to
give rise to misleading IRT levels and thus be very critical, especial
ly during the neonatal period when the IRT test is used for a diagnostic purpose.
    The aim of this study was to assess the time related evolution in
IRT levels and TBIgG incidence in CF and non CF children within each
of the following periods of life : (I) from birth to 6 weeks, (II) 6
weeks to 6 months, (III) 6 months to 3 years, (IV) 3 to 17 years.
    RESULTS
    (I) - As shown in table, IRT levels in CF remain high and fairly
constant, while they slowly decrease in NHT.

| weeks of life | 1st | 2nd | 3rd | 4th | 5th | 6th |
|---|---|---|---|---|---|---|
| CF (n = 37)[*] | No significant variation range : 900 - 3500 $\mu$g/l | | | | range : 700-2500 $\mu$g/l | |
| NHT (n = 438) | x $\mu$g/l = 1120 (x+3 $\sigma$ = 1820) | 400 (1000) | 285 (765) | 260 (700) | 245 (635) | 220 (550) |

[*] CF children with meconium ileus and one CF with persistent normal
levels are not included in these data.
    None of CF and NHT newborns had TBIgGs, which, interestingly,
were found in 5 % of 1000 randomly selected neonates.
    (II) - Blood IRT slowly decreases in CF children (n = 33) ; in
most cases, levels remain above the normal range (0 - 500 $\mu$g/l) -
TBIgG is found in 6 % of 52 age matched controls, but not in CFs.
    (III) - In 13 of 35 CF children IRT falls down to undetectable ; a
sharp decrease is observed in all cases and associated with TBIgG in
16 (46 %), while in normal children (n = 42) TBIgG's incidence is 12 %
    (IV) - IRT levels are (or become) undetectable in 32 out of 48 CF
children and TBIgG is found in 34 (71 %), compared to 18 % in 45 age
matched controls.

**POSTER GROUP ONE No. 1.29b**

SPECIAL FEATURES OF THE TIME RELATED EVOLUTION IN IRT BLOOD LEVELS, IN SIX OUT OF SEVEN NEWBORNS WITH CYSTIC FIBROSIS COMPLICATED BY MECONIUM ILEUS.

J.F. DUHAMEL, G. TRAVERT, P. DELMAS, J. BROUARD, R. VENEZIA : C.H.U. de CAEN - 14040 CAEN - FRANCE.

For four years now, neonatal screening for CF has been systematically performed in 80500 babies born in Basse-Normandie, using IRT assay in dried blood specimens collected between 4 and 6 days of life.

During this period, among 29 CF children who were early diagnosed, seven had meconium ileus (MI) at birth. In six out of these seven children, Day 5 IRT levels were normal (range : 160 - 750 µg/l) ; and only one CF child had both MI and D5 hypertrypsinemia (> 900 µg/l)

A detailed study of the time related evolution in IRT, from birth to four weeks of age, clearly showed a different profile for 6 out of 7 CFs with MI as compared to other CF children :
- when measured on the $1^{st}$ or $2^{nd}$ day of life IRT levels were found abnormally high (> 1000 µg/l) within the MI group.

- Following management of the functional or organic occlusion, IRT decreased under 500 µg/l within a few hours.

- Then, levels slowly increased again over 1000 µg/l in 3 cases, while they remained "normal" for the other ones.

- In the same time, in all (but one) CF children without MI, IRT levels remained high and fairly constant.

This study helps understanding how and why CF newborns with MI are potentially false negatives in IRT screening. However the results show that trypsin levels are always high at birth and thus prompt us to measure IRT before medical or surgical management in every case of neonatal occlusion.

Understanding of these results could be clarified by further studies of IRT levels and IRT molecular forms in normal and CF meconium samples, as well as daily variations of blood IRT in all neonates with occlusion.

**POSTER GROUP ONE No. 1.29c**

NEONATAL SCREENING FOR CF USING IRT ASSAY IN DRIED BLOOD SPOTS :
A FOUR YEARS' EXPERIENCE IN BASSE-NORMANDIE.

G. TRAVERT, J.F. DUHAMEL
C.H.U. de CAEN - 14040 CAEN - FRANCE

Neonatal screening for cystic fibrosis in Basse-Normandie started on February 1980, and it is now an essential part of a region
wide CF program including follow-up and treatment of the early diagnosed patients, clinical and biological research.

From the beginning of our experience to December 1983, 80500
five day old babies have been screened. The upper limit of normal
range (cut-off) for blood IRT level was  set at 900 µg/l and this
choice resulted in a 0.33 % positive rate ; so during this study, 267
tests were considered positive. In these cases a second heel prick
blood sample was requested in order to appreciate the evolution of
IRT level during  the first weeks of life. Only those children with
persistently elevated IRT were sweat tested.

During this study, CF was confirmed in 29 by positive sweat tests
With respect to their Day 5 IRT levels, these CF children can be divided into three groups : a) 22 babies had hypertrypsinemia and thus
were detected by screening ; b) 6 had normal IRT levels and all of
them were born with a meconium ileus ; c) one CF newborn had normal
IRT (200 µg/l) on the 5th day as well as later in life.

According to these results, the incidence of cystic fibrosis in
Basse-Normandie is 1/2770.

**POSTER GROUP ONE No. 1.30a**

BLOOD TRYPSIN IN PRETERM BABIES

R. Dinwiddie,[1] D. Padelis,[3] J. Davey,[2] P. Quartey-Papafio,[2] M. Hjelm,[2]

Departments of Respiratory Medicine[1] and Clinical Biochemistry[2] The Institute of Child Health/The Hospitals for Sick Children/ Queen Charlottes Maternity Hospital, 3)   LONDON

Trypsin in blood (Plasma) was assayed in preterm babies (n=63) with a radioimmunological method. The gestational ages of the babies at birth ranged from 25 to 34 weeks, birth weights from 530 - 2440 g. Blood specimens were collected at intervals for a period varying between 3 to 10 weeks. The result indicates that the intra-individual trypsin level remains fairly constant throughout the observation period and that the reference interval for the period is the same as for full term babies after the first days of life 5 - 20 µg/l. Blood trypsin in preterm babies with the lowest gestational age was marginally higher than in babies with the highest age (mean values 13.0 and 11.5µg/l, respectively). The enzyme level was the same in surviving and non-surviving babies. Thus it is concluded that blood trypsin could be used as a screening parameter for CF also in preterm babies though this suggestion needs positive confirmation.

PLASMA PROTEINS IN CYSTIC FIBROSIS

M. Hjelm,[1] J. Davey,[1] R. Dinwiddie,[2] P. Quartey-Papafio[1]

Departments of Clinical Biochemistry[1] and Respiratory Medicine[2]
The Institute of Child Health/The Hospitals for Sick Children
LONDON WC1N

Patients with established CF, based on several pathological
sweat tests and varying in age from neonates to 18 years, were
selected for the study (n=73). Plasma proteins were examined
qualitatively by agarose electrophoresis and quantitatively by
immunoelectrophoresis and the results related to the age of the
patients.

Plasma protein electrophoresis, did in general, indicate an acute
phase response as evidenced by a decreased albumin band and increased alpha-1 and alpha-2 globulin fractions. The gammaglobulin
band showed no consistent trend. Plasma prealbumin and albumin
levels tended to be decreased on average by 30% and 10% respectively, whereas the concentration of the acute phase protein and
protease inhibitor alpha-1-antitrypsin was increased on average by
30%. C-reactive protein averaged 12 μg/l compared to normal of
less than 1 μg/l. No variation with age was observed for these
proteins. The alpha-2-macroglobulin level was markedly decreased
in many of the younger patients, the lowest values corresponding to
about 30% of the mean value for healthy children of the same age.
Later in childhood and adolescence the values were within or above
the reference intervals. The plasma protein pattern was not
related to a specific type of CF.

It is concluded that the acute phase response in CF is similar to
that in many other chronic disorders. The decreased concentration
of a major plasma protease inhibitor, alpha-2-macroglobulin, indicates increased elimination of the protein due to increased
release of proteases into the circulation during the age period
when lung infections appear as a characteristic feature of the
disease. Serial measurements of some of the proteins could provide
a sensitive indicator of the degree of activity in CF and the
effectiveness of treatment.

**POSTER GROUP ONE No. 1.31**

LONGITUDINAL STUDY OF BLOOD PANCREATIC ENZYMES IN CF FROM BIRTH TO 24 MONTHS. Pederzini F., Armani P., Barlocco E.G., Canciani M., Olivieri D Rizzotti P.,Zanchetta M.,and Mastella G.(CF Research Center and Clinical Enzymology Center, Ospedale B.Trento,Verona.Statistics Institute,Verona University, Italy).

34 CF patients early diagnosed (30 by newborn screening, 4 by symptoms within 6 mo.life)entered in a longitudinal study of the blood pancreatic enzymes, with blood samples taken every 3-4 months. Pancreatic function was studied by fat balance and secretin-pancreozymin test. Blood spot (TRY-SPOT) and serum immunoreactive trypsin (CIS-Sorin reagent), serum lipase (Turbidimetric-colipase method and immunoenzymatic method),serum isoamylase (electrophoretic separation and visualization by a chromogeni starch substrate) have been studied. The results were compared with an age-matched control group. A marked variability of the results for individual patients and for single periods was observed. TRY levels were, on the whole, elevated at birth, with a rapid decline in the first months, remaining slightly higher than normal at 24 months. Lipase activity (LIP Act.) showed constant high levels. Pancreatic Iso-Amylase levels (I-AMY) in CF did not differ on average from the controls at this age but its variability was much higher. The mean levels tended to rise slowly after 3-4 months. The theoretical pattern of each enzyme was studied. In addition, the serum enzymatic trend was correlated with the pancreatic function, with the aim of determining the prognostic value of each serum enzyme (particularly TRY and lipase) and the diagnostic valu of the enzyme pannel in discerning the extent of the underlying pancreatic damage during the first 2 years of age.

| | | | 0-10d | 11-30d | 2mo | 3-4mo | 5-6mo | 7-9mo | 10-12mo | 13-18mo | 19-24mo |
|---|---|---|---|---|---|---|---|---|---|---|---|
| TRY | CF | X̄ | 126.5 | 110.6 | 104.5 | 69.1 | 107.1 | 52.6 | 35.1 | 28.1 | 29.5 |
| SPOT | | SD | 54.6 | 45.7 | 74.1 | 28.3 | 89.1 | 35.1 | 31.3 | 32.8 | 32.2 |
| µg/l | | n | 84 | 16 | 17 | 12 | 15 | 12 | 15 | 28 | 17 |
| | CONTROLS | X̄ | 20.1 | | | | 10.4 | | | | |
| | | SD | logn.distr. | | | | 6.3 | | | | |
| | | n | 7274 | 99thp.60 | | | 103 | | | | |
| LIP | CF | X̄ | 5.0 | 196.1 | 116.9 | 159.4 | 223.0 | 158.4 | 131.1 | 170.0 | 245.9 |
| ACT. | | SD | 0.0 | 122.8 | 70.4 | 133.3 | 204.5 | 100.7 | 95.9 | 137.8 | 203.9 |
| U/L | | n | 1 | 7 | 12 | 16 | 13 | 13 | 17 | 21 | 11 |
| | CONTROLS | X̄ | 18.0 | | | 30.3 | | | | 50.6 | |
| | | SD | 16.3 | | | 26.2 | | | | 24.1 | |
| | | n | 31 | | | 96 | | | | 111 | |
| I-AMY | CF | X̄ | 0.5 | 0.09 | 0.03 | 1.55 | 3.13 | 1.90 | 6.69 | 6.71 | 8.81 |
| µg/l | | SD | 0.0 | 0.21 | 0.08 | 2.53 | 4.26 | 2.90 | 10.42 | 7.88 | 7.92 |
| | | n | 1 | 7 | 12 | 15 | 12 | 14 | 14 | 21 | 14 |
| | CONTROLS | X̄ | 0.40 | | | 3.6 | | | | 10.3 | |
| | | SD | 2.1 | | | 3.2 | | | | 5.2 | |
| | | n | 77 | | | 54 | | | | 111 | |

**POSTER GROUP ONE No. 1.34**

PLASMA SERINE PROTEASES IN CYSTIC FIBROSIS

Picci L., Masiero D., Giunta A.M.*, Amoretti M.*, Marcadella I., Ferrari V., Chiandetti L., Zacchello F.
Dept. of Pediatrics, University of Padua, Via Giustiniani, 3, 35128 Padua, Italy; *II Pediatric Clinic, University of Milan, Via Commenda, 9, 20122 Milan, Italy.

Previous studies in our laboratory did not show any difference in the esterolytic activity of plasma from cystic fibrosis (CF) homozygotes and control subjects, employing 4-MUGB and fluorescein isothiocyanate di-guanidinobenzoate as substrates. Since both methods lack specificity, we have studied plasma serine proteases in CF, by means of affinity chromatography and isoelectric focusing techniques.
MATERIALS AND METHODS.
Citrated plasma (1 ml) from 6 CF homozygotes (3 males and 3 females; age 4-15 years) and 8 healthy children (5 males and 3 females; age 2-10 years) was first desalted by passing through a column (1.5 x 5 cm) of Bio-Gel P2, and then albumin was selectively removed by applying 2 ml of the eluate to a column (1.0 x 5 cm) of Blue Sepharose CL-6B.Each eluate was then dialyzed against 0.04 M Tris-HCl buffer pH 8.5, and passed through a column (1.0 x 5 cm) of Arginine-Sepharose 4B. Serine proteases were eluted with 0.04 M Tris-HCl, pH 8.5, containing 0.1 M NaCl and concentrated utilizing Minicon B/15 concentrators. Protein content of each eluate was determined by the method of Böhlen (1973). Aliquots corresponding to 60 µg of proteins were applied to a 0.3 mm thick polyacrylamide gel and focused utilizing a Pharmacia isoelectrofocusing apparatus (carrier ampholytes: Servalyt, pH range: 4.0-6.0). The gels were stained with Coomassie Blue R-250.
RESULTS:
The selective removal of albumin from plasma samples permits a clear separation of several protein bands focusing in the pH range of 4-6. The resulting patterns are heterogeneous and no consistent difference in protein bands is apparent in CF homozygotes as compared to control subjects. No attempts have been made to further elucidate the nature of each single protein, but these results seem to agree with previous reports according to which CF primary defect is not related to a serine protease deficiency.

**POSTER GROUP ONE No. 1.35**

USEFULNESS OF A MATHEMATICAL APPROACH TO INCREASE SPECIFICITY OF CEN-
TRALIZED SQ-RID TEST FOR CF NEONATAL SCREENING.

D. Faraguna, I. Cigui, F. Uxa, A. Luchesi. Istituto ci Clinica Pedia-
trica, Cattedra di Puericultura e di Genetica Medica, Università di
Trieste; Laboratorio di Analisi Cliniche - Istituto per l'Infanzia -
Trieste - (Italy) - .

This report concerns the results of CF screening, based on meconium analysis, which was performed in the region Friuli-Venezia Giu-
lia (Italy) from March 1982 to December 1983. During this period 17838
neonates were born in this area and 17201 of them (96,4%) were screened at the regional CF Center of Trieste.

Semiquantitative radial immunodiffusion technique for albumin
(SQ-RID test)[1] was performed on meconium samples smeared and dried on
filter paper and mailed daily to the central laboratory. A mathematical formula has been used to reduce the number of screening false positive subjects before submitting them to sweat test. The multivariate discriminant analysis formula

MULTIVARIATE INDEX (M.I.) = (0,125 X albumin) + (5,75 X gestational
age) + (2,34 X lactase) + (2,29 X $\frac{albumin}{antitrypsin}$ ) - 132,38    (M.I.    115)

correlates four parameters: i.e. meconium albumin (RID), albumin/anti-
trypsin ratio, lactase and gestational age.

In this way 77(0,45%) SQ-RID positive samples was screened. Only
15(0,09%) of them resulted positive at RID analysis. M.I. formula application reduced the positive number to 6(0,03%). Only these newborns
were selected for the sweat test, and 3 of them were confirmed as suffering from CF. Up today, only one child, born in Friuli-Venezia Giu-
lia during the same period and proved negative at the screening test (meconium albumin and serum trypsine included) has been subsequently
identified as suffering from CF on clinical grounds.

Our data suggest that by performing analysis for CF in subse-
quents steps on the same sample can reduce to a minimum the number of
children to be tested with sweat test.

Reference: 1 Mastella G. at al.:  Newborn screening for CF. Two me-
           thods compared on 229.626 newborns tested in 8 years in
           Veneto. It.J.Ped. 9,1983 (in press).

**POSTER GROUP ONE No. 1.36**

NEUROBLASTOMA AND CYSTIC FIBROSIS.   J.Blessing, T. Zwerling,
S.Rubinstein, N.Lewiston, R.Moss.   Children's Hospital at Stanford,
Palo Alto, CA.

We are presently following a 6-month-old child who has congenital
neuroblastoma, malabsorption, and a positive sweat chloride.  This
child was the product of a full term, normal vaginal delivery,weighed
2.38 kg at birth and developed stridor with respiratory distress
within the first few minutes after birth.  The initial chest x-ray
revealed a mediastinal mass which on pathology after resection was
reported to be a congenital neuroblastoma.  The child initially did
well, except for insufficient weight gain and at 3 months of age was
readmitted to the hospital for a work-up of malabsorption.  The VMA
and urine catecholamines were normal.  The sweat chloride was 126,
stool trypsin was negative, stool Sudan stain revealed >60 fat
globules per hpf.  The child was started on Pancrease, Pregestamil
24 calories per ounce and MCT oil.  There was a notable weight gain
with a decrease in the number of stools.

At 5 months of age the child was noted to be wheezing and started
on theophylline.  The sputum at this time grew scant Staph and
Klebsiella.  Subsequent cultures have grown out Pseudomonas.  At this
time the child has had 2 additional sweat chlorides which were 83 and
100mEq/L.A follow-up CT scan of the chest has revealed no change in the
size of the mass.  No metastases were noted on bone scan. Liver function tests were initially mildly abnormal, but at this time the SGOT
is 23, the SGPT 27, alk. phos. 584.  The electrolytes, glucose,
calcium, phosphorus, albumin and CBC are normal.  The chest x-ray
reveals prominent bronchial markings at the lung bases, as well as
the anterior mediastinal density.

At this time the major problems for this child are (1)poor weight
gain despite pancreatic enzymes and supplements, (2)intermittent
respiratory stridor which is unrelated to the size or position of the
mass, and (3)intermittent bronchospasm.  Because this tumor has not
regressed, chemotherapy and/or radiation therapy has been considered
and discussed with the family.  However, because of the diagnosis of
cystic fibrosis as well as neuroblastoma, the family is reticent to
consider aggressive tumor therapy.

We present this case for discussion as we are not aware of other
cases of neuroblastoma with a positive sweat chloride and malabsorption.  The catecholamines have remained normal in this child.  We are
in the process of evaluating other possible vaso-active amines that
might be released by this tumor, as well as evaluating the sweat
chloride in other newly diagnosed patients with neuroblastoma.

**POSTER GROUP TWO No. 2.01**

ATTITUDE OF PARENTS AFTER INITIAL DIAGNOSIS OF CF TO
REPRODUCTION, FAMILY PLANNING AND NEONATAL SCREENING
Perobelli S., Barlocco E.G., Borgo G., Braggion C.,
Canciani M., Forno S., Oliveri D. and Mastella G.
CF Center, Verona and Statistics Inst., Verona Univ.

A self-administered questionnaire was sent to 300
families who received the first diagnosis of CF at the
Verona CF center in the period 1973-80, to study the
effect of diagnosis and consequent genetic information
and counselling on the parents' reproductive behaviour.
The first data includes a sample of 118 couples residing
in an area of north-east Italy partially covered by CF
neonatal screening programmes. 29.6% of the children
were diagnosed by screening or meconium ileus, the rest
by symptoms. The proband child died in 19 families. The
mean age of the couples was 31.5y at diagnosis, 38.5y
now. 42.3% of them had only primary school education; in
37.9% both parents are employed. 84% of the couples
don't want further children; anxiety over the possibility
of a further CF child is the main reason in 77% of the
cases. The presence of at least one non-CF child
supports this attitude. The dread of "child loss" seems
to be more important motivation to wish new children than
the death itself (77% of the couples with at least one
dead child have not had any more children; but only 17%
of the couples who have had another child after diagnosis
experienced the death of their child). 67% of the
couples use contraception, in 58% only after diagnosis.
Elective abortion occurred in 24 couples, 58% after
diagnosis. The couples who received the first CF
diagnosis by neonatal screening (N=35) were compared with
those whose child was diagnosed by symptoms (N=38). The
mean age of the mothers is 33.8 years in the screening
group and 38.7 in the symptoms one. New children after
diagnosis were born to 11.4% of the screening mothers and
to 21.6% of the others, even though use of contraception
before and after diagnosis was the same in the two
groups. Contraception was started after diagnosis by
42.8% of the screening couples but by only 16.8% of the
others; among the couples who don't want more children,
78% practice contraception in the screening group and 44%
in the symptoms one. Dread of another CF child was
present in 83% of the screening group and 65% of the
symptoms groups. It seems that neonatal CF screening is
in some way helpful for a better understanding of the
genetic implication of CF.

**POSTER GROUP TWO No. 2.02**

EXPERIENCE OF A YOUNG ADULTS' CF CLINIC

C.A. Smalley and I.D. Green. Selly Oak Hospital, Raddlebarn Road Birmingham, B29 6JD. England.

Increasing numbers of CF children are reaching adolescence and young adult life, at which time their medical care is transferred, not always successfully, from paediatricians to adult physicians. In order to minimise the difficulties of this transition period, we established in April 1980 a young adults' CF clinic run jointly by physician and paediatrician. Our first $3\frac{1}{2}$ years experience is described.

Patients 21 patients (13 male and 8 female) aged between 15 years 5 months and 25 years were referred.

At referral they were noted to be shorter than average (18/21 < 50th centile height), often very thin (11/21 < 3rd centile weight), nearly half (9/21) moderately or severely affected by their disease (Shwachman scores)[1], nearly half (9/21) with an $FEV_1$ > 2 SD's below the mean for height and age, half (11/21) culturing pseudomonas from sputum, and a quarter (5/21) with a very reduced life-style (special school, home teaching or invalidity pension).

Follow up 5 patients (4 male and 1 female) died. No death was unexpected. All 5 patients had been in very poor health at referral. They died after a total of 24 admissions (range 1-9). Mode of death was respiratory failure in 4 and massive haematemesis in one. Of the 16 survivors 10 have been followed up for a minimum of 2 years. In these 10 there was a tendency to deteriorate (Schwachman score, $FEV_1$, and weight) but values did not reach statistical significance. The 16 survivors have been admitted on 26 occasions, predominantly for intravenous antibiotics.

Complications seen in 21 patients have included delayed puberty (3), insulin dependent diabetes mellitus (2), glycosuria (further 3), hyperglycaemia (10/15 tested), meconium ileus equivalent (1), portal hypertension and varices (1), haematemesis (1), pneumothorax (2), major hemoptysis (2), nasal sinusitis requiring surgery (2), major psychiatric illness (2).

Conclusions This is a very vulnerable group of patients who reach adult life often in a precarious state of health. The joint (physician and paediatrician) approach may offer a more acceptable transition period for these patients.

1.  Shwachman, H., Kulczycki, L.L. (1958) Long term study of 105 patients with cystic fibrosis. Am.J.Dis.Ch. 96, 6 - 15.

**POSTER GROUP TWO No. 2.03**

PSYCHOLOGICAL AND PSYCHOMETRIC COMPLETE STUDY ABOUT 30 CF PATIENTS

M.A. Villamira, R. Nobili, D. Costantini, R. Padoan, A. Giunta
CF Centre, Dept. of Paediatrics, University of Milan, Via Commenda 9,
Milan, ITALY

Aim of investigation: Our purpose is to point out the most important
and frequent psychological features of CF subjects treated in the CF
Centre of Milan in order to prevent and/or treat, in the best way we
can, eventual psychological problems related to CF.
Materials and Method: We studied 30 subjects out of the 180 treated
in the CF Centre of Milan following these criteria: 1) the age: we
considered subjects from 6 years at least; 2) the availability in ha
ving some talks with the psychologists and carrying out some psycholo
gical tests. A comprehensive follow-up of all patients was performed
during a period from 1 to 2 years. We proposed to all subjects the fol
lowing projective tests, which offer a rich picture about the persona
lity of CF patients and their relationships within the family: 1) hu
man figure drawing; 2) drawing of a tree; 3) drawing of a family; 4)
drawing of a family of animals. Moreover to the subjects older than 15
years we also proposed two questionnaires of personality, the Sixteen
Personality Factor Test (16 PF) and the Anxiety Scale Questionnaire
(A.S.Q.). The human figure drawing and the drawing of a tree were also
proposed to some parents. Each subject had, at least, 4 meetings with
the psychologists.
We compare, analyzing both the personal situation of each patient and
the group data, the results pointed out by psychological tests and
those emerged during the interviews with parents and patients.
Results and Conclusions: Regarding group data we found that these
subjects do not differ significantly from an omogeneous group of sub
jects without CF. Furthermore it was pointed out that problems of com
prehension and communication, related to cultural background of each
family, often make more heavy and difficultly manageable the onerous
burden imposed by the disease. Moreover adolescence problems make a)
very distressing, for CF subjects, the ambivalence of adults towards
the disease and the fears evoked by CF and b) more and more difficult
the conquest of autonomy as far as these patients are concerned.

THE DEVELOPMENT OF INDEPENDENCE IN ADOLESCENTS WITH CF

G.Sinnema

University Children's Hospital
Nieuwe Gracht 137, 3512 LK Utrecht, The Netherlands

In cystic fibrosis (CF), a slowing down of growth and maturation is quite common. Likewise, the literature often suggests that adolescents with a chronic illness such as CF, show a delay in the development of independence.However, clear-cut evidence is lacking.
In our study 3 major psychological elements of CF are considered: its chronic nature, its fatal outcome, and the visibility of the handicap (retarded growth). In order to study the influence of these variables on adolescent independence, 3 reference groups have been chosen besides the CF-group (n=64): adolescents with asthma (chronic, but not fatal; n=36); healthy, but small adolescents (n=47), and normal healthy controls (n=71). Eight forms of independence have been measured by an extensive questionnaire.
Some of the main results: At younger ages (13-14) CF-adolescents clearly show a delay in "dating and mating", but in general they do not have less social activities outside the home than their healthy peers. At ages 15-17 CF-adolescents do have a smaller social range. Younger CF-adolescents seem to be less independent in handling social conflicts. They bear less responsibility for their own body hygiene. Responsibility for living according to health rules seems to be less in CF-adolescents only at ages 15-17. There are no differences between the groups regarding the formation of ideals and the development of own ideas in politics, religion and ethics. CF-patients are surprisingly optimistic about their personal happiness in the future, in spite of possible set-backs. The influence of factors such as a small stature and the severity of the illness on the development of independence will be discussed in some detail.
To conclude, in future research it will be necessary to avoid general labels such as "immature" or "dependent", and to differentiate further between different types of independence. Whether a delay in development is (dys)functional in coping with the disease will be discussed.

**POSTER GROUP TWO No. 2.05**

SOCIAL AND ORGANIZING ASPECTS IN A SWISS HOLIDAY CAMP WITH
INTENSIVE THERAPY FOR PATIENTS WITH CYSTIC FIBROSIS

H.-P. Müller*, M.H. Schöni** and R. Kraemer***

Swiss Association for Cystic Fibrosis, Hubacherweg 12, CH-3097 Liebe-
feld*, Inst. for clin. & exper. Cancer Research, Berne** and Department of Paediatrics, University of Berne, Switzerland***

Since 1981 summer holiday camps with intensive therapy for patients
with cystic fibrosis (CF) have been organized in a mountain rehabilitation clinic(Montana, Wallis, 1500 m above sea level). The aims of
these three weeks lasting stays are: Application of intensive physiotherapy by a professional team, activation of patients for a selected
physical training, instruction and control of methods for independent
physiotherapy, clinical evaluation with set-up of adequate drug
therapy, promotion of self-control and self-confidence by exchange
of experience between each other, relief of parents from the daily
therapy. The number of attending patients has increased every year
(1981: 21; 1982: 37; 1983: 44). Children from all parts of Switzerland independent of their native language are accepted. The patients
are medically pre-evaluated by their own physician in the view of
their degree of disease, their age and their possible profit of such
a stay. Patients from the age of 7 throughout the adolescence as
well as young adults attend the camps. Severely ill children confined
to bed are accepted in exceptional cases only because of organizing
problems. Each patient competes in the daily morning inhalation and
physiotherapy sessions and receives its own personal physiotherapy
under strict control (conventional clapping, self-clapping, autoge-
nous drainage). The take of drugs as well as the selection of meals
are controlled by the physicians. As far as possible no I.V. drug
therapy is administered. Every day up to two hours of swimming in an
indoor swimming-pool are allowed. Several physical training
possibilities, ball games, running and jogging in the forest, riding,
tennis, skating (even in summer) as well as attractive facilities
for constructive hobby, painting, needlework, music an theatre
playing are provided. One to two day trips with walking, cooking
and eating in the open air are organized every week. The patients can
select and perform most of these activities on a voluntary basis.
About 20 persons, in part as volunteers (2 physicians, nurses,
physiotherapy professionals, social workers) are required to take
care or the patients. The costs are raised from different sources:
Parents 10%, the Swiss Insurance for disable people 75%, the Swiss
Association for Cystic Fibrosis 15%.

**POSTER GROUP TWO No. 2.06**

EFFECTS OF INTERPERSONAL SKILLS TRAINING FOR PARENTS OF CF CHILDREN

Adrianne B. Casadaban, PhD, Keith H. Schroder, PhD, & Brian Davis,MD
Cystic Fibrosis Center, Rm. M-687, University of California, San Fran.
San Francisco, Ca. 94143 USA

The paper reports a pilot research project on the acceptability and benefit of workshops on communication and problem-solving skills for parents of children with Cystic Fibrosis. Previous studies have indicated higher levels of marital distance, separation, and divorce in families with CF children compared to U.S. national norms and documented high levels of tension and overwork occasioned for parents of CF children. Concommitantly, reports indicate a reticence of CF parents to use mental health resources. These factors indicate the need for interventions specifically aimed at alleviating stress on the marital relationship in CF families. Moreover, these must be 1) free of the stigma of psychological or interpersonal pathology, 2) provide a clear educational benefit, and, 3) include safeguards to prevent parents being confronted with issues which are beyond their emotional capacity to consider. Finally, they must also be brief to allow parents with strict time demands to attend.
The workshops in this study were designed with these factors in mind and occurred over two week-end days. They were a structured, skill-learning experience which focused on well-researched methods of inter-personal communication and mutual problem-solving. The present study is the first application of these methods specifically to Cystic Fibrosis. The skills to be learned were generic in nature, and did not force couples to deal specifically with Cystic Fibrosis, itself, except as they so chose. Couples were assessed two months before and after the workshop with measures of marital satisfaction, family functioning, self-esteem, and communication and problem-solving skill. Over the four months surrounding the workshops they made weekly ra-tings of family tension. Over periods of six months before and after training, indices of events indicative of family breakdown were ga-thered, as well as ratings of ill children's medical status. Finally, participants completed questionnaires evaluating their response to the training immediately after the workshop, and at two and six months thereafter.
Twenty couples completed pre-measures; thirteen then participated in the workshop. Immediate post-workshop evaluations reveal that all parents found the workshops acceptable, and all but one individual found the skills useful. Complete results will be available in April, 1984 (except four families' long-term data which will be available for inclusion in June). While more complete conclusions await final data analysis, preliminary conclusions point to the efficacy of this ap-proach, which is also the first quantitative study of psychosocial interventions to be done in Cystic Fibrosis.

**POSTER GROUP TWO No. 2.07**

PRESCHOOL YEARS INTO ADULTHOOD:  A PSYCHOSOCIAL SURVEY OF CF PATIENTS
AND THEIR FAMILIES.  <u>Leslie Cowen</u>, M.S.W., <u>Robert Simmons</u>, M.D.,
<u>Mary Corey</u>, M.Sc., <u>Nancy Keenan</u>, B.A., <u>Henry Levison</u>, M.D.  Cystic
Fibrosis Clinic, The Hospital for Sick Children, 555 University Avenue
Toronto, Ontario, Canada.

In order to assess how psychological and social factors affect or
are affected by the chronic disease process in patients with cystic
fibrosis (CF) and their families, a survey of the CF population at the
Hospital for Sick Children (HSC) was undertaken.  Four hundred and
thirteen of the 530 CF patients and their family members completed
questionnaires appropriate to age, sex, and family position assessing
social competence, behavior problems, self concept, extent of
emotional disturbance, and family function.  Psychosocial measures
were merged with patients' physical parameters in the CF clinic data-
base and family demographic variables.  There were no significant
differences between the patients who responded (78%) and those who
did not (22%).  The large patient population made possible study of
the impact of CF upon developmental stage and the variation of the
effect by gender.
A general lack of relationship between disease severity and
psychosocial function and demographic characteristics was seen in all
developmental stages.  Male patients demonstrated increased behavior
problems peaking in early adolescence and improving during later
years.  Female CF children showed few behavior problems using more
denial than males.  In the adolescent females denial was less
effective and emotional symptomatology more prominent, disturbance
increasing with age.  Self concept was normal or better in patients
6 years and over with adequate social competence clearly demonstrated.
Overcompensation and minimization were found to support the good
psychosocial function with distortion of reality, in older patients,
likewise enhancing adaptation.  CF patients above 6 years somatize
stress which may be related more to their necessary pre-occupation
with body function than to pathophysiological process.
Family dysfunction was found to be greater in older patient groups
and parents of older children had more difficulty maintaining
defenses.  Family profiles of parents revealed a high degree of
cohesion.  Non CF sibs demonstrated adequate social competence, a
lack of behavior problems and had a defended self concept revealing
elevated self criticism.

**POSTER GROUP TWO No. 2.08**

ERRONEOUS DIAGNOSIS OF CYSTIC FIBROSIS PSYCHOLOGICAL
ASPECTS

Percy Bray, University Hospital of Wales, Heath Park, Cardiff

The diagnosis of Cystic Fibrosis is an event of such
magnitude in the life of a child and the family that
it necessitates the optimum accuracy in laboratory
tests and clinical appraisal. The psychosocial impact
of cummunicating the diagnosis has been reported by
Dodge and Burton (1979) Sibinga (1980) and Barbero (1981).

Like JANUS, "Erroneous Diagnosis" has two faces:
one giving false positive diagnosis of C.F., the other
giving false negatives. A sub-group which has been studied
by Warwick (1981) and Wilcken (1983) includes those
instances where an unacceptable delay in positive diagnosis
has occurred.

This review comprises 45 false positive cases and
35 false negative diagnoses, and in a group of 22
families an attempt has been made to quantify the effects
of having to reverse the original diagnoses: the problems
were many and various, grouped as (a) Cognitive
(b) Affective (c) Adaptive. In group 1 (false positive)
Cognitive problems were found in 85%, affective in 100%,
adaptive in 15%. Group 2 (false negatives) produced
Cognitive problems in 9%, affective in 100%, and adaptive
in 9%. The problems are also grouped as:-
(i) Immediate (ii) Delayed (iii) Resultant
The duration of erroneous diagnosis ranged from 4 weeks
to 14 years in Group 1 and from birth to 15 years in
Group 2.

**POSTER GROUP TWO No. 2.09**

SELF CARE IN CYSTIC FIBROSIS

Mary Jo McCracken, RN; Marianne O'Carroll, PhD; Warren Warwick, MD
University of Minnesota Hospitals & Clinics
420 Delaware St SE, Box 603 Mayo
Minneapolis, MN  55455
USA

The implementation of a self care approach to health care was identified as a coping strategy for adolescents with Cystic Fibrosis (CF). The philosophy of self care was adopted for the purpose of achieving an effective level of independence and facilitating a positive adaptation to adolescence and CF. An adolescent CF self care program was designed and implemented as an intervention aimed at developing the adolescent's self care capabilities and providing a social support system through group involvement.

A two week, multifaceted, inpatient program was undertaken  with adolescents with CF. The program focused on:  (1) intensive education regarding CF, (2) developing self care skills with home cares and health maintenance cares, and (3) providing a social support system. Program content included individual assessment of self care potential and capabilities, educational and group therapeutic sessions, as well as practical skills workshops. Several tools were developed and utilized which assisted the multidisciplinary care team in implementing the philosophy of self care. These tools include a self care data base, teaching flow sheet, patient contract and evaluation outcome criteria.

It was hypothesized that an increased understanding of CF, mastery of self care skills and the opportunity to share concerns through group interactions would have numerous positive outcomes. Outcomes of the program included:  (1) a significant increase in knowledge regarding CF, (2) the development of effective self care skills and activities, (3) increased independence, (4) an increase in feelings of control over health maintenance and self mastery, (5) increased ability to verbalize and discuss CF related issues and (6) an increase in decision making regarding health care needs and appropriate priority setting.

In summary, a self care approach to health care in CF promises to provide an effective means of promoting independence and facilitating a positive adaptation to adolescence and CF. It provides the adolescent, family and health care team with a viable solution to solving some of the long term hardships imposed by CF.

**POSTER GROUP TWO No. 2.10**

"GROUP INTERVENTION TECHNIQUES WITH PARENTS OF CHRONICALLY ILL CHILDREN"

Marguerite M. Bryce, ACSW, Denise Rodgers, MS, Joan B. Rodnan, M.D.
Children's Hospital of Pittsburgh, 125 DeSoto Street, Pittsburgh,
Pennsylvania  15213 USA

Much information has been written about the use of groups in working with families.  This paper will focus on the specific application of group technique to developmental stages of families as they attempt to manage a chronic, life-threatening illness.

Discussion will focus on

1.  Developmental stages of families following the diagnosis of an illness.
2.  Considerations in the application of group technique to the different stages of parenting groups.

    a.  impact of chronic illness (non-resolvibility)
    b.  attempts to gain control of illness
    c.  predictability of disease management
    d.  ability to invest energy in therapeutic involvement

3.  Evolution of Parenting Group Models in Chronic Illness.
    (Newly Diagnosed, Parenting, Grandparenting, Bereaved)

Conclusion
Professionals working with families must have flexibility in the application of group technique skills.  No single technique is effective in meeting the range of family needs through the course of an illness.  The therapeutic focus which is appropriate to some stages is too intense for others.  Supportive or educational groups which sustain families in coping and focusing on normal living become ineffective in the demands of a crisis or intense illness.

Using flexibility in group technique fulfills the primary goal of maintaining continuity of emotional/psychological care for these families.  This allows the professional to support coping techniques and to shift to more intensive techniques as the family needs change.

**POSTER GROUP TWO No. 2.11**

THE PROBLEM OF CYSTIC FIBROSIS IN EGYPT

EKRAM ABDEL SALAM
PEDIATRIC & GENETIC DEPT. CAIRO UNIVERSITY, EGYPT

The utopian principle calling for prevention and management of cystic fibrosis in Egypt cannot equally follow similar programs in other counteries. The degree of success is directly correlated to the degree of conviction of the population as to the value of such programs specially in developing countries where malnutrition, endemic parasitization and infections diseases are still widely prevalent. In Egypt the prevalence of gastroenteritis and chest infection in children interferes with proper detection of CF. Maldigestion which follows gastroenteritis promotes nutritional deficiencies in CF. Pancreatic enzyme replacement proved to be helpful in CF cases specially those uncomplicated with diarrheal diseases. Similarly control of chest infection ameliorates respiratory symptoms and helps patients to achieve an acceptable rate of growth. Patients with advanced lung disease need extraordinary amount of calories and need high caloric supplemental feeding. Supplementation of fat soluble vitamines improves the quality of life or longevity. Bronchodilators helps to establish a reversible airway obstruction. This must be complemented with specific antimicrobials treatment. Corticosteroids are not favourable therapy due to frequent chest infection. This chest infections usually trigger exacerbations of lung disease in CF.

**POSTER GROUP TWO No. 2.12**

EVALUATION OF SELF-PERCUSSION DURING POSTURAL DRAINAGE
USING THE FORCED EXPIRATION TECHNIQUE (FET).

Barbara A. Webber, Rosemary A. Parker, Janet L. Hofmeyr
and Margaret E. Hodson*, Physiotherapy Department and
Cardiothoracic Institute*, Brompton Hospital, London.

The FET is commonly used in conjunction with self-
percussion of the chest wall and thoracic expansion
breathing exercises while lying in appropriate gravity
assisted positions.   The importance of percussion in
this context has not been studied, so we have compared
the effects of self-postural drainage with and without
self-percussion.

16 adolescent and adult CF patients (ages 13-35 yrs.) were
studied over 4 days prior to discharge from hospital.   On
2 days treatment included thoracic expansion exercises
and self-percussion interspersed with the FET (treatment P).
On the other 2 days self-percussion was omitted
(treatment A). Treatment days were randomised.   Recordings
were made of sputum weight produced during treatment
periods and 24 hour periods, and lung function before and
after the first treatment each day.

Self-percussion showed no advantage in weight of sputum
produced.   With treatment A the mean daily sputum weight
in treatment periods was 57.1g and with treatment P 52.0g.
These results were not statistically significant. In the
24 hour non-treatment periods there was no significant
difference in weight of sputum produced.   Comparing $FEV_1$
and FVC before treatment each day there was an improvement
in lung function following both treatment days A and P.

Many patients will wish to continue doing self-percussion
if they feel it is beneficial, and unless studies prove
satisfactorily that it is detrimental, there is no reason
to stop them doing percussion.   Those who dislike doing
percussion and find it tiring can be advised to omit
percussion provided breathing exercises and FET are
carried out effectively.

These results should not be extrapolated so that
percussion is omitted from the treatment of the infant
and small child.   Until a child is old enough to do
breathing exercises and huffing effectively, coughing
must be stimulated to clear secretions and percussion,
clinically, is an effective means.

**POSTER GROUP TWO No. 2.13**

EVALUATION OF THREE INDIVIDUAL COMPONENTS OF A POSTURAL
DRAINAGE TREATMENT

R.A. Parker, B.A. Webber, P.P. Sutton*, S.P. Newman*,
N. Garland*, M.T. Lopez-Vidriero*, D. Pavia* & S.W.Clarke*
Physiotherapy Department, Brompton Hospital, London, and
*Department of Thoracic Medicine, Royal Free Hospital,
London.

The individual components of a postural drainage treatment
are:-
gravity assisted position, percussion, shaking, breathing
exercises, coughing and more recently the forced
expiration technique (FET).  FET has been shown to be
of benefit when combined with a postural drainage
treatment but the benefit of each component of treatment
has not been assessed.

The present study was designed to compare three of the
individual components of a postural drainage treatment
namely, FET  a gravity assisted position, and coughing.

10 Patients (5 with bronchiectasis, 4 cystic fibrosis
and 1 chronic asthma) with copious sputum (mean 63.3ml/
 24 hr) were studied using the inhaled radioaerosol
method and dry and wet weight of sputum recorded.   Each
patient received four 30 min.treatments in random order
over two weeks.   Treatment included:-
(a)  Control with the subject sitting upright
(b)  4 double coughs in each 3 min. period, sitting
     upright
(c)  4 forced expirations (FET) in each 3 min. period,
     sitting upright
(d)  4 forced expirations (FET) in each 3 min. period in
     an appropriate postural drainage (PD)   position.

Radioaerosol clearance following FET and FET + PD   was
significantly greater than directed coughing and the
control period (P< 0.01).

Sputum production following FET, FET + PD  and directed
coughing was significantly greater than the control
period (P< 0.01).

FET + P.D. produced significantly more sputum than FET
alone (P< 0.05).   It is suggested therefore that both
these manoeuvres should be included in a treatment.

**POSTER GROUP TWO No. 2.14**

THE VALUE OF A DETAILED COMPREHENSIVE PHYSIOTHERAPY ASSESSMENT IN THE MANAGEMENT OF CYSTIC FIBROSIS

Mrs Fiona Henry, Senior Paediatric Physiotherapist, St. James' University Hospital, Leeds LS9 7TF.

St. James' Hospital is now a CF centre for the Yorkshire region. Eighty-four new patients throughout the region had had a full physiotherapy assessment as part of an overall CF evaluation.

1. Visual assessment: the following were noted: thoracic measurements during respiration, rate, pattern and embarrassment of breathing, including a measure of finger clubbing, rib recession, audible wheezing etc.
2. A full physiotherapy session was performed by the therapists including; postural drainage, percussion, the forced expiration technique and relaxed controlled breathing. The following were noted: areas of the chest yielding more sputum than others, its quantity, texture, colour volume and ease of removal. The parent or patient then demonstrates their usual physiotherapy routine. Their understanding of the reasons for regular physiotherapy is ascertained.
3. Enquiries are made about physiotherapy at home: who performs the physiotherapy, how many times per day (or week), understanding of the nebuliser in relation to physiotherapy times, do they regularly attend an out patient physiotherapy department? Is the frequency and technique altered with the state of the chest. What happens at school or on holidays?

Effectiveness was judged by consideration of the following:
1. Knowledge 2. Technique 3. Compliance 4. Psychosocial Attitudes and scored as: Good (3) Satisfactory (2) Poor (1). A simple scoring scheme was used to permit general use of the system.

From these assessments we found that almost 40% of patients were having ineffective physiotherapy. The reasons ranged from complete lack of knowledge to total non-compliance. This study demonstrates a widespread need for more teaching and education of CF patients and their parents in the theory and practical application of chest physiotherapy.

**POSTER GROUP TWO No. 2.15**

COMPARISON OF PHYSIOTHERAPY TECHNIQUES EMPLOYED IN CYSTIC FIBROSIS

D. Rogers, J. Tottle, D.M. Pickering, E. Plews, V. Davies, R.G. Newcombe, M.C. Goodchild, J.A. Dodge, Departments of Physiotherapy, Medical Computing and Statistics and Child Health, Welsh National School of Medicine, Cardiff, U.K.

Physiotherapy is the least controversial of the treatments of cystic fibrosis (CF) and yet its efficacy varies, as does patient compliance. This study was an attempt to assess and compare statistically, three types of physiotherapy: forced expiration technique (FET) alone; FET with percussion; FET with postural drainage.

Patients were studied in groups of four, according to a prearranged balanced treatment schedule. Each patient received physiotherapy on four occasions each day for four days and each group of four patients was treated by the same physiotherapist. Four groups, that is 16 patients, completed the trial.

Assessment was by respiratory function tests ($FEV_1$, FVC, $FEV_1$ as % FVC, PFR) and sputum weight.

Analyses were of two types, employing analyses of variance and took into account order of treatments and the best transformation of data.

Results showed no significant differences, at the 5% level, between the three types of physiotherapy.

Consequently FET alone was as effective as the therapies requiring an assistant or a tipping frame or bed, and would allow the older CF patient to conduct his physiotherapy independently.

Reference   J.A. Pryor et al. (1979). Evaluation of forced expiration technique as an adjunct to postural drainage in the treatment of cystic fibrosis. British Medical Journal, II, 417-418.

**POSTER GROUP TWO No. 2.16**

PROLONGED USE OF FORCED EXPIRATION TECHNIQUE IN CYSTIC FIBROSIS

J. van der Laag, H. Steenbergen, P.J.M. Helders
University Children's Hospital "Het Wilhelmina Kinderziekenhuis",
Nieuwe Gracht 137, 3512 LK Utrecht, The Netherlands.

Forced Expiration Technique (FET) is a new method of physiotherapy
which appears to be especially convenient for adolescents and adults
with Cystic Fibrosis (CF), since these patients are not any longer
dependent on physiotherapists, parents and friends daily.
In May 1981 we started to introduce this technique to our patients.
All were hospitalized for three days for a special training-course.
Up till November 1983 74 patients (aged 6 - 25 years, mean 14) have
been taught FET. Follow-up results of lungfunction (VC, FEV1, PEFR)
of 51 patients reveal a slight but not significant deterioration
over 2 years (table). In spring 1984 more results of these parameters
will become available.

| Lungfunction % pred. value | Start FET | $\frac{1}{2}$ year | 1 year | $1\frac{1}{2}$ year | 2 years |
|---|---|---|---|---|---|
| VC | 74,5 | 72,2 | 76,2 | 69,5 | 68,8 |
| FEV1 | 56,4 | 51,6 | 56,0 | 47,9 | 42,9 |
| PEFR | 70,3 | 70,0 | 74,8 | 62,9 | 61,0 |
| n | 51 | 35 | 38 | 21 | 15 |

At present we believe these data show a natural course of lungfunction in CF independent on the method of physiotherapy (clapping
or FET). The big advantage of FET is independency, but it needs a
great deal of self-discipline.

**POSTER GROUP TWO No. 2.17**

EFFECT OF THE FORCED EXPIRATION TECHNIQUE AND POSTURAL DRAINAGE IN ADULTS WITH CYSTIC FIBROSIS.

J.M.L. Verboon[1], W. Bakker[2] and J.H. Dijkman[2].
Department of Physiotherapy[1] and Pulmonology[2], University Hospital Leiden, Rijnsburgerweg 10, 2333 AA Leiden, the Netherlands.

This study was designed to measure the effect of the Forced Expiration Technique (FET) with or without postural drainage (PD) on pulmonary function and sputum production and to examine whether an additive effect of postural drainage using the FET could be established. Eight patients with Cystic Fibrosis (age 17 to 43 years) took part in the study. Each subject was investigated one day a week for 4 consecutive weeks. Two times they performed FET in the upright position (FET) and two times FET with postural drainage including sleeping the night before in the head-down position (FET + PD), in a randomized order. Before physiotherapy, immediately afterwards and after 45 minutes FVC, $FEV_1$, PEFR and $MEF_{50}$ were recorded on a computerpneumotachograph (Pneumoscreen[R], Jaeger & Koellisch MBH). The sputum was collected over a $22\frac{1}{2}$ hours period before physiotherapy and during the $1\frac{1}{2}$ hours treatment session, including physiotherapy, lungfunction tests and rest.

The studied lungfunction tests showed no improvement after FET and FET + PD, nor was there any difference in the lungfunction values between FET and FET + PD. The sputum of patients with more than 30 mg sputum per $22\frac{1}{2}$ hours during FET + PD was significantly more than during FET. The weight of sputum collected during the physiotherapy session of FET and FET + PD showed no statistical difference.

The results of this study demonstrate that sleeping in the head-down position is effective in aiding the expectoration in CF patients with more than 30 mg sputum per day. Due to very small sample size no statistical difference in lungfunction parameters were found.

**POSTER GROUP TWO No. 2.18**

AUTOGENIC DRAINAGE (A.D.)

Jean CHEVAILLIER - ZEEPREVENTORIUM - DE HAAN (BELGIUM)

Principle
The model of MEAD et al. (J. of Applied Physiol. 1967, 22) makes us
understand what happens in obstructive lung diseases when exhaling is
performed with reduced expiratory pressure.  The correct localisation
of the E.P.P. (equal pressure point) gives the minimal needed air-
stream acceleration to move the mucus, without causing too much obstruction  neither downstream nor upstream.  Therefore, their must be
an exact correlation between the inspiratory volume, the expiratory
force, the mechanical properties of the bronchial tubes, the degree of
obstruction, the compression phenomena and the frictional resistance.

Technique
Mostly the ventilated volume is reduced, to localize the E.P.P. in the
peripheral airways during the forced expiration which is done as
"sighing".  Thus the needed decrease in bronchial diameter is obtained
both in the small and medium sized bronchi.  The airflow increases
without secondary effects, and the mucus is simultaneously transported
through the largest parts of the bronchial tree.  As the loosened mucus
travels to the upper airways, and gathers, the inspiratory volume is
progressively increased to localize the right airvelocity in the more
central airways.  This brings the mucus to the throat, wherefrom it
can be driven into the mouth with an accelerated exhalation. This progressive procedure helps, after training, to suppress the coughing reflex so that coughing is usually no longer necessary.  The drainage
can be devided into three phases :
1. loosening the mucus by very low lung volume breathing (ERV)
2. gathering the mucus by low lung volume breathing (ERV + TV)
3. evacuating the mucus by higher lung volume breathing ($\pm$ VC)
To avoid the effects of ventilatory asynchronism, inhalátion through
de nose, occurs slowly.  At the end of inhalation follows a short
breathing stoppage, glottis held open, so that all lung segments, including the obstructed ones, can fill up equally. During the next exhalation the alveolar pressure will be the same in most of the lung
segments and this will avoid paradoxical airflow.

General remarks
After an initiation period, the patient works independent, from a
seated position, with straight back and slightly raised head.  He uses
a diaphragmatic breathing.  Ventilation is determined by continuous
information the patient receives through auditive, sensory and proprio
  ceptive channels.  It is essential, for many reasons, to have chronic bronchorrhea patients follow a complete and intensive respiratory
reeducation program.

236

## CF - PATIENTS IN MARATHON

Johan Kvalvik Stanghelle, ·Sunnaas Hospital, 1450
Nesoddtangen & Dag Skyberg, the Department of Paediatrics,
the Central Hospital of Aust-Agder, Arendal, Norway.

Metabolic consequences of prolonged, severe exercise were
investigated in a 16-year-old boy with CF who completed
Oslo Marathon in 1982 and New York Marathon one year later
In the latter event the same studies were also performed
in another 17-year-old CF-marathoner.

The boy who completed two marathon races(in 3 hours 51
min and 3 hours 47 min) is mildly affected of CF. His
maximal oxygen uptake was 63 ml/kg/min one week prior
to both races. The other boy is severely affected by CF,
with pseudomonas infection the last 9 years, pancreatic
achylia and severelung changes. During the last 3 years
he had trained endurance activities regularly 3-6 times
weekly, and his Schwachman score raised from 45 to 60.
His maximal oxygen uptake was 38 ml/kg/min prior to New
York Marathon, in which he completed in 7 hours 12 min.

Several blood, urine and lung function parameters as
well as body weight, fluid intake and rectal temperature
were measured. No changes were found in the serum concentrations of electrolytes. Besides elevated sweat electrolytes, none of the findings differed from those reported
in healthy marathoners.

These CF-patients demonstrate that some of these patients
may participate in strenuous physical training regimes
and strenuous prolonged exercise.

**POSTER GROUP TWO No. 2.20**

PHYSICAL TRAINING OF CHILDREN WITH CF.

B. Andréasson, R. Kornfält, E. Nordmark, B. Jonson.
From the Departments of Pediatrics and Clinical Physiology,
University Hospital, Lund, Sweden.

Patients with cystic fibrosis who are physically active have a
better prognosis than inactive cystic fibrotics. Physical training
in specialized camps has been proven to raise their working capacity and to improve their pulmonary function (Zach et al, 1982,
Skyberg, 1983). This study was designed to investigate whether
cystic fibrotics of different age and disease severity are capable
of completing a daily exercise program over a period of two years
and to see if physical training can replace traditional physiotherapy. Seven children with cystic fibrosis, aged 6 - 21 years
were given an exercise program which should be carried out daily
during one entire year together with their traditional physiotherapy. The following year the same children continued their
physical training, but excluded the traditional physiotherapy.
Spirometry tests and exercise tolerance tests were performed before,
during and after the two year long study.

The effects of the exercise program on pulmonary function working
capacity and the patient's general wellbeing are reported.

**POSTER GROUP TWO No. 2.21**

PHYSICAL EXERCISE, A SUBSTITUTE FOR POSTURAL DRAINAGE AND PERCUSSION

K.W. Mittenzwey, W. Leupold, B. Gottschalk and D. Paul, Children's Hospital, Medical Academy "Carl Gustav Carus", Fetscherstrasse 74, 8019 Dresden, German Democratic Republic

During a four week summer camp for CF children we tried to determine whether physical exercise is a possible alternative to postural drainage and percussion. We selected 55 children between 10 and 14 years of age and prepared a special physical training programme in co-operation with specialists for sport medicine. Our training programme consist of a run over 2000m, gymnastics and games.

After an ergometer test and estimation of lactate in 11 patients, and the examination of lung function (FVC, FEV1%FVC, PFR, MMEF, MEF50%FVC, MEF25%FVC) we started a cross-over study with two groups, each with 22 children.

With regular monitoring of pulse rate and frequency of breathing, and under supervision of a doctor, one group of children were exposed to this load for a fortnight while withdrawing postural drainage and percussion.

The other group was treated with postural drainage and percussion for 20 minutes. After a fortnight the two groups were changed after lung function testing. In a third group of children the postural therapy and percussion were substituted for the entire four weeks by physical exercise. In this group we monitored lung function continously.

The results give us a positive answer to our primary question, and give us hope that lung function will stablilise at a higher level during exercise. We observed an autodrainage effect, especially during running, and a more positive attitude towards physical activity and psychological behaviour.

**POSTER GROUP TWO No. 2.22**

CONTROL OF BREATHING AND VENTILATORY PATTERN DURING EXERCISE IN
PATIENTS WITH CYSTIC FIBROSIS.

R. Kraemer, B. Perren, M. Schoeni and E. Rossi.

Dept. of Pediatrics, University of Berne, Inselspital, CH-3010 Berne,
Switzerland.

Control of breathing and ventilatory pattern at rest and during the
steady-state-phase of progressive exercise was studied in 32 patients
with cystic fibrosis (CF), aged between 8 and 22 years. Breathing
pattern (ventilation (VE); O2-uptake (VO2) and CO2-production (VCO2))
as well as "central respiratory output" (mouth occlusion pressure
(P.1); mean inspiratory flow (Vt/Ti) and inspiratory time as fraction of total respiratory time (Ti/Ttot)) was measured at rest and
during bicycle-ergooxymetry, up to a working capacity at a heart rate
of 180/min. This workload was stepwise increased with increments of
0.5 watt/kg lean body mass (LBM) in at least 4 phases of 4 minutes.

VE, VO2 and VCO2 increase with progressive workload linearly and
dependent of lung involvement judged by pulmonary functions and
X-ray scores. Central respiratory drive (P.1) and mean inspiratory
flow (Vt/Ti) increase age-dependently steeper in respect to healthy
controls, whereas Ti/Ttot, representing the respiratory timing remains in a constant range for any age and any workload. VE and Vt/Ti
also increase linear and similar to controls with increasing VCO2
(the unit of metabolic load). In order to evaluate the effectiveness
of the thoracopulmonary system to convert the central respiratory
signals, the relationship between P.1 and Vt/Ti, VE resp. is considered as the "effective" inspiratory impedance. Whereas this relationship increases in healthy children curvilinear, in patients with
CF a plateau is reached for high P.1, indicating a higher thoracopulmonary impedance in patients with CF due to increased work of
breathing.

We conclude that ventilatory pattern during exercise in CF is characterized by increased impedance and respiratory drive, both related to the degree of reduced compliance and increased visco-elastic
work of the lung, which seems to be the major factor to limit physical performance in CF.

**POSTER GROUP TWO No. 2.23**

EXERCISE TESTING IN ASSESSING THERAPY FOR RESPIRATORY INFECTIONS

M. Harris, D.M. Cooper, I. Mitchell. Alberta Children's Hospital, University of Calgary, Calgary, Alberta, Canada. T2T 5C7.

Measured changes in pulmonary function tests (PFT's) are often small when compared to reported changes in lifestyle before and after acute pulmonary infections (API) in patients with Cystic Fibrosis (CF). We compared exercise testing (ET) pre and post therapy for API with conventional PFT's.

Ten patients with CF, aged 7 to 15 years, followed regularly in the CF Clinic and familiar with PFT's were studied during API associated with deteriorating PFT's and clinical status. All had significant cultures of Pseudomonas aeruginosa in their sputum. Pulmonary disease ranged from moderate to severe, but $PaO_2$ was >40 mmHg in air at the time of admission.

PFT's were measured using forced expiratory indices derived from maximal expiratory flow volume loops (Gould CPI 5000IV) and static lung volumes by plethysmography, both pre and post bronchodilator. Progressive treadmill stress testing to exhaustion was performed, monitored by ECG, clinical status, expired $O_2$, $CO_2$ and workload, at 20 second intervals (Gould CPI 7000III) prior to bronchodilator. All tests were performed before, immediately after and at 2 & 4 weeks post intensive antibiotic therapy.

Changes in PFT's showed a uniform trend of improvement in all indices, but none proved statistically significant. Larger improvements were noted in ET, particularly maximum work, peak work and $\dot{V}O_2$ max. The improvement in ET corresponded with the patient's and their families subjective assessment of well being.

| | initial | post therapy | 2 weeks post | 4 weeks post |
|---|---|---|---|---|
| $\dot{V}O_2$MAX+ | | | | |
| mean | 62.88* | 85.25* | 81.00 | 97.17 |
| range | 31-101 | 50-115 | 50-90 | 56-133 |
| MAXIMUM WORK COMPLETED+ | | | | |
| mean | 63.0# | 81.0# | 84.6 | 80.7 |
| range | 22-104 | 38-112 | 38-114 | 43-111 |

+ percent predicted normal
\* paired t test p< 0.005          #paired t test p< 0.001
No statistical difference between immediate and late results.

This study demonstrates that dynamic tests (ET) can be safely performed and can add significantly to static measurement (PFT's) in the assessment of progress during therapy in CF children. ET adds a new and seemingly more realistic dimension to assessing response to antibiotic therapy in CF.

**POSTER GROUP TWO No. 2.24**

EXERCISE TESTING IN CYSTIC FIBROSIS (CF) CHILDREN. G. BELLON,
SO SATTA, R. GILLY, Clinique Médicale Infantile A, Université Lyon I,
Centre Hospitalier Lyon–Sud, 69310 Pierre Bénite, FRANCE.

Exercise tolerance and cardiorespiratory adjusments were determined at peak
work capacity (PWC) during progressive exercise and at submaximal power
(Sub P) (PWC 50 % and PWC 66 %, 6 minutes each)on a cycle ergometer in
14 CF patients aged $12.0 \pm 2.4$ years (7 males) and 19 matched controls (C),
aged $11.2 \pm 2.9$ years (10 males).
The results were related to resting lung function tests (in all) and resting blood
gases (in CF). All CF had significant obstructive disease (CF versus C, % predicted) : FVC $75.6 \pm 20.34$ vs $97.6 \pm 12.4$ p$<$0.05, $FEV_1$ $61.3 \pm 23.6$ vs $97.5 \pm$
$9.4$ p$<$0.05, PEFR $71.8 \pm 22.6$ vs $102,2 \pm 15.0$ p$<$0.001, MMEF $39.3 \pm 25.2$
vs $97.1 \pm 16.3$ p $<$0.01. Most of them (12 of 14) had resting hypoxemia (PO 2$<$
80), but only 2  had resting hypercarbia (PCO2$>$40).
Although the maximum oxygen consumption ($\dot{V}O2$ max) showed no statistical
difference ($39.55 \pm 8.61$ ml.mn$^{-1}$. kg$^{-1}$ vs $43.44 \pm 6.67$), there was a respiratory
exercise limitation in CF : lower PWC ($3.055 \pm 0.639$ W.kg$^{-1}$ vs $3.654 \pm 0.593$
p$<$0.02), positive correlation between spirometric values and $\dot{V}O 2$ max in CF
only (FVC r = 0.72  p$<$0.01, $FEV_1$ r = 0.70 p$<$0.01, PEFR r : 0.55 p$<$0.05,
MMEF r = 0.57 p$<$0.05, PO 2 and PCO 2 Ns). A wasted ventilation was a
general observation : at exhaustion the CF ventilation (VE) averaged 112 %
of the predicted maximum ventilation ($112 \pm 32$ vs $71 \pm 12$, p$<$0.01), $\dot{V}E/PWC$
was elevated ($0.516 \pm 0.103$ l.mn$^{-1}$. w$^{-1}$ vs $0.417 \pm 0.057$ p$<$0.02) as VE/
$\dot{V}O 2$ max ($40.45 \pm 10.12$ l ml$^{-1}$ vs $34.99 \pm 6.53$ p$<$0.05). The peak heart
rate was lower ($181 \pm 8$  vs $192 \pm 8$  p$<$0.01).
However 3 CF including the 2 with resting hypercarbia showed individual
significantly abnormal $\dot{V}O 2$ max, became increasingly hypercarbic with PO 2
lowering  and had a significantly low oxygen pulse at PWC suggesting a cardio
vascular intolerance. Only 2 of them had significant abnormalities (increased
hypercarbia, lowered hypoxemia, abnormal oxygen pulse) at subP.
In most patients with CF, exercise remains possible and well tolerated. A
training program to improve their physical ability, and perhaps their entire
prognosis can be envisaged. Only the severely affected patients (spirometric
values less than 50 % of predicted, with or without hypercarbia) should engage
with caution in exercise training programs and strenuous physical activity.
But in all patients, the cardiorespiratory adjustments to exercise need be
evaluated to adapt the training program or/and objectively judge the results.

242

EXERCISE TESTING IN HOSPITALIZED CF PATIENTS

J.C. Kramer and M.L. Henly
St. John's Medical Centre, 1923 S. Utica, Tulsa,
Oklahoma 74104, USA.

We present what may be a sensitive method of
documenting improvement in acute endobronchial and
pulmonary relapse of chronic infection in CF. From May
to Dec. 1983 we studied 14 admissions of 9 CF patients
(6 male, 3 female; ages 5 to 20 years), using a
modification of the Bruce Multistage Exercise Test
(treadmill speeds from 1.5 to 5.5 mph, without
elevations). Heart rate (max. allowable 200/min), and
ECG were monitored. Oxygen saturation was monitored by
a Biox digital readout ear oximeter (max. allowable
fall from a resting state 10%). Of 45 tests, one was
discontinued because of tachycardia 200/min; 5 tests
were discontinued because of increasing hypoxia ($\leq$10%
fall). Half of these occurred in the presence of
hypoxia at rest (71% and 84% sat.); no lasting ill
effects were noted. Patients returned to within 30% of
resting state in 8 min. ECG monitoring did not
disclose any significant rhythm disturbances or cardiac
ECG changes of increasing RVH or RB strain. One
seriously ill patient failed to respond to treatment
and died 8 days after the test. Eight patients
responded to high dose IV antibiotic treatment. All
were offered aerobic exercises, with variable
complicance. Improvement in work output (speed x time)
varied from -14% to +200%, mean +74%, measured from
near beginning of hospitalization to near end of stay.
Exercise produced a change in oxygen sat. in 8
patients, range -16% to +8%, mean -1%. Starting sat.
improved little (except for one patient), range -2% to
+19%, mean +3%. Heart rate increase during exercise
varied from +9% to +146%, mean: +55%. The mean %
maximum predicted heart rate achieved was 76%, range of
64% to 91% at the beginning of hospitalization, and
within 5% at end of hospitalization. Improvement in
FVC (N=13) varied from -40% to +101%, mean +39%; FEV1
(N=13) range -29% to +152%, mean: +52%; PEF (N=11)
range -14% to +163%, mean +55%; RV (N=11) range -8% to
-51%, mean -23%; $PO_2$ (N=6) range +12% to +31%, mean
+21%; $PCO_2$ (N=6) -27% to +42%; mean -1%. Eight
readmissions showed +18% to -51% change in work output,
mean -25%, and a beginning $O_2$ saturation from +2% to
-10%, mean -4%.

**POSTER GROUP THREE No. 3.01**

LUNG FUNCTION AND OXYGEN UPTAKE DURING EXERCISE IN
16 - 17 YEAR OLD BOYS WITH CYSTIC FIBROSIS

Johan Kvalvik Stanghelle, Nils Hjeltnes & Dag Skyberg,
Sunnaas Hospital, 1450 Nesoddtangen and the Department
of Paediatrics, the Central Hospital of Aust-Agder,Norway.

As a part of prescribing individual training programs
and in evaluating their effects, eight out of totally
nine Norwegian boys with CF about 16 years old were
subjected to pulmonary function and bicycle exercise
testing. Eight healthy boys of the same age performed
the same tests.
  The CF boys showed large individual variations. However,
the two groups showed great differences in mean body height
and weight, pulmonary function variables and maximal
oxygen uptake. Increased ventilatory equivalent for
oxygen was a characteristic finding during rest and exercise for the CF boys, and their oxygen uptake was higher
during rest and corresponding work loads compared with
the controls. The maximal oxygen uptake for the CF boys
ranged from 40 to 125 % (mean 79 %) of predicted values.
  We have found the results from these exercise tests
valuable when we prescribe individual training programs,
and when repeated the tests will be of great value in
the evaluation of such programs.

**POSTER GROUP THREE No. 3.02**

TECHNETIUM-99M DTPA AEROSOL IMAGING WITH VIDEO-SUPERPOSITION
TECHNIQUES IN PATIENTS WITH CYSTIC FIBROSIS. G.R. Elliott, S.A. Sirr,
R.L. Morin, R.J. Boudreau, R.P.Chandler, W.J. Warwick, and M.K. Loken.
University of Minnesota Hospitals, Minneapolis, Minnesota, U.S.A.

This study was undertaken to evaluate the use of aerosol for
measuring regional ventilation and clearance patterns in patients with
cystic fibrosis (CF). Using a mixture of 10% concentration ethanol
added to Tc-99m DTPA solution, 0.5u particles were given with a
SynteVent aerosol delivery device. Count rates of 8-10 K/sec were
achieved in a supine position after 5 min. Gamma camera images were
obtained immediately after breathing the aerosol and at 30 and 90 min.
A video based prototype image processing system (Measuronics Corp.)
was used to superimpose the gamma camera images on current PA chest
radiographs as an aid in regional delineation of disease. Krypton-81m
ventilation scans correlated well with aerosol ventilation.
Clearance in CF patients with mild pulmonary disease was more
rapid than controls or CF patients with severe bronchiectasis. T-1/2
were 86, 48, and 33 min for controls, patients with severe and mild
pulmonary disease, respectively. Deposition and retention of
Tc99m-DPTA particles occurred in areas which were superimposible on PA
radiograph bronchectatic segments. In mild cases, small airway
plugging was evident by peripheral ventilation defects determined by
superpositioning techniques. Initial areas most often affected were
the apical and posterior segments of the upper lobes. Bronchial
drainage enhanced the clearance from bronchiectatic segments. A scan
pre and post bronchial alveolar lavage showed increased deposition in
the area lavaged. Figures A and B are scans with superposition
techniques in a control and severe CF lung respectively. Dark areas
represent non-ventilated areas, red areas (///) represent initial
deposition, and yellow areas (\\\) represent retention after 90 min.
At 90 min. the patient imaging revealed high intensity counts in areas
of bronchiectasis compared with uniform clearing in the control.

A 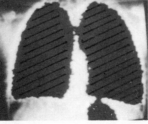 B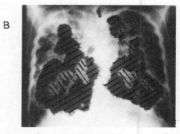

These techniques may be useful in the study of the pathogenesis and
evolution of small airway disease and development of bronchiectasis in
CF. They also appear helpful in assessing various treatment
modalities in CF and the early detection of small distal plugs.

**POSTER GROUP THREE No. 3.03**

ONCE A DAY THEOPHYLLINE (UNIPHYL) IN PATIENTS WITH CYSTIC FIBROSIS AND ASTHMA. J. Blessing, R. Leong, S. Machtinger, B. Hindi, S. Rubinstein, N. Lewiston, and R. Moss. Children's Hospital at Stanford Palo Alto, CA. 94304.

Nine patients with cystic fibrosis 6-37 years of age (average = 27 yrs) and 17 patients with asthma 12-22 years of age (average = 15 yrs) with reversible bronchospasm participated in a study to determine the efficacy of single daily theophylline dosing (Uniphyl - Pardue Fredrick Co.). Serum theophylline levels were evaluated over 24 hours after patients had been on a minimum of 5 days of a.m. medication. The study was repeated after the patients had been on 5 days of p.m. medication. Patients who had only been on prn theophylline were started on a low dose and advanced to maximum tolerated dose. The average tolerated dose for the cystic patients was 13 mg/kg/day and for the asthmatics 15 mg/kg/day. The following theophylline levels were obtained using the Pharmacia method:

|  |  | Cystic Fibrosis | | Asthma | |
|---|---|---|---|---|---|
|  |  | Day | Night | Day | Night |
|  | n= | 9 | 5 | 16 | 15 |
| Hr | 0/24 | 5 | 4 | 6 | 7 |
|  | 3 | 7 | 6 | 12 | 9 |
|  | 6 | 12 | 7 | 13 | 12 |
|  | 12 | 9 | 9 | 11 | 11 |
|  | 15 |  |  | 9 | 12 |
|  | 18 | 9 | 9 | 8 | 10 |

In conclusion, this form of theophylline was well tolerated in patients who had been on regular theophylline and provided relatively good levels and control of bronchospasm.

246

A DOUBLE-BLIND PLACEBO CONTROLLED TRIAL WITH AMBROXOL AND
N-ACETYLCYSTEINE FOR MUCOLYTIC TREATMENT IN CYSTIC FIBROSIS
Ratjen,F., Posselt,H.-G., Wönne,R., Stöver,B., Bender,S.W.
J.W. Goethe-University, Center of Paediatrics
D-6000 Frankfurt/M., FRG.

A rational basis for mucolytic therapy in CF is missing.
The effect of ambroxol (30 mg, 3 times daily) and N-acetylcysteine (200 mg, 3 times daily) was tested in a randomized prospective double-blind study, in which both therapy
groups were compared with placebo. The groups consisting
of 12 CF patients each (age >5 years, cooperative for lung
function testing) with mild to moderate disease (scored
according to Crispin and Norman, not exceding 15) were
matched for both age and severity of lung damage. Patients
on longterm antibiotic and bronchodilator therapy were
excluded.

A washout period of two weeks preceded the actual trial
of 12 weeks of treatment. Patients were evaluated at time
0, 6 and 12 weeks during climatically stable months (June
to September 83). Physiotherapy was constant during the
trial and uniformly performed by a physiotherapist two
hours before lung function testing.Assessment of therapeutic
efficiency consisted of a thorough history, physical examination and pulmonary function testing. In addition to
conventional spirometric measurements (FVC, VC, FEV, $FEV_1$/
VC, PEFR, V max at 75, 50 and 25 % of VC) body plethysmography was performed (TGV, Raw, SRaw, ERV, RV, TLC).
Trapped gas was determined from the difference between
TGV minus helium FRC.

No clinical differences were verified in the three therapy
groups. Concerning pulmonary function parameters, a significant impairment was found in the placebo group for both
$FEV_1$ (p < 0.05) and trapped air (p < 0.01) as compaired -
with the treatment groups. Differences between ambroxol
and N-acetylcysteine could not be observed. These data
suggest therapeutic effects in CF but should stimulate
further therapeutic trials on larger patients groups,
longer treatments periods and perhaps higher mucolytic
dosage.

Informed consent on this ethically approved study was
obtained in all patients.

**POSTER GROUP THREE No. 3.05**

NON-INVASIVE MONITORING OF BLOOD GAS PARAMETER IN PEDIATRIC AND
YOUNG ADULT PATIENTS WITH CYSTIC FIBROSIS

M. Alley, A. Spock, Department of Pediatrics, Duke University Medical
Center, Durham, North Carolina 27710

Evaluation of respiratory function in patients with cystic
fibrosis usually encompasses clinical evaluation, pulmonary function
testing, blood gas analyses and chest radiography. Non-invasive
methods of evaluating blood gas parameters have been utilized for
inpatients but they have not been studied in depth for outpatient
usage. Due to the lack of discomfort, such techniques would be much
more acceptable to patients, particularly those in the pediatric age
range. In this study, we prospectively compared the results of non-
invasive techniques, as measured by an IL capnograph for $PECO_2$ and
a BIOX oximeter for oxygen saturation ($SoxO_2$) with arterialized
blood gas values ($SaO_2$, $PaO_2$, $PaCO_2$) in 22 consecutive cystic
fibrosis patients, 5 of whom had multiple tests, resulting in a
total number of 31 comparisons. There were 21 caucasians with 1
black, 11 M and 11 F, with an age range of 6 to 31 years (mean 20.4).
The following results were obtained:

|       | $PaO_2$ | $SaO_2$ | $SoxO_2$ | $PaCO_2$ | $PECO_2$ |
|-------|---------|---------|----------|----------|----------|
| Range | 54-82   | 86-96   | 87-96    | 30-52    | 30-52    |
| Mean  | 65.1    | 91.5    | 91.6     | 41.0     | 40.9     |

|                      | Coefficient of Correlation |
|----------------------|----------------------------|
| $SoxO_2$ v $SaO_2$   | 0.789*                     |
| $PaO_2$ v $SoxO_2$   | 0.782*                     |
| $PECO_2$ v $PaCO_2$  | 0.964*                     |

*significance $p < 0.001$

These data indicate that $SaO_2$ and $PaO_2$ are both predictable from
$SoxO_2$ in cystic fibrosis patients, although there was a suggestion
of less accuracy in the black patient. The $PaCO_2$ is highly predictable from the $PECO_2$ in all instances. We suggest that the
capnograph and oximeter can be effectively used to monitor blood gas
parameters non-invasively in patients with cystic fibrosis. Any
abnormalities or variations from previous studies can be confirmed
by blood gas analysis. Further evaluations remain to be done in
black patients to determine the accuracy of the oximeter results.

**POSTER GROUP THREE No. 3.06**

INFLUENCE OF CHEMOTHERAPY ON AIRWAY REACTIVITY IN CYSTIC
FIBROSIS (CF) PATIENTS WITH CHRONIC PSEUDOMONAS AERUGINOSA
INFECTION.

Dawid Kramarz[1], Vibeke Johansen[1], Christian Koch[1], & Allan Bundgaard[2].
1 Cystic Fibrosis Centre, Department of Pediatrics, and
2 Laboratory of Respiratory Physiology, Department of Internal
Medicine B, Rigshospitalet, Copenhagen, Denmark.

Airway obstruction, responsive to $\beta$-2 agonists is frequent
in CF but the pathogenesis is unclear. We studied the relation
to activity of chronic Pseudomonas aeruginosa infection in 24
CF patients, without clinical asthma, being hospitalized for
14-day courses of anti-Pseudomonas treatment. Peak expiratory
flow rate (PEFR), forced expiratory volume in 1 second ($FEV_1$)
and mid-expiratory flow at 50% vital capacity ($MEF_{50\%}$) were
recorded on days 1, 7, and 14 of treatment, both before, and
15 minutes after inhalation of salbutamol, 15 µg per kg body
weight. Mean pre-inhalation values increased during treatment,
whereas the mean response to salbutamol was unaffected. On
days 1, 7, and 14 the $\triangle PEFR$ was + 5.8%, + 5.4%, and + 5.3% -
$\triangle FEV_1$ was + 6.4%, + 6.4%, and + 5.9%, - $\triangle MEF_{50\%}$ was + 18.8%,
+ 13.1%, and + 17.9%. Thirteen patients responded on one or more
occasions with + 15% in PEFR, + 15% in $FEV_1$, or + 30% in $MEF_{50\%}$.
Four patients responded with + 25% in PEFR, + 25% in $FEV_1$, or
+ 60% in $MEF_{50\%}$. However, positive responses were inconsistent
and poorly correlated to anti-microbial treatment. Furthermore,
the correlation between changes in individual lung function
parameters (PEFR, $FEV_1$, and $MEF_{50\%}$) was poor. None of the
patients responded with airway obstruction to the salbutamol
inhalation.

In conclusion: in CF patients, without asthma, airway reactivity,
as measured by response to inhaled $\beta$-2 agonists is highly
variable and influenced by chronic infection in an unpredictable
manner. Repeated tests must be done to.determine the therapeutic
value of $\beta$-2 agonists in individual patients.

**POSTER GROUP THREE No. 3.07**

CHANGE OF LUNG VOLUMES DURING POSITIVE EXPIRATORY PRESSURE
(PEP-MASK) PHYSIOTHERAPY IN CYSTIC FIBROSIS

S. Groth (2), G. Stafanger (3), H. Dirksen (2), J.B. Andersen (1),
M. Falck (3), M. Kjelstrup (3), The Depts. of Anaestesiology (1),
Herlev Hospital, The Depts. of Clinical Physiology (2), Paediatrics (3)
and Physiotherapy (4), The Finsen Institute, Rigshospitalet,
Strandboulevarden 49, DK- 2100  Copenhagen, Denmark.

To investigate changes of lung volumes during PEP-physiotherapy in
cystic fibrosis, the PEP resistance tube of the PEP-mask was
inserted into the expiratory outlet of our lung function equipment.
This enabled us to measure a variety of lung function variables,
while the lung function equipment functioned as a PEP-mask. We
studied 12 patients and found that during PEP-mask physiotherapy
functional residual capacity increased significantly ($P < 0.02$).
A decrease of wash-out volume ($P < 0.05$), lung clearance index
($P < 0.001$) and volume of trapped gas ($P < 0.05$) were registered,
whereas the total lung capacity, vital capacity, tidal volume and
residual volume did not change. Fifteen minutes after the termination
of the PEP-mask physiotherapy, the lung function of the patients
did not differ significantly from base line values. It is concluded
that during PEP-mask physiotherapy ventilation becomes more evenly
distributed and that some closed-off regions are opened.

**POSTER GROUP THREE No. 3.08**

IS BRONCHIAL HYPERREACTIVITY A SPECIAL FEATURE OF CF?

H.G. Wiesemann, U.Stephan and T. Lehnert
Univ. Kinderklinik Essen, Hufelandstrasse 55, Germany

Bronchial hyperreactivity is reported to have a high incidence in patients with CF. The reported incidence rates vary between 21% and 68% (Haluzska et al 1975; Mitchell et al 1978; Holzner et al 1981; Mellis et al 1981; van Asperen et al 1981).

We measured the reaction to inhaled histamine in a group of 22 patients between 10 and 26 years of age. The patients inhaled an aerosol containing concentrations of histaine up to 8 mg/ml. The control parameter was specific airway conductance.

Histamine challenge was postive only in those patients who had an acute exacerbation (increased cough/sputum production, fever, raised sedimentation rate/WBC). There was no correlation between the histamine threshold and the Shwachman score, or vital capacity, or FEV. In three children we determined the histamine threshold before and after antibiotic treatment; in all of them there was a marked decrease of histamine sensitivity. We conclude that the decrease of the histamine threshold in CF patients is related to acute exacerbations or acute lower respiratory tract infections. Bronchial hyperreactivity is not a special feature of CF. The discrepancies between the different incidence figures may be explained by different proportions of patients with acute exacerbations within the cohorts studied.

**POSTER GROUP THREE No. 3.09**

Pulmonary Mucociliary Clearance In Cystic Fibrosis: Changes Between Two Examinations In An 2 Weeks Interval.

Sandor Gonda*, Thom, K.*, Steinkamp, G.**, Müller, W.** and von der Hardt, H.**
Abteilung Nuklearmedizin und spezielle Biophysik* und Zentrum für Kinderheilkunde und Humangenetik** der Medizinischen Hochschule, D-3000 Hannover 61, FRG

The determination of the mucociliar clearance (MC) has been proposed as method to estimate the effect of mucolytic agents in cystic fibrosis (CF).
We have performed a study to prove the effect of an oral mucolytic agent on the MC and compared it with an untreated group. The second examination eas performed 2 weeks after the first one.
All these 6 patients were receiving antibiotics and/or bronchodilators, and were inhalating saline solution (NaCl 9 %). The MC was studied by 99m-Tc-labeled millimicrospheres delivered by a compressed air nebuliser. The patients habe been examined in the supine position. The regional activities have been measured by a gamma camera in the dorsal position. The time activity curves were obtained for the total lung, for the peripheral and for the central hilair zones. We have also measured the penetration of the particles.
The intraindividual variations were studied for all these parameters. The penetration showed very low changes between both measurements. A significant change was observed only in one patient. Important changes of the total lung MC were observed in 3 patients. The MC of the peripheral zone were not significantly modified. On the other hand, the modifications in the central zone were very important. In two patients, we have observed an important improvement of the MC in the central zone; slight impairements have been observed in 3 patients. The clinical data have also confirmed these intraindividual changes. The MC of the central zone, i.e. the great bronchi, showed the most important changes in two following measurements. In the assessment of the effects of mucolytic agents, it must be considered, that MC can spontaneously change between two examinations with an interval of 2 weeks. The MC can improve in untreated patients and, in other hand, can not improved in treated patients, because other factors (infection) act against a waited improvement.

**POSTER GROUP THREE No. 3.10**

MAXIMUM STATIC RESPIRATORY PRESSURES IN CYSTIC FIBROSIS AND ASTHMA.

J. Marks, F. Leahy, S. O'Neill, A. Tal, H. Pasterkamp, V. Chernick, Section of Pediatric Respirology, University of Manitoba, Children's Hospital, Winnipeg, Manitoba.

We have measured maximal static inspiratory and expiratory pressures (PiMax and PeMax) in 26 asthmatic patients (ages 5 - 20). We compared the asthmatic group to a group of 25 CF patients and 80 normals previously reported (S. O'Neill et al, ARRD Dec 1983) using the same method to determine if a difference in nutritional status (Body Mass Percentile, BMP) affects PiMax and PeMax in patients with chronic hyperinflation. The asthmatic patients were hyperinflated (RV/TLC .40 ± .1(SD), RV 214 ± 92% predicted) but had Pi and PeMax similar to normals. Asthmatics compared to CF patients were significantly better nourished (mean BMP 104% vs 78%, p<.001), less hyperinflated (mean RV/TLC .40 vs .50, p<.01) and less obstructed (mean $FEV_1$ % predicted 78% vs 35%, p<.001). In spite of these differences the mean PiMax and PeMax was similar in both groups (p>.05). The mean age of the 2 groups was different (Asthma - 11.0y vs CF - 14.5y, p<.01) and there was a positive correlation between age and PeMax in both groups and normals (CF:r=.614, p<.001, Asthma:r=.475, p<.02) We therefore examined asthmatic and CF patients of similar age (Asthma 12.3 ± 1.1y n=10, CF 12.7 ± 1.1y n=7). In this age group asthmatic patients had significantly higher PeMax than CF patients (mean 117.1 vs 91.4 cm $H_2O$, p<.05). Pi Max was not significantly different. In the asthmatic patients there was no correlation between hyperinflation (RV/TLC) and PiMax or PeMax. There was a negative correlation between PiMax and the degree of airflow obstruction ($FEV_1$ % predicted: r=-.472, p<.02). Asthmatics with airflow obstruction ($FEV_1$ 60.1 ± 5.5% predicted, n=9) had significantly higher PiMax than those without obstruction ($FEV_1$ 88 ± 8.9% predicted, n=15), 127.7 ± 27.2 cm $H_2O$ vs 97.8 ± 23.1 cm $H_2O$ (p<.01). There was no correlation between PiMax and $FEV_1$ with CF patients. We conclude 1) nutritional status does affect expiratory muscle strength in patients with chronic airflow obstruction. 2) inspiratory muscle strength may improve due to a training effect secondary to chronic airflow obstruction in well nourished patients.

(Funded by the Children's Hospital Research Foundation, Mead-Johnson and Organon (Canada).

**POSTER GROUP THREE No. 3.11**

BRONCHIAL RESPONSIVENESS TO ISOCAPNIC HYPERVENTILATION OF COLD AIR AND

HIGH DOSE SALBUTAMOL IN CYSTIC FIBROSIS

J. Marks, A. Tal, H. Pasterkamp, R. D. Pagtakhan, Section of Pediatric
Respirology, University of Manitoba, Children's Hospital, Winnipeg,
Manitoba.
We have studied bronchial responsiveness of CF subjects using isocapnic hyperventilation with cold air (IHCA).  We then correlated the
subjects' response to IHCA with their response to a high dose of a
$\beta_2$-adrenergic agent and with their history of atopy. We studied 8
males and 1 female ranging in age from 9 to 28 (mean 15.8). Cold air
challenge was done as previously reported (A. Tal et al, J Pediatr
Mar 84).  On a separate day flow volume curves and lung volumes were
measured before and after 0.03 ml/kg salbutamol respiratory solution,
diluted to 2 ml with normal saline and delivered by face mask.
Clinical scores (NIH Scoring System) of the subjects ranged from 63
to 95.  They had no acute pulmonary exacerbations in the preceding
3 mo.  Chest physiotherapy was done 1-2 hr. prior to testing.  Mean
maximal change (max $\Delta$ %) in $FEV_1$ post IHCA was -5.8% ± 4.3 (SE).  Only
3/9 subjects had a max $\Delta$ % in $FEV_1$ of $\geq$-15%.  There was no correlation
between the max $\Delta$ % in $FEV_1$ post IHCA and the response after high dose
salbutamol, or with a history of atopy.  Mean % change after bronchodilator was +11.3% ± 3.9 for $FEV_1$, +31.4% ± 8.1 for PEFR, and +13.9% ±
9.2 for $FEF_{50}$.  Three subjects had no change after bronchodilator.  We
compared each subject's previous best response after 2 puffs of salbutamol aerosol (Ventolin) with their response after high dose
salbutamol.  Four subjects with no previous response to Ventolin
showed a significant increase in PEFR after high dose salbutamol
(p<.02).  Two subjects with previous response to bronchodilator
showed a better response after high dose salbutamol.  The 3 subjects
with no response to high dose salbutamol had shown no response to
bronchodilator in the past.  In conclusion, cold air hyperventilation
does not produce bronchospasm in most CF patients although many of
them show bronchial responsiveness after $\beta$-adrenergic treatment.
Higher doses of $\beta$-sympathomimetic drugs may be needed in patients with
cystic fibrosis.

**POSTER GROUP THREE No. 3.12**

BIDIRECTIONAL CHANGES OF FORCED EXPIRATORY VOLUME IN 1 SEC.(FEV$_1$) INDUCED BY COLD AIR CHALLENGE (CACh) IN PATIENTS WITH CYSTIC FIBROSIS (CF).

Linda L. Darga, George Polgar, Maximilian Zach and Larry A. Eason. Departments of Pediatrics, Wayne State University, Children's Hospital of Michigan, 3901 Beaubien Blvd., Detroit, Mi. 48201 and University of Graz, Austria.

Controlled challenges with pharmacological agents have resulted in high frequencies of bronchial hyperreactivity in children with CF [1]. In asthmatic children CACh proved to be comparably useful for testing hyperreactivity [2]. Twelve patients with CF (mean age 15 years, range 8-27), who had mild to severe lung diseases, but no respiratory exacerbation for at least three weeks and no bronchodilator treatment for at least 24 hours, breathed room air <-15°C at 75% MVV for four minutes under eucapnic conditions. Based on reference intervals established for healthy and asthmatic children [2], 3 of 12 patients had FEV$_1$ values at 5 minutes post-CACh which were below baseline by 12, 14 and 28%, within the range for asthmatics. However, in 5 of 12 patients FEV$_1$ increased by 4-27% above baseline, exceeding the +2SD reference limit for healthy children. Values of those responding with decreased FEV$_1$ tended to reverse by 15 minutes post-CACh, but in all those with increased FEV$_1$ values remained 4-29% above baseline. Four of 5 patients with this paradoxical response had the lowest baseline FEV$_1$s in % predicted. These results indicate that in CF the effect of CACh might be different from that of pharmacological agents. The few results of decreased flow could have been due to true bronchospasm, but also to a decreased contribution of volume from the now less unstable downstream segment of anatomical dead space. The paradoxical increases of FEV$_1$ post-CACh in the most severely diseased patients were probably related to the prevention of a collapse of large, unstable airways allowing for a more complete contribution of the alveolar air volume to the first second of forced expiration. This would be the reverse situation of the observed paradoxical decrease of end-expiratory flow after an inhaled bronchodilator in children with CF [3]. In view of the possible bidirectional changes induced by airway instability, the effects of both natural causes of airway hyperreactivity and of bronchodilators in CF must be further explored.

REF.: 1. Mellis, C.M., Levison, H.: Bronchial reactivity in cystic fibrosis. Pediatrics 61:446, 1978.
        2. Zach, M., Polgar, G., Kump, H. and Kroisel, P.: Cold air challenge of airway hyperreactivity in children: practical application and theoretical aspects. Pediatric Research (in press).
        3. Zach, M., Kump, H., Oberwaldner, B., Polgar, G.: Bronchodilator-induced alterations of supramaximal expiratory flow transients in children with cystic fibrosis. 12th Annual Meeting of the EWGCF, Athens, Greece, October 3-4, 1983.

**POSTER GROUP THREE No. 3.13**

INHIBITION AND REVERSIBILITY OF EXPERIMENTAL 'BRONCHITIS'
Duncan F. Rogers and Peter K. Jeffery
Department of Lung Pathology, Cardiothoracic Institute,
Brompton Hospital, London SW3 6HP.

Secretory cell hyperplasia with a shift to a predominance of acidic secretory cells is an histological change characteristic of chronic bronchitis and cystic fibrosis. Whole tobacco smoke (TS) given daily for two weeks induces similar histological changes in the airways of specific pathogen-free rats. Counting the number of secretory cells, containing neutral or acidic mucin, allows the degree of hyperplasia to be quantified. The present studies assess whether secretory cell hyperplasia is inhibited by a 'mucolytic' agent or a number of anti-inflammatory drugs and whether the time course of recovery after cessation of TS can be shortened by their administration. Secretory cell hyperplasia is as high as 207% above control values when 'middle to high tar' cigarettes are used.

Inhibition: Secretory cell hyperplasia was inhibited to varying degrees by indomethacin (indo), flurbiprofen (flur), dexamethasone (dexa), prednisolone (pred), hydrocortisone (hydro) and a mucolytic drug, N-acetylcysteine (Nac) given during the period of exposure to TS:

DEGREE OF INHIBITION (%) OF SECRETORY CELL HYPERPLASIA

| Airway | Drug (daily dose, mg/kg, and administration) | | | | |
|---|---|---|---|---|---|
| | indo (4,ip) | dexa (2,ip) | pred (4,ip) | hydro (4,ip) | Nac (973,oral) |
| TRACHEA | 110* | NS | NS | NS | 36 |
| LUNG: proximal | 82* | 79* | 65* | 77* | 61 |
| peripheral | 70 | 120* | 55 | 35 | 76* |

ip = intra peritoneal injection, oral = 1% of drinking water
* = complete inhibition, NS = inhibition not significant

Recovery: The time for the increase in secretory cell number to return to control values (ie. recovery) took between 21 and 84 days depending on airway level. Indomethacin and flurbiprofen (4 mg/kg,ip) had no effect on recovery time in the trachea but shortened recovery to between 4 and 9 days in the intrapulmonary airways.

All the drugs tested inhibited TS-induced secretory cell hyperplasia. Nac and flurbiprofen were the least toxic. Thus, the drugs may have a clinical role in the treatment of hypersecretory conditions.

**POSTER GROUP THREE No. 3.14**

NOCTURNAL HYPOXEMIA IN PATIENTS WITH CYSTIC FIBROSIS

From the Departments of Lung Medicine, Infectious Diseases, Clinical Physiology, Neurophysiology and Pediatrics, University Hospital, Lund, Sweden.
B. Midgren, I. Atterholm, K. Petterson, P. Airikkala, D. Elmqvist and R. Kornfält.

CF-patients with severe hypoxemia, which is not relieved by conventional treatment (e.g. antibiotics, physiotherapy) shall be recommended oxygen therapy. Casual blood gas measurements during the day do not give adequate information about the degree of hypoxemia or hypercapnia throughout the day or information about the blood gases during the night, when hypoxemia often worsens.
In this study are presented the results of continous measurements of blood gases with non-invasive methods during an entire night's sleep with a simultaneous registration of sleep stages. Two male CF-patients aged 16 and 19 years and with very advanced lung disease were examined with polygraphic sleep recordings including EEG, EOG, EMG of chin muscles and ECG. Oxygen saturation was measured with a Hewlett-Packard ear oxymeter HP 47201A and cutaneous $pCO_2$ with a Hewlett-Packard cutaneous capnometer HP 47210A A10. The results of the registration are presented in diagrams. The 16-year old boy showed a considerable and progressive lowering of oxygen saturation during the night. The cutaneous $pCO_2$ increased with onset of sleep to reach a stable plateau during the rest of the night. During a second night's recording, supplemental oxygen, 0.8 l/min, was given via nasal prongs. The sleep induced hypoxemia was greatly reduced. Only during the REM sleep period there was a marked desaturation. This was associated with a large increase in cutaneous $pCO_2$, which reached very high levels during the REM sleep. The 19-year-old boy was hypoxemic and hypercapnic in the awake stage, but showed no further aggravation of his blood gas disturbances during sleep.
The study shows that it is impossible to predict the nocturnal blood gases from the diurnal. The capnometry makes it possible to detect the potentially dangerous hypercapnia during oxygen therapy and to adjust oxygen flow to the appropriate level.

**POSTER GROUP THREE No. 3.15**

SURVIVAL RATES IN CYSTIC FIBROSIS:  THE INFLUENCES
OF ALLERGY AND PSEUDOMONAS INFECTION OF THE
LUNGS

Robert W. Wilmott, Saba L. Tyson, Duncan J. Matthew and John
F.   Soothill. The Respiratory Unit, The Hospital for Sick
Children, Great Ormond Street, London, and The Department of
Immunology, The Institute of Child Health, Guilford Street,
London, England.

Most cystic fibrosis (CF) patients eventually die from
progressive obstructive pulmonary disease and respiratory
failure.   Allergy and  chronic Pseudomonas aeruginosa (PA)
infection are two factors which possibly affect the clinical
severity of CF pulmonary disease, although the role of allergy
is controversial.  We therefore examined the effects of these
factors on CF survival rates.  Actuarial survival analysis for the
period 1974 to 1979 was performed with data from 117 CF
children who were skin tested in 1974 and classified as allergic
(A+) or non-allergic (A-) by their reactions to 12 prick tests
with common environmental allergens.   Patients were also
classified according to whether or not they had chronic
pulmonary infection with PA in 1974 (PA+, PA-). Survival rates
in A+ patients were not significantly different from those in the
A-group (% survival to 16 yr. 67% vs 80% $p > 0.05$).  Whereas
the PA+ group had significantly worse survival rates than the
PA-group (% survival to 16 yr. 53% vs. 84%, $P < 0.05$) by Desu
rank sum test.  There was no significant interaction between
allergic skin reactions and either age of onset of chronic PA
infection or subsequent duration of survival.   Chronic
pulmonary PA infection is an important factor related to
severity of pulmonary disease in CF whereas the effect of
hypersensitivity to common environmental allergens appears to
be insignificant.

**POSTER GROUP THREE No. 3.16**

ELECTRON MICROSCOPY OF THE LUNG IN CYSTIC FIBROSIS.

Delia Beju and John C. Kramer. The William and Natalie Warren
Medical Institute and the University of Oklahoma Tulsa Medical
College, 6465 South Yale, Suite 1010, Tulsa, Oklahoma  74136, U.S.A.

The ultrastructure of the pulmonary alveoli was investigated in
lung from patients who died with cystic fibrosis.  The morphology
was dominated by atelectasis, bronchiectasis, edema, interstitial
fibrosis, and diminished alveolar space.  One case showed severe
necrosis and numerous microorganisms trapped in the cellular
debris.  Electron microscopic examination revealed extensive
interstitial accumulation of elastic and collagenous fibers.
Intraalveolar and interstitial edema were noted.  There was
alteration of the capillary wall manifested by swollen endothelial
cells, intraluminal cell processes, numerous pinocytotic vesicles
and blisters, and rare intracytoplasmic myelin figures.  The
capillaries were often tortuous, measuring over $30\mu m$ in diameter,
and contained frequent neutrophils, platelets and fibrin.
Occasionally the capillaries bulged into the alveolar space.
Modifications of the alveolar lining epithelium were seen involving
primarily the type II cells, which showed irregular topographic
distribution, a reduced number of luminal microvilli, and an
inconsistent number of cytoplasmic lamellar bodies and cell
processes penetrating the basal lamina.  Intraalveolar and
intercellular accumulation of lung surfactant was also demonstrated.
The results show ultrastructural changes of the alveoli
underlying the pulmonary dysfunction in cystic fibrosis.
Morphological evidences of lung surfactant involvement in cystic
fibrosis are presented.  Considering that neither the type II cells
nor the amount of intracellular surfactant show an increase in our
material, the intraalveolar accumulation of tubular myelin may be
the result of a faulty clearance mechanism or altered physiochemical
properties.  The disturbance of the lung surfactant function could
account for some of the pulmonary condition manifested in cystic
fibrosis.

**POSTER GROUP THREE No. 3.17**

ORAL HIGH FREQUENCY OSCILLATION IMPROVES LUNG AND MUCOCILIARY
CLEARANCE IN NORMAL SUBJECTS.

R.J.D. GEORGE, M.A. JOHNSON, D. PAVIA, J.E. AGNEW, S.W. CLARKE,

D.M. GEDDES,  London Chest Hospital, Bonner Road, London, E2 9JX.

The effects of oral high frequency oscillation (OHFO) on
mucociliary clearance (MCC) was studied in 7 normal subjects by
comparing clearance of radiolabelled aerosol particles from the lung
during OHFO with control.  The control run and OHFO run were
carried out on separate days and delivered in random order.  OHFO
was applied to the air column by an 8" loudspeaker delivering sine
waves (mean frequency 10 Hz) through a mouth piece.  Following
inhalation of $^{99}$Tc  labelled polystyrene particles (diameter 5$\mu$)
a background count was measured by scintillation counters.
Additional counts were then made half hourly over the ensuing 6
hours with a final count at 24 hours.  During the HFO limb
30 minutes oscillation alternated with 30 minutes rest to coincide
with the scintillation counts.  Between 3 and 4.5 hours OHFO
cleared approximately 10% more particles than control ($p < 0.05$).
Overall MCC as expressed by the time taken to clear 90% of the
deposit was 130% that of control ($p < 0.05$).

The technique which was comfortable and well tolerated, may be of
therapeutic benefit in those with chronic sputum retention and
merits further investigation.

**POSTER GROUP THREE No. 3.18**

THE CHANGING BRONCHODILATOR RESPONSIVENESS IN CYSTIC FIBROSIS (C.F.)

Nancy L. Hordvik, B.S., R.R.T., Peter König, M.D., Ph.D., Cynthia
Kreutz, B.S., Debra Morris, M.S., R.N., Giulio J. Barbero, M.D.,
Department of Child Health, University of Missouri Health Sciences
Center, Columbia, Missouri, 65212, USA

Previous cross-sectional studies have shown widely differing
responsiveness to bronchodilators. A longitudinal, 2 year study
was performed in 20 CF patients. Bronchodilator (B.D.) responsiveness was repeatedly tested by spirometry before and 10 minutes
after the administration of 0.5ml isoetharine 1% solution by
nebulizer. Significant bronchodilation was considered an increase
of 10% in FVC, 15% $FEV_1$ or 49% $FEF_{25-75\%}$. During hospitalizations
for i.v. antibiotic therapy, all but one patient had significant
b.d. response at least once. Only 5/15 tested had positive skin
tests for allergy. The highest number of significant b.d. tests
were found with $FEF_{25-75\%}$ (23% of tests on admission as opposed to
5% with $FEV_1$ and 7% with FVC). % b.d tended to increase during
hospitalization along with improving baseline.

% bronchodilation during hospitalization (mean±SEM)

| | Days of hospitalization | | | | | |
|---|---|---|---|---|---|---|
| | 1–3 | 4–6 | 7–9 | 10–12 | 13–15 | 16–18 |
| FVC | 6.6±3.7 | 4.6±1.4 | 4.2±2.4 | 5.0±2.9 | 6.2±3.3 | 12.8±5.7 |
| $FEV_1$ | 4.9±3.2 | 11.6±6.0 | 12.2±4.0 | 6.3±3.7 | 10.6±4.4 | 15.2±6.9 |
| $FEF_{25-75\%}$ | 24.8±8.3 | 28.0±6.3 | 50.0±8.4 | 32.6±10.9 | 41.6±11.5 | 59.6±10.0 |
| n | 20 | 14 | 15 | 12 | 16 | 6 |

% b.d. $FEF_{25-75\%}$ increased significantly from 24.8% on admission
to 59.6% on day 16-18 (p<0.0025). $FEV_1$ and FVC showed similar ten-
dencies, but the change did not reach statistical significance. On
day 16-18 57% of all tests performed showed significant b.d. The
pattern during hospitalization reversed after discharge with gradual
decrease in % b.d. parallel with decrease in baseline. Conclusions:
1) The prevalence of significant b.d. responsiveness is much higher
at certain stages of the disease than previous studies indicated; 2)
A post- bronchodilator measurement can be useful for routine testing
of CF patients as a potential guide for bronchodilator therapy and an
indicator of the real level of pulmonary function; 3) b.d. responsiveness changes with disease stage, apparently increasing with
clearing of infiltrates and/or improved clearance of mucus
secretions.

**POSTER GROUP THREE No. 3.19**

INFLAMMATION OF THE BRONCHIAL MUCOSA IN CYSTIC FIBROSIS:
CORRELATION BETWEEN BRONCHOSCOPIC, MICROSCOPIC AND
ULTRASTRUCTURAL FINDINGS

P.Wunderlich[1], R.Fischer[2], Christa Kemmer[2],
H.-J.Dietzsch[1] and B.Gottschalk[1]

1) Children's Hospital, Dept. of Bronchopneumology,
   Medical Academy "Carl Gustav Carus" Dresden
2) Institute of Pathology, Medical Academy
   "Carl Gustav Carus" Dresden
   German Democratic Republic
   8019 Dresden, Fetscherstrasse 74

22 patients (14 boys and 8 girls, 7 to 17 years old)
with cystic fibrosis underwent a special bronchological
investigation in general anaesthesia with muscle relaxation using a ventilation bronchoscope (Friedel's
type). The endoscopic picture of the mucous membranes
was compared with the state of the bronchial secretions,
its bacteriology and content of acid mucopolysaccharides
and DNA fibers (semiquantitative estimations). In all
patients small biopsies of the mucous membrane (central
part of the bronchial tree) were taken for light and
electron microscopy. The degree of reddening, swelling
of the mucous membrane and hypersecretion was in some
agreement with the intensity of the cellular infiltration and the production of pus (microscopic investigation). Secondary ultrastructural changes were
detected in nearly all children: cellular oedema,
swelling of mitochondria, dilatation of the endoplasmic
reticulum, protrusion of cells and fusion of cilia,
enlarged intercellular spaces, thickening of the epithelial basal membrane, increased number of goblet
cells, microtubular abnormalities of the cilia, lesions
of the apical cell membranes with loss of cilia and
microvilli. These changes of ultrastructure were not
correlated to the above mentioned signs of inflammation.

**POSTER GROUP THREE No. 3.20**

SURVIVAL WITH CYSTIC FIBROSIS IN NOVA SCOTIA:    1950-1983

C.T. Gillespie, A.C. Irwin, I.M. O'Kane, V.T. Belgaumkar
Departments of Pediatrics and Preventive Medicine, Dalhousie
University and The Izaak Walton Killam Hospital for Children, Box
3070, Halifax, Nova Scotia, B3J 3G9   Canada

The survival of 207 patients from Nova Scotia (NS) with cystic
fibrosis (CF), consecutively diagnosed and treated from 1950 to 1983,
was calculated using life table methods.  Patients were divided into
3 cohorts based on therapy prevailing during specific periods:
Cohort I, 47 patients diagnosed from January 1, 1950 to June 30, 1958,
before a CF clinic was established in the fall of 1958; Cohort II, 67
diagnosed during the first 8 years of clinic operation from July 1,
1958 to June 30, 1966; and cohort III, 93 diagnosed between July 1,
1966 and December 31, 1983 and treated under a new protocol.

Before the clinic began, diagnosis was based on clinical history
and duodenal trypsin levels and treatment was provided by various
physicians throughout the province.  After the clinic began all
patients in NS were registered there and received treatment under its
auspices.  From 1959 onward, pilocarpine iontophoresis was used for
confirmation of diagnosis.  Inhalation therapy (mist tents,
intermittent aerosols) was undertaken for prominent respiratory
complaints, and antibiotics given more frequently in relatively low
doses for prolonged periods.  Depending on clinical status some were
admitted to hospital but most were placed on daily home treatment.

Cohort III therapy, governed by new therapeutic guidelines
emphasizing more comprehensive preventive therapy for all patients,
included hospitalization at diagnosis and provision of mist tents,
intermittent aerosol therapy, postural drainage, and specific,
intensive but intermittent antibiotic therapy, high protein high
carbohydrate diet, water-soluble vitamins, rehospitalization early
and "PRN" to avoid or limit complications, full activity and frequent
clinic followup.

There were 2 survivors from cohort I, 28 from cohort II and 86
from cohort III.  Survival for cohorts II and III combined was 71%
and for cohort III 93%.

We conclude that comprehensive preventive therapy started in all
patients at diagnosis and consistently maintained thereafter is
effective and offers reasonable expectation of survival into
adulthood for the majority of patients with CF.

**POSTER GROUP THREE No. 3.21**

STORAGE, RETRIEVAL AND COMPARISON OF DATA. THE USE OF A
MICROCOMPUTER AT ST JAMES'S TERTIARY REFERRAL CENTRE.

MILLER M G, LITTLEWOOD J M.
CYSTIC FIBROSIS REGIONAL TERTIARY REFERRAL CENTRE
ST JAMES'S HOSPITAL, LEEDS.

Since early 1980 the concept of regular, full assessment of
patients with cystic fibrosis has been developed. This has led
to the accumulation of much data on over a hundred patients.

The Royal Variety Club of Great Britain paid for a Sirius computer
for this centre and a Software Package was developed with the help
of Baron systems.

120 items of information from each assessment is filed onto a
diskette. A diskette holds 3 full assessments for each of 160
patients. Use of another programme transfers up to 16 fields
per patient, in addition to Patient Name, Age and Assessment Number,
to a commercially available data base programme D Base II. Easy
and rapid computation can then be made on the data.

Further files have been built up to help in running our Day Unit and
monitoring our treatment of in-patients.

This poster is presented to stimulate discussion between cystic
fibrosis centres on the use of microcomputers and on the exchange
of suitable data on treatment, complications and associated
factors.

**POSTER GROUP THREE No. 3.22**

A COMPARISON OF THE SHWACHMAN, CHRISPIN-NORMAN AND BRASFIELD METHOD
FOR SCORING OF CHEST RADIOGRAPHS OF PATIENTS WITH CYSTIC FIBROSIS.

Dankert-Roelse J.E. , A. Martijn, G.J. te Meerman, H. van Woerden.
Departments of Pediatrics and Human Genetics,
State University of Groningen, The Netherlands

Aim of study. The aim of this study was to investigate the
instrumental qualities of the three methods available for scoring of
chest radiographs of Cystic Fibrosis patients.
Materials and methods. Three systems have been described for
scoring of Chest Radiographs in Cystic Fibrosis patients: The
Shwachman-Kulczycki, the Chrispin-Norman and the Brasfield method.
Divided over 6 evenings 60 radiographs of 39 patients were scored
independently according to the three methods, using separate
evenings for all methods. Scoring was done independently in
separate rooms and in a counterbalanced order.
Results and discussion. The different scoring methods are not
systematically different: the intercorrelation within the methods
is not higher than the correlation between methods. The standard
error of measurement is in all methods rather large: The average
standard error of measurement is 57% of the sample standard
deviation, equivalent with 3.3 points on the 25 point Shwachman
scale, 3.2 points on the 22 point Brasfield scale and 4.0 points on
the 38 point Chrispin-Norman scale. The correlation between a
combined score is significantly higher (.94) than the Z-transformed
mean correlation of .84 between tests. Evaluation of scoring
differences indicated that specific observer training on the
relevant discrimination may improve both the inter- and
intra-observerreliability.
Conclusions. A substantial improvement of the measurement error
can be obtained by combining the scores of the three methods. The
standard error of measurement for each method is so large that
clinical evaluations should never be made on the basis of absolutely
scored Chest Radiographs. Independent rescoring with a different
method of the same photographs gives a significant improvement of
the precision. New scoring methods should be introduced only when a
specific difference or advantage compared with other methods can be
demonstrated.

References:
Shwachman H. Kulczycki L.L. Long term study of one hundred five
patients with cystic fibrosis Am. J. Dis. Child. 1958,96:6-15
Chrispin A.R. Norman A.P. The systematic evaluation of the chest
radiograph in Cystic Fibrosis. Pediatric radiology 1974,2:101-106
Brasfield D. Hicks J. Soong S. Tiller R.E. The chest roentgenogram
in Cystic Fibrosis: a new screening system. Pediatrics 1979,63:24-29

## CYSTIC FIBROSIS IN ADULTS IN THE UNITED KINGDOM

Penketh, A.R.L., Wise, A., Hodson, M.E. and Batten, J.C.
Cardiothoracic Institute, Brompton Hospital, London SW3 6HP.

A significant number of cystic fibrosis patients now survive into adult life. Many older patients have complications of the disease not always seen in childhood and it is recommended that they should be cared for in specialised units. A marked improvement in survival of CF patients in such units has been reported from the USA and Denmark. We report our experience at the Brompton Hospital CF Unit, to provide information for physicians who may in the future become involved in the care of CF adults.

286 patients were seen between 1965 and 1982, 164 males (57%) and 122 females, aged 16 to 50 years. The majority of patients presented classically in infancy with respiratory problems and malabsorption, but 17 were diagnosed in adult life, four in their thirties. Pulmonary disease was almost universal, (99%) and responsible for 94% of all deaths and two thirds of hospital admissions. All patients had a chronic productive cough by the age of 20, half before the age of five. Many complained of wheezing, but reversible airflow obstruction (a greater than 10% increase in $FEV_1$ with salbutamol) was present in only 37% of those tested. Minor haemoptysis was very common (60%) but major episodes less so (8%). Pneumothorax was seen in 19% and was often recurrent. Right heart failure occurred in 15%. Thirty-four patients (12%) had no symptoms of malabsorption and seven were able to stop pancreatic supplements altogether. Acute meconium ileus equivalent was seen in 15% and a chronic partial obstruction with episodic symptoms in a further 20%. Diabetes mellitus developed in 33 cases, 11 of whom were insulin-dependent. Hepatomegaly was common (32%), often without biochemical abnormalities, and only 1% of patients developed portal hypertension. 109 patients have died, 94% from infection or other pulmonary complications - 177 were alive in December 1982, mean age 26 years. 78% of patients were in full time education, full or part-time employment or housewives, and only 12% were unemployed for reasons of health. Many patients are married and nine women have borne children. The average time between hospital admissions was seven months, but 40% were admitted less than anually.

The incidence of other complications and features of the disease and aspects of treatment will be discussed; in particular the social and psychological problems of the transition from adolescent to independent adult. The improvement in survival and quality of life for CF adults should encourage a positive attitude in those caring for them.

**POSTER GROUP THREE No. 3.24**

COMPREHENSIVE CLINICAL AND LABORATORY ASSESSMENT IN CYSTIC FIBROSIS

Littlewood J M, Kelleher J, Losowsky M S, Page R, Crollick A J,
Miller M G, Conway S P, Firth J, MacDonald A, Henry F.
Cystic Fibrosis Referral Centre
St James's University Hospital, Leeds

One hundred and three C.F. patients from the Yorkshire Region had a
comprehensive clinical, laboratory, radiological, dietetic and
physiotherapy assessment. In a further five patients,previously
considered to have C.F. the diagnosis was not confirmed and an
alternative diagnosis established.

There were 55 males and 48 females; the average age was 8.2 years,
the mean Shwachmann score 74 (range 100 - 30) and the mean Chrispin-
Norman x-ray score 9. At the time of initial assessment 57 patients
were attending our C.F. clinic and 46 referred from clinics of 20
other paediatricians and chest physicians.

Delays in diagnosis were common (20% 7 1 year, 27% 7 6 months and
40% 7 3 months). Ten families had no knowledge of the C.F. Trust,
22 siblings had not had a sweat test.

Detailed clinical, laboratory and x-ray evaluation revealed evidence
of active chest infection in 34 patients. 34 had inflammatory
infiltration on chest x-ray, 24 had an absolute neutrophil count
greater than 7,500 per cu.mm., 9 patients were growing staph. aureus
or haemophilus influenzae or both and not on an appropriate
antibiotic. 23 patients had an ESR more than 25. 27 had a total
white blood cell count more than 12,000. These results not
infrequently resulted in more aggressive management of the chest
infection. Significant malabsorption persisted in 78 treated patients
and evidence of gastro-intestinal involvement was invariable. Sub-
normal fat soluble vitamin levels were present; Vit A - 68%, Vit E -
88%. Mineral levels were normal except for iron which was low in 43%.
Despite the usually recommended daily energy intake of 120% R.D.I.
only 21 patients (out of 86) achieved this in practice. In many
patients total energy intake was compromised by the traditional
"low fat diet".

In the majority of patients there were multiple areas where changes
in therapy were indicated. Expectations of doctors and parents was
often low by modern standards.

Regular comprehensive assessment by a team experienced in C.F. will
significantly improve the management and quality of life of C.F.
patients in the U.K. A "tertiary referral service" appears to be
accepted and used by the majority of paediatricians in our region.

**POSTER GROUP FOUR No. 4.01**

Effectiveness of prolonged antibiotic treatments against
Pseudomonas aeruginosa (PA) in patients with cystic fibrosis (CF), during acute exacerbations of pulmonary infection.

B. SABLAYROLLES, G. DUTAU. Unité de Pneumologie et d'Al-
lergologie - Sce Pr ROCHICCIOLI - CHU Rangueil 31054 Tse.

Taking into account the results of antibiotic treatments
against PA, we wanted to know their effectiveness, as respiratory functions (RF) were concerned.
MATERIAL AND METHODS : I2 CF children with acute exacerbation due to PA were studied : 6 boys and 6 girls aged I3 $\pm$
4 years ; their pulmonary status was serious. These children had an antibiotic treatment against PA intravenously
for 2I $\pm$ 7 days, (with, depending on the antibiogram, semi
syntethic penicillin derivative, or aminoglycoside). Detai
led clinical, biochimical, bacteriological and respiratory
data were obstained immediately before and after antibiotic therapy : spirometric tests, maximun expiratory flow
volume curves, diffusing capacity, gasometry). The statistical analysis uses the calculation of the mean $\pm$ SD and
the Student's tests.
RESULTS : This antibiotic treatment is efficient in the
whole children group : (I) for clinical data : decrease of
fever and tachycardia, improvement in the aspect and quantity of sputum, and increase of weight. (2) for biologic
data : inflamatory syndromes disapear ; decrease of white
blood count. (3) for bacteriological data : important decrease of the PA quantity in the sputum. These results
mean a very significant improvement of the functional respiratory data : increase of FRC, TLC and VC, decrease of
airway obstruction, improvement of $FEV_I$ and MEFR at 75, 50
and 25% VC, amelioration of gasometry. As a conclusion the
effectiveness is very good in 7 patients/I2, good in 4/I2,
null in I/I2. There is a narrow link and the increase of
the RF (respiratory functions), especially $FEV_I$, MEFR $_{75}$,
50, 25% VC ( $p < 0,0I$).
COMMENT : A rather prolonged antibiotherapy against PA
seems to be efficient in acute exacerbation of pulmonary
infection in the CF children (even in serious cases). The
very significant decrease of the amount of PA allows a
true improvement of the clinical and biological signs. The
(respiratory function) RF seems to an excellent data of
survey and theses results during the treatment seems to be
directly linked to the evolution of the amount of PA in
the airways.

**POSTER GROUP FOUR No. 4.02**

MICROBIOLOGICAL EFFICACY OF THREE DIFFERENT THERAPEUTICAL REGIMENS IN THE TREATMENT OF RESPIRATORY INFECTIONS DUE TO PSEUDOMONAS IN PATIENTS WITH CYSTIC FIBROSIS.

W.Cambisano,P.Bergamo,A.Boccazzi,R.Padoan,M.G.Piovan,G.Trezzi, A.Giunta.
Centre for therapy of Cystic Fibrosis,Department of Pediatrics, University of Milan,via Commenda 9 -20122 Milano, Italy

The series studied in the present trial consist of 45 CF patients with pulmonary exacerbations randomly allocated to one of the following treatment regimens:1)Ceftazidime (CAZ),2)CAZ plus Sisomicin(SIS),3)Piperacillin(PIP)plus SIS. A quantitative evaluation of the bacterial strains(Pseudomonas aeruginosa cfu/ml count)present in sputum at the start of the therapy,at the end,and not later than a month since the end,makes us to asses the microbiological efficacy of the treatments and the persisting in the time of the obtained results.The microbiological success has been considered as the eradication of Pseudomonas aeruginosa strain or in any case as the decrease in its concentration of $\geqslant 10^4$ cfu/ml.A microbiological success has been obtained in a satisfactory percentage of sputum samples at the end of all three therapeutical regimens:the larger percentage(78.6%) of eradication and significant decrease in concentration is obtained in patients treated with CAZ alone.Strains that showed a significant decrease in sputum count have been found after a month in concentration similarto that at start,not related to the treatment carried out:for the eradicated strains, instead,the larger percentage of reapperance has been shown in the sputum of patients which have received CAZ in monotherapy The susceptibility to the more common antipseudomonal drugs was evaluated with Kirby-Bauer disc method.The development of direct and cross resistance following antibiotic therapy appears acceptable for all three regimens.The M.I.C. of CAZ and PIP has been evaluated by a broth-diluition method. The course of M.I.C.g both of CAZ and PIP for PA is almost similar in the three different regimens: an increase of M.I.C. values was noticed constantly at the end of therapy with return to the previous values after a month.

**POSTER GROUP FOUR No. 4.03**

THIENAMYCIN TREATMENT OF MULTIRESISTANT PSEUDOMONAS AERUGINOSA
INFECTION IN CYSTIC FIBROSIS.

Svend Stenvang Pedersen, Tanja Pressler, Niels Høiby and
Christian Koch.
Department of Paediatrics, Rigshospitalet and Statens Seruminsti-
tut, Department of Clinical Microbiology, Rigshospitalet.
Copenhagen, Denmark.

At the Danish Cystic Fibrosis Center more than half of the CF-
patients with Pseudomonas aeruginosa infection of the lungs
harbour strains resistant to tobramycin, cefsulodin, ceftazidime
and carbenicillin. All the strains are sensitive to the new carbapenem antibiotic, thienamycin.

Ten CF-patients with multiresistant P. aeruginosa entered an open
study, where they received 45 mg/kg/24h of thienamycin intravenously for two weeks.

The drug was well tolerated, only two patients complained of adverse reactions, one with slight nausea during infusion and one
with mild glossitis.

There were no signs of hepato- or nephrotoxicity nor changes in
hematology parameters.

Although, P. aeruginosa was not eradicated in any of the patients,
they all improved during treatment with increase in lung function
parameters.

Data on susceptibility of P. aeruginosa to thienamycin and on
pharmacokinetic studies will be presented.

In conclusion, thienamycin seems to be a promising new agent for
the treatment of Pseudomonas aeruginosa infection in CF-patients.

**POSTER GROUP FOUR No. 4.04**

IMMUNOLOGICAL RESPONSES FOLLOWING VACCINATION WITH PSEUDOMONAS
AERUGINOSA VACCINE

A.J. Day, P.H. Weller, R.J. Jones* and E.A. Roe*
Institute of Child Health, Birmingham. B16 8ET and MRC Vaccine
Research Unit, University of Birmingham. B15 2TT*.

Assessment of immunological responses have been undertaken in a
double blind controlled trial of a polyvalent pseudomonas aeruginosa
vaccine (BA 4162, Wellcome), in cystic fibrosis patients, not
colonised with pseudomonas aeruginosa.  21 children were recruited,
matched for age, sex and severity of lung disease: 10 received
vaccine and 11 placebo.  Ages ranged from 18 months to 9 years.
2 subcutaneous injections were given on day 0 and 14.  Blood was drawn
on day 0, 14 and 28 and investigation of leucocyte and antibody
fuction undertaken.  Antibody responses were measured using immunoassay (ELISA), passive haemagglutination (PHA) and mouse passive
protection tests.  Vaccinated patients showed raised titres against
all 16 components of the vaccine, as measured by ELISA and PHA.
Only vaccinated patients showed a significantly high antibody titre
which passively protected mice against lethal challenge with
pseudomonas aeruginosa serotype 6.  Children of both groups showed
active phagocytosis, but limited ability to kill ingested pseudomonas
aeruginosa.  Phagocyte activity in the vaccinated group showed no
enhancement over that of the placebo group in respect of their ability
to ingest and kill mucoid and non-mucoid pseudomonas aeruginosa
strains.

This study has shown an enhanced humoral response following
pseudomonas vaccination, but no  alteration of phagocytic activity.
It is too early to know whether these findings have clinical
significance and we are closely following the progress of the
children.

**POSTER GROUP FOUR No. 4.05**

THE NEPHROTOXICITY OF AMINOGLYCOSIDES IN CYSTIC FIBROSIS.

M. G. MILLER, L. WHITTAKER, J. T. BROCKLEBANK, J. M. LITTLEWOOD
CYSTIC FIBROSIS REGIONAL TERTIARY REFERRAL CENTRE
ST JAMES'S HOSPITAL, LEEDS.

Over two years, 14 patients known to have cystic fibrosis were
given 56 courses of aminoglycosides to treat exacerbations of
their chest condition.

Single urine samples were collected before, during and after
treatment. To estimate renal tubular damage the N-acetyle-
glucosaminidase:creatinine (NAG:CRE) ratio was measured on each
sample and proximal tubular reabsorption was estimated by the
$alpha_1$-microglobulin:creatinine $(A_1M:CRE)$ ratio. Glomerular
function was estimated by serum creatinine measured before and
after each treatment.

The NAG:CRE ratio rose throughout each course. The mean levels
during each final week were significantly correlated to the total
dose of aminoglycoside given. The mean NAG:CRE ratio for the
second week of treatment was higher for second and third courses
but was not higher in subsequent courses. For each patient the
NAG:CRE ratio returned to normal within 8 weeks.

The $A_1M:CRE$ ratio rose a mean of eight times greater than pre-
treatment levels within a day of starting treatment. Levels
remained constant during treatment, falling to normal within two
days of stopping. No cumulative effects were seen.

No significant changes occurred in serum creatinine and minor
changes did not correlate with either ratio. These results suggest
that although aminoglycosides cause tubular damage in C.F.
patients detectable by sensitive methods, this damage is reversible
and not cumulative.

**POSTER GROUP FOUR No. 4.06**

IMIPENEM TREATMENT OF PATIENTS WITH CYSTIC FIBROSIS

B Strandvik, H Alfredsson, A-S Malmborg, Departments of Paediatrics and Clinical Microbiology, Karolinska Institutet, Huddinge University Hospital, Stockholm, Sweden.

Imipenem is a carbapenem antibiotic with a broad spectrum of activity on Gram-positive and Gram-negative bacteria, including Pseudomonas aeruginosa. The drug was used in the treatment of patients with cystic fibrosis colonized with P. aeruginosa and hospitalized due to lower respiratory tract infections. The concentration in serum and sputum of Imipenem DPI was followed at regular intervals. The antibiotic was given intravenously in a dose of 45 mg/kg/day divided in 6 hours intervals and with a maximum dose of 4 g/day. Antibiotic concentration was determined in serum after the 1st and the 9th dose during 4-5 hours after administration. The concentration in sputum was analyzed parallel to serum after the 9th dose. Imipenem was always detectable in sputum and the maximum concentration was obtained after 30-60 minutes. The concentration was usually low, 0.1-0.7 µg/ml and only occasionally values above 1 µg was found. All except one patient improved clinically but P. aeruginosa was seldom eradicated from the sputum. In some patients pseudomonas persisted in spite of being fully sensitive to the antibiotic in vitro. No adverse effects were seen except a small transient increase of the serum transaminases.

PROSPECTIVE STUDY ON THE EFFECT OF DAILY AND INTERMITTEND
ANTIBIOTIC TREATMENT IN CYSTIC FIBROSIS

K.F. Kerrebijn, coordinator of a multicentre study, Dept.
paediatric respiratory diseases, Erasmus University and
University Hospital Rotterdam/ Sophia Children's Hospital,
Gordelweg 160, 3038 GE Rotterdam.

The value of daily antibiotic treatment (a.b.) on the development of symptoms, X-ray abnormalities, sputum flora
and respiratory function was studied in a prospective
multicentre investigation. Children below the age of 6
months with proven CF were admitted between 1977 and 1980.
Assignment to either daily a.b. or a.b. on clinical indication only (intermittend a.b.) was done by the physician
and hence not random. A p.a. and lateral chest X-ray,
sputum culture (if possible), respiratory function (in
the older children) and standardised registration on signs
and symptoms were completed every 6 months. X-rays were
coded by the coordinator according to the Chrispin-Norman
score. The number of children in the study is about 200.
5 year follow-up data on 31 patients with daily a.b. and
64 with intermittend a.b. were available for analysis.
Height and weight increment were equal in both groups.
Cough frequency did not differ between groups and did not
increase during follow-up. The number of periods with
exacerbations was lower in the daily than in the intermittend a.b. group during the second but not during the
first 2½ years period. X-ray scores increased significantly during follow-up but between groups no differences were
present. Insufficient data on sputum cultures and pulmonary function were present. Death rates in both groups
were small and not different.
It is concluded that, except for fewer exacerbations in
the daily a.b. group in the second half of the follow-up
period, no differences were found between the effect of
daily and intermittend a.b. in the first 5 years of age.
The implications of these findings will be discussed.

**POSTER GROUP FOUR No. 4.08**

A COMPARISON OF INHALED THERAPIES IN CHILDREN WITH CYSTIC FIBROSIS.

D.P. Heaf., S. Tyson., R. Dinwiddie., D. Matthew.
Respiratory Unit, The Hospital for Sick Children, Great Ormond
Street, London WC1N 3JH.

A double blind cross over study to examine the effect of inhaled
Azlocillin versus inhaled mucolytic (Mercaptoethane sulphonate
'Mistabron') versus a combination of Azlocillin and Mistabron was
performed in 21 C.F. children with chronic Pseudomonas aeruginosa
infection.  Each treatment module lasted 4 months and the modules
were separated by 2 month fallow periods.  Effect of therapy was
evaluated by serial respiratory function measurements, chest
radiographs, lung ventilation and perfusion scans and diary card
scores.  The results will be presented.

THE EFFECT OF 2-MERCAPTOETHANE SULPHONATE 'MISTABRON' ON
PSEUDOMONAS AERUGINOSA GROWTH AND AZLOCILLIN ACTIVITY IN VITRO.

D.P. Heaf., G.T. Webb., D.J. Matthew.
Respiratory Unit and Department of Microbiology, The Hospital for
Sick Children, Great Ormond Street, London WC1N 3JH.

The combination of inhaled mucolytics and antibiotics is used in
the treatment of C.F. patients with Pseudomonas lung infections.
To investigate if the mucolytic agent Mistabron would alter the
anti-pseudomonal activity of Azlocillin we performed in vitro
studies. The minimum inhibitory concentration 'MIC' and minimum
bacteriocidal concentration 'MBC' of Azlocillin were determined
for 20 Pseudomonas aeruginosa isolates using Azlocillin alone and
in combination with 1% Mistabron. MIC was significantly lower
when the Azlocillin was combined with Mistabron. This bacteriostatic effect was also observed with 1% Mistabron alone but was
not seen with lower concentrations of Mistabron, either alone or
in combination with Azlocillin. Mistabron did not alter the
bacteriocidal activity of its own.

We conclude that Mistabron does not reduce the anti-pseudomonal
activity of Azlocillin and should be safe to use in combined
inhalation therapy with Azlocillin. Our in vitro study suggests
that Mistabron may have some anti-pseudomonal activity of its own
which may help in the treatment of C.F. patients with Pseudomonas
lung infections.

**POSTER GROUP FOUR No. 4.10**

EDTA    AEROSOL    IN    PSEUDOMONAS    LUNG    INFECTION

J. Brown, C.M. Mellis and R.E. Wood, Royal Alexandra
Hospital for Children, Sydney, Australia and Rainbow Babies
and Children's Hospital, Case Western Reserve University,
Cleveland, Ohio, U.S.A.

In 1980 Wood presented in vitro and animal experimental
data suggesting a beneficial effect of EDTA by aerosol when
used in conjunction with antimicrobial therapy in pseudomonas
bronchitis. Animal studies in Cleveland, involving extended
periods of exposure to EDTA aerosol in sheep and rhesus monkeys,
failed to show any toxic effects. We found an excellent
clinical response in a CF child with chronic pseudomonas
infection when given regular EDTA inhalations by ultrasonic
nebulization, with oral tetracycline, for 3 weeks.

Consequently, we selected ten Sydney children, aged
between 8 and 15 years, with sweat test-proven cystic fibrosis,
for a double blind cross-over study. The selection criteria
were as follows: Shwachman-Kulczycki clinical score at least
70. Pulmonary function: VC at least 70% predicted, $FEV_{1.0}$
at least 60% predicted, no significant improvement in $FEV_{1.0}$
following bronchodilator inhalation. No significant fall
in $FEV_{1.0}$ following inhalation of EDTA or buffered saline
aerosol. Not requiring continuous antibiotics, productive of
sputum, sputum-positive for pseudomonas at least three times
in last 6 months. Each patient was studied for a six-month
period during which time tetracycline was taken orally in a
dose of 30 mg/kg/day (maximum/day = 1.25 g) in three divided
doses. Each patient received EDTA aerosol (50 mM) for half of
the study period and buffered saline (50 mM) for the other half,
the type of aerosol being allocated randomly by a pharmacist
and known only by him. The aerosols were generated by ultrasonic
nebulizers running at maximum capacity and inhalation was
continued for 10 minutes per session, twice daily. One of the
divided doses of tetracycline was given 45 minutes before each
of the aerosol treatments. Progress was assessed by measurement
of pulmonary function, physical examination and sputum cultures
at 4-weekly intervals. Chest radiographs were taken on entry
and each 3 months.

Two patients could not complete the study, one because of
severe clinical relapse, the other because of antibiotic
side-effects. Of the remaining 8 patients, none showed any
consistent improvement in pulmonary function, none showed any
growth acceleration and none was rendered free of pseudomonas
lung infection. Semiquantitative assessment of colony growths
from sputa showed no change. Diary cards showed no significant
change in cough frequency, sputum volume nor sputum thickness
in any patient and none showed radiological improvement.

We conclude that a combination of EDTA by aerosol and
tetracycline by mouth over a short (3 months) period does not
modify the clinical course nor the pulmonary flora of a group
of young CF patients with chronic pseudomonas lung infection.
Nevertheless, in view of the animal and in vitro results,
further controlled clinical trials using higher concentrations
of EDTA for more prolonged periods are indicated.

**POSTER GROUP FOUR No. 4.11**

INDIVIDUALIZED DOSAGE REGIMENS FOR PATIENTS WITH CYSTIC FIBROSIS
(C.F.), UNDERGOING INTRAVENOUS AMINOGLYCOSIDE THERAPY. G. Delage,
R. Lasalle, L. Desautels, S. Legault, J.G. Lapierre, A. Lamarre,
P. Masson, S. Spier. Hôpital Sainte-Justine, Montréal, P.Q., Canada.

It is well known that aminoglycoside serum levels in the individual patient cannot be reliably predicted on the basis of simple
dosage formulae. Furthermore it has recently been shown that patients
with C.F. require increased aminoglycoside dosages. Therefore, we
established a program for individualizing dosage regimens in patients
with C.F.

Individualized dosage regimens were calculated from serum concen-
tration-time data in 48 patients with C.F. undergoing 64 courses of
intravenous aminoglycoside therapy (tobramycin, 49; gentamicin, 12;
amikacin, 3).[1] Pharmacokinetic parameters were calculated for each
patient on a programmable pocket calculator (TI-59, Texas Instruments) using the method of Sawchuk and Zaske (J. Pharmacokin. Bio-
pharm. 1976; 4: 183-195) modified by Loertscher (Drug Intell. Clin.
Pharmacy 1982; 16: 563-568). The elimination rate constant and the
volume of distribution varied greatly from one patient to the other
with both gentamicin and tobramycin. Calculated dosage regimens varied from 7 to 21.8 mg/kg/day for tobramycin, from 8.6 to 17.5 mg/kg/
day for gentamicin, and were 30 mg/kg/day for the two patients who
received amikacin. Desired peak levels at were 10 $\mu$g/ml for gentamicin and tobramycin, and 25 $\mu$g/ml for amikacin; the corresponding
trough levels were 1 $\mu$g/ml for gentamicin and tobramycin, and 4 $\mu$g/
ml for amikacin. All patients had normal renal function. Predictability of the system was assessed by follow up blood levels in 47
cases. Observed peak levels were within 2 $\mu$g/ml of the predicted level in 78% of cases, and observed trough levels were within 0.5 $\mu$g/
ml of predicted level in 66.6% of cases. No nephrotoxicity or ototo-
xicity was noted.

Twelve patients undergoing a second course of therapy with the
same aminoglycoside were reanalysed: differences of up to 42% between the two calculated regimens were noted reflecting important variations in time of the same patient's pharmacokinetic parameters.
Therefore, individualized dosage regimens seem necessary to optimize
systemic aminoglycoside therapy, and patients undergoing a subsequent
course of the same aminoglycoside should be reanalyzed.

[1] All patients received combined antibiotic therapy that included an
antistaphylococcal and an antipseudomonal penicillin. Blood levels
were determined with the use of both a microbiological and a fluo-
rometric assay in all patients.

**POSTER GROUP FOUR No. 4.12**

SELF ADMINISTERED HOME ANTIBIOTIC THERAPY IN ADULT CYSTIC FIBROSIS

R.J.D. WINTER, R.J.D. GEORGE, C.D. SHEE, S.J. DEACOCK, D.M. GEDDES
London Chest Hospital, Bonner Road, London, E2 9JX.

9 adult patients with cystic fibrosis (mean age 19.4 SD 4.2 years) have been taught to administer their own intravenous antibiotics at home to treat infective exacerbations due to pseudomonas aeruginosa.

Antibiotics were administered via an indwelling cannula (Venflon, Viggo products). Following a variable period in hospital (mean 4 SD 2.6 days) for instruction, initiation of treatment and to establish adequate antibiotic levels, a total of 11 courses of intravenous antibiotics have been continued for at least 5 further days at home (mean 5.5 SD .9 days). In two patients complete courses of antibiotics have been given without hospital admission.

Subjective well being improved and sputum volume fell during treatment. $FEV_1$ and FVC rose from 0.64 SD 0.06 and 1.09 SD 0.12 l prior to treatment to 0.81 SD 0.12 and 1.38 SD 0.46 l respectively when assessed after completion. Response to treatment was assessed by temperature, body weight, lung function and relapse time, defined as the interval between completion of treatment and subsequent antibiotic therapy. There was no difference between home and previous hospital inpatient treatments.

Self administered home intravenous therapy for adult cystic fibrosis leads to shorter hospital admissions and does not appear to be associated with an increased rate of recurrent infection.

NEBULISATION OF GENTAMICIN SOLUTION.

S.P.Newman, P.G.Pellow, M.M.Clay  and S.W.Clarke.
Department of Thoracic Medicine, Royal Free Hospital, Pond St.,
London NW3 2QG.

Nebulised antibiotics are useful for treating respiratory
tract infections in patients with cystic fibrosis (Hodson et al.
Lancet 1981;2:1137-1139, Wall et al. Lancet 1983;1:1325), although
little is known about the output characteristics of nebulisers
used with antibiotic solutions. We have measured nebulisation time,
aerosol mass output and droplet size from 4 well-known brands of
jet nebuliser (Upmist, Inspiron, DeVilbiss and Bird) used with
80 mg (2ml) of gentamicin solution (Garamycin, Kirby-Warrick)
nebulised to dryness at 4 compressed air flow rates (6,8,10 and 12
l/min - the range of flows generated by most electrically driven
compressors). The mass of gentamicin released was calculated from
the mass of drug solution retained in the nebuliser and from the
increase in concentration of this solution brought about by
preferential evaporation of solvents (Advanced Instruments
Digimatic Osmometer). The droplet size distribution was measured
30 sec after commencement of nebulisation using a Malvern
Instruments 2600 laser droplet and particle analyser.
Nebulisation time decreased ($P < 0.01$) as gas flow rate was
raised from 6 to 10 l/min, but then increased with a further rise
in flow rate to 12 l/min. The longest mean nebulisation time
(11 min 3 sec)was found for Bird at 6 l/min and the shortest mean
nebulisation time (3 min 59 sec) for Upmist at 10 l/min. The mass
of gentamicin released varied by more than 2-fold from $22.8 \pm 3.9$
(mean $\pm$ SEM) mg for Bird at 8 l/min to $55.8 \pm 1.6$ mg for Upmist
at 8 l/min. There was a significant ($P < 0.001$) negative correlation
between droplet size and flow rate. Consequently the mass of
gentamicin contained in droplets $< 5 \mu m$ (the respirable range)
was approximately doubled ($P < 0.01$) as flow rate was increased
from 6 to 12 l/min, being as follows: Upmist $11.4 \pm 0.8$ mg to
$24.2 \pm 2.9$ mg; Inspiron $7.0 \pm 0.5$ mg to $15.6 \pm 1.8$ mg; DeVilbiss
$9.4 \pm 1.0$ mg to $25.9 \pm 2.2$ mg; Bird $7.6 \pm 0.8$ mg to $13.3 \pm 2.2$ mg.
These results show that both the nebulisation time and the
mass of respirable gentamicin aerosol vary widely according to the
type of nebuliser and the compressed gas flow rate. Past
unfavourable reports of antibiotic aerosols may have arisen partly
from incorrect choice of nebuliser and/or inappropriate operating
conditions.

**POSTER GROUP FOUR No. 4.14**

Effect Of Longterm Continuous Anti-staphylococcal Antibiotic Treatment In Young Children With Cystic Fibrosis

Elisabeth Schlesinger*, Müller, W.*, von der Hardt, H.*, Schirg, E.** and C.H.L. Rieger°

Zentrum für Kinderheilkunde und Humangenetik* und Zentrum für diagnostische Radiologie** der Med. Hochschule Hannover, FRG und Zentrum für Kinderheilkunde°, Universitätskinderklinik Marburg, 3550 Marburg FRG

In a prospective randomised study on 28 children with CF and mildly advanced pulmonary disease (1 to 7 years of age; 12 males, 16 females) the effect of continuous anti-staphylococcal antibiotic treatment (CASAT) was compared to intermittent anti-staphylococcal antibiotic treatment (IASAT) over one year. 14 children received CASAT (8 males, 6 females) and 14 children received IASAT (8 males, 6 females) during episodes of infection. The two groups were comparable with respect to mean age (CASAT: 42 months, range 10-81; IASAT: 53 months, range 16-81), SDS scores for weight and height (- 1,2, - 0,5; -1.4, -0.6), clinical-(Berne) score (22.1, 21.4), radiologic score (4.9; 7.1) and treatment. Nor were there differences at the beginning of the study in ESR (18 mm/h; 16 mm/h), leucocyte count ($11x10^3$/ul; $11x10^3$/ul) or degree of hypergammaglobulinemia (IgG), expressed as % deviation from values of normal age-matched controls (+ 31%; + 49%). As only throat-cultures could be obtained in this age-group these cultures revealed Staph. aureus in 2 CASAT-children and 7 IASAT-children at the beginning. Antibiotic tratment consisted of TMP/SMZ, Cefadroxil and Dicloxacillin in three-monthly changes or one of these drugs intermittently. Patients were seen every two months in the outpatient clinic and venipunctures were done. Significantly better results (p < 0.05, Mann-Whitney U-Test) were found in CASAT-children for SDS-score for weight (-0.7; -1.5), ESR (10; 14) and IgG (+ 10%; + 38%). These differences between the group became statistically significant after 6 months (ESR), 10 months (IgG) and 12 months (SDS-score for weight). At that time no CASAT-child grew Staph. aureus compared to 5 IASAT-children.
Our results suggest that CASAT may be usefull at least in some children with CF and only mildly advanced pulmonary disease but further studies involving larger groups of young CF-children are urgently needed.

**POSTER GROUP FOUR No. 4.17**

BACTERIOLOGICAL AND CLINICAL EVALUATION OF CEFTAZIDIME IN THE
TREATMENT OF CHRONIC LUNG INFECTIONS IN CYSTIC FIBROSIS (CF).

Quattrucci S., Bertasi S., Bravo E., Chiodi R., Antonelli M.
Dept. Pediatrics and Cystic Fibrosis Center,
"La Sapienza" UNIVERSITY OF ROME - ROME  ITALY

Chronic respiratory infection with Pseudomonas aeruginosa
(Pa) and staphilococcus aureus (Sa) represents the main cause of
morbidity and mortality in C.F. These pathogens are more and more
resistens to specific antimicrobial agents. Ceftazidime (a new
cephalosporin) has been used to assess its "in vitro" activity
against Pa and Sa and value in the control (Beaudry score) of severe
lung infections in C.F. Twenty patients (13♀ - 7♂) aged 2 - 31 years
received one or more courses of Ceftazidime (CAZ) (mg 100-200/Kg/day
i.v.). Each course lasted 15-21 days. In 21 sputum samples was
coltured Pa alone and in 13 it was associated with Sa. In 7 of 34
courses  CAZ was associated to tobramycin. In the first course  all
patients received  CAZ alone wich showed a good antimicrobial  actvity
"in vitro" and caused  a marked clinical improvement. In further courses  the bacteriological activity and improvement of clinical conditions resulted less marked . CAZ totally cleared 5 out of 21 Pa
coltures containing Pa e Sa associated . Therefore also if all
patients showed remarkably clinical benefit, Pa, when present only
rarely and temporarily could be totally eradicated.

No. side effects were observed except in one patient who presented abdominal pain and vomit after three days of treatment.

REFERENCES
1) Beaudry P.H. et al. J. PED. 97, 144, 1980.
2) Gordts B. et al.  Proceedings 11th annual meeting EWGCF Brussels
   171, 1982.
3) Mastella G. et al. J. ANTIMICROB. CHEMOTHER. 12, suppl A, 297, 1983.

**POSTER GROUP FOUR No. 4.18**

FURTHER EXPERIENCE WITH CEFTAZIDIME IN CYSTIC FIBROSIS

R.T. Cullen[1], W.M. McCrae[2], J. Govan[3], M. Grant[1],
R. Sutherland[1], and J.A. Raeburn[1].
Host Defence Laboratory, University Depts. of Medicine[1],
Child Life & Health[2], and Bacteriology[3], Royal Hospital
for Sick Children, Sciennes Road, Edinburgh, U.K.[1].

Ceftazidime therapy of pseudomonas infection in
cystic fibrosis (CF) has been studied clinically and
with respect to host defence functions.  36 courses have
been given in doses of up to 250mg/kg intravenously daily
for 4 weeks.  The antibiotic is effective in reducing the
counts of pseudomonas in sputum during treatment,
particularly in the first course, but within a few days
of stopping therapy the counts have increased.  Clinical
improvement is maintained longer but repeated courses of
ceftazidime are usually necessary.Since ceftazidime is
relatively free from toxic effects, multiple courses are
feasible, often in high doses.

Ceftazidime effects on phagocytic cell function were
studied in a few patients and also in vitro using
leukocytes from healthy volunteers.  Phagocytosis and
killing of Staphylococcus aureus by neutrophils were
unaffected by ceftazidime given in vivo or used in vitro.
Neutrophil myeloperoxidase activity was also unaffected.
The more sensitive assay of phagocyte function, chemiluminescence, provided evidence that in some patients
neutrophil responses to opsonised zymosan could be
enhanced.  Monocyte responses were either depressed or
unaffected.  Incubation in vitro with a range of
therapeutically relevant ceftazidime concentrations
provided variable data which mirrored that obtained
in vivo.

In conclusion, it would appear that ceftazidime is a
useful anti-pseudomonal in cystic fibrosis and does not
grossly interfere with neutrophil antibacterial activity.
In some individuals the antibiotic may be associated with
a transient elevation in chemiluminescence response.  We
are now using a modified chemiluminescence technique,
which utilises less than 0.5ml whole blood, to study the
clinical significance of such variations in patients'
responses to ceftazidime or other antibiotic therapy.

OUT-PATIENT TREATMENT OF ACUTE INFECTIVE RESPIRATORY EXACERBATIONS OF CYSTIC FIBROSIS WITH CEFTAZIDIME

J.A. Kuzemko, R.S. Jobanputra, K.J. Williams
Departments of Paediatrics, Public Health Laboratory Service, District Hospital Peterborough and Glaxo Group Research Ltd, Greenford.

Thirteen cystic fibrosis patients, six males and seven females, aged 20 months to 19 years received 21 courses of ceftazidime including two patients who had three courses, for the treatment of acute infective episodes of their chest infections. The mean dose of ceftazidime was 124 mg/kg/day (range 94-213, s=43.1). The maximum dose of 2.4g of ceftazidime was given in one severe pulmonary exacerbation three times daily and on three separate occasions. A single patient aged 20 months received twice daily doses of 600mg intramuscularly. All of the patients had previously received oral flucloxacillin. One of the main advantages of ceftazidime in this study was that the patients' schooling and social life were disrupted minimally. In this centre daily home or school visits by a physiotherapist are part of the routine management of cystic fibrosis.

In all 21 courses of therapy a pre-treatment pathogen was isolated from the sputum and in six subjects two pathogens were found. The 27 pathogens included 13 pseudomonas aeruginosa of which seven were eradicatd, one cleared with immediate relapse post-treatment, three failed to clear and in two instances no post-treatment sputa were taken. Of the eight staph aureus isolates five were cleared, one cleared with relapse, one failed and one was unassessable. Six haemophilus influenzae isolates were cleared but one relapsed first week post-treatment. There was one patient who became colonised with staph aureus. All of the pathogens isolated pre-treatment were sensitive to ceftazidime. All patients improved with ceftazidime treatment and the symptoms of the acute exacerbation resolved within 1-5 days (mean 3 days). Laboratory parameters were assessed before, during and immediately post-treatment and the only adverse drug related finding was a rise of SGPT which had risen marginally outside the normal range.

Sputum levels of ceftazidime were assayed in 74 separate samples. Ceftazidime levels of 0.2 to 10.2 mg/l (mean 2.2 mg/l) were recorded which suggested that the sputum penetration of the antibiotic was adequate to control most of the infective episodes.

In conclusion ceftazidime because of its activity against pseudomonas species and also its excellent tolerance is a useful additional antibiotic for treating acute pulmonary exacerbations of cystic fibrosis and if local facilities are available, can be given on an out-patient basis.

**POSTER GROUP FOUR No. 4.20**

CLINICAL AND MICROBIOLOGICAL EVALUATION OF CEFTRIAXONE (ROCEPHIN) IN THE TREATMENT OF PSEUDOMONAS CHEST INFECTION IN CYSTIC FIBROSIS

A. Paull, M.C. Goodchild, H.M. Tyler, J. Dodge & J.R. Morgan, Departments of Medical Microbiology and Child Health, Welsh National School of Medicine, Cardiff, U.K.

Ceftriaxone is a new extended spectrum cephalosporin with activity against Pseudomonas aeruginosa (Ps.aer.) and a long serum half life which permits once daily dosage. Five cystic fibrosis (CF) patients were treated with Ceftriaxone in hospital for 10 days and reviewed at 6 weeks. Ceftriaxone dosage was 50mg/kg/day given as a single intravenous bolus injection. Clinical evaluation, respiratory function tests ($FEV_1$, FVC, PFR) and body weight showed improvement in all 5 patients at 10 days but with some reversal of this trend at 6 weeks. Mean values of percentage increase were:- $FEV_1$, 36% (5/5 patients at 10 days) and 13% (4/5 patients at 6 weeks); FVC, 36% (5/5 patients at 10 days) and 10% (5/5 patients at 6 weeks); PFR, 21% (4/5 patients at 10 days) and 17% (3/5 patients at 6 weeks); body weight, 4.3% (4/5 patients at 10 days) and 3.4% (5/5 patients at 6 weeks). There were no significant differences between colony counts of Ps.aeruginosa strains in pre-treatment and post-treatment sputa in 4/5 patients. Ps.aer. was not eliminated from any patient. Ceftriaxone sputum concentrations 23 hours post dose ranged between <0.5 and 3.7 mg/l. Serum ceftriaxone concentrations were 264-357 mg/l one hour post dose and 13-39 mg/l 23 hours post dose. Ceftriaxone M.I.C.s against Ps.aer. strains in pre-treatment sputa were 0.78-12.5 mg/l. In the sputum of two patients after treatment, Ps.aer. strains appeared with M.I.C. values of 50-100 mg/l. Ceftriaxone in single daily doses appeared clinically effective in the treatment of Ps.aer. chest infections in cystic fibrosis. However, the emergence of antibiotic resistant strains in 2/5 patients necessitates caution if ceftriaxone is used as a single antibacterial agent.

**POSTER GROUP FOUR No. 4.21**

PSEUDOMONAS PULMONARY INFECTIONS IN CYSTIC FIBROSIS: CEFTAZIDIME VS CEFTAZIDIME PLUS SISOMICIN VS PIPERACILLIN PLUS SISOMICIN.

R.PADOAN, W.CAMBISANO, D.COSTANTINI, R.CROSSIGNANI, A.GIUNTA

Center for Therapy of Cystic Fibrosis, Department of Pediatrics, University of Milan, via Commenda, 9,20122 MILANO i(Italy)

Our previous clinical trial demonstrated the efficacy of Ceftazidime (C) in the treatment of pulmonary exacerbations due to Ps.aeruginosa (PA) in patients with Cystic Fibrosis (CF). Nevertheless, the combined therapy with an aminoglycoside and an antipseudomonal penicillin is indicated as the first choice by many authors, in these patients. This study has been done to compare the monotherapy treatment with C (150 mg/kg/day) to the two associations C plus Sisomicin ( 150 mg/kg/day + 9 mg/kg/day) and Piperacillin plus Sisomicin (300 mg/kg/day + 9 mg/kg/day) in CF patients with chronic infection due to PA and acute pulmonary exacerbations. The antibiotics were administered i.v. in three divided doses every 8 hours. 26 CF patients entered into the study, they were randomly assigned to one of the three regimens for a total of 45 therapeutic courses, for 14 days. The three groups are similar respect to age, sex, clinical status and chest x-ray score. Most of our patientsare in the severe and moderate classes according to Shwachman score. All the patients had normal renal and hepatic function. None had previous allergic reactions to $\beta$-lactam drugs. Clinical and radiological efficacy of the three schedules was blindly assessed with a clinical score (from Beaudry modified) and a chest x-ray score (Chrispin-Norman). Microbiological evaluation with quantitative sputum cultures was also performed. We used for statistical analysis: Student's t tests, $x$ square test, covariance analysis. Statistically significant improvement in clinical and radiological score was obtained at the end of any therapeutic regimens, as well as micro biological results. Covariance analysis showed no difference among the three treatments. Slight and transient elevation of AST and ALT was seen during therapy with Piperacillin. 50% of the patients treated with Piperacillin developed hyperpirexia up to 40°.
In conclusion our data show that:
1. Ceftazidime alone gives good clinical results as the combination antipseudomonal penicillins plus aminoglycosides in the treatment of pulmonary infections due to PA in CF patients.
2. aminoglycoside's combination to Ceftazidime does not increase its clinical efficacy.

288

IN VITRO ACTIVITY OF TICARCILLIN, CEFSULODIN, AND CEFTAZI-
DIME, IN COMBINATION WITH TOBRAMYCIN, AGAINST ISOLATES OF
PSEUDOMONAS AERUGINOSA FROM PATIENTS WITH CYSTIC FIBROSIS.

Horrevorts A.M.[1], de Ridder R.[1], Degener J.E.[1], Dzoljic-
Danilovic G.[1], Michel M.F.[1], Kerrebijn K.F.[2].

Departments of Clinical Microbiology and Antimicrobial
Therapy[1] and Paediatric Respiratory Diseases[2], Erasmus
University Rotterdam, The Netherlands.

In this study, the in vitro activity of ticarcillin, cefsulodin, and ceftazidime, in combination with tobramycin
was determined against 15 isolates of Pseudomonas aeruginosa. Organisms were cultured from sputa submitted from 15
patients with cystic fibrosis. Synergy between tobramycin
and the β-lactams was studied by both checkerboard and
timed killing curve techniques. For the checkerboard studies dilutions of antibiotics were prepared using a modified twofold dilution scheme. The degree of interaction
was calculated as described by Elion[1]. The interaction was
defined as synergistic if the fractional index was < 0.75.
For the time-kill curves synergy was defined as at least
100-fold increased killing at 24 hr by the combination compared with the most efficacious of individal drugs. Statistical analyses were carried out using the Wilcoxon Rank-
sum test. Based on the fractional inhibitory concentration
indices (bactericidal concentration indices), in the checkerboard studies the combination tobramycin + ticarcillin
was synergistic against 8 (4) strains, tobramycin + cefsulodin against 5 (2) strains, and tobramycin + ceftazidime
against 9 (7) strains. In the killing curve studies 8
strains were synergistically affected by the combination
tobramycin + ticarcillin. Synergy by the combination tobramycin + cefsulodin was demonstrated with 8 strains, by
the combination tobramycin + ceftazidime with 13 strains.
Conclusion: Synergy was observed significantly more often
when tobramycin was combined with ceftazidime than it was
combined with ticarcillin or cefsulodin.

[1]Elion G.B. et al. Antagonists of Nucleic Acid Derivatives
J. Biol. Chem. 1954; 208: 447-488

**POSTER GROUP FOUR No. 4.23**

Comparative antibacterial activity of ciprofloxacin, ß-lactams and
aminoglycosides against P. aeruginosa.

A. Dahlhoff, G. Döring and W. Goldstein
Hygiene Institut der Universität Tübingen
Silcherstr. 7, D 7400 Tübingen

The antibacterial activity of ten drugs differing in their molecular
structure as well as their mode of action was assessed by means of the
determination of their minimal inhibitory concentrations (MIC) against
100 clinical isolates of P. aeruginosa; strains were predominantly isolated from the respiratory tract of patients suffering from cystic fibrosis. A broth microdilution method was employed. In addition to the well
established penicillins, cefalosporins and aminoglycosides two quinolones
(ciprofloxacin and norfloxacin) were studied. Quinolones interfere with
DNA synthesis and thus may affect protein metabolism, too. Therefore we
also analyzed in one strain the effect of a constant concentration of
ciprofloxacin, sisomicon and cefsulodin respectively on the synthesis
of extracellular proteases being regarded as pathogenicity factors.

Following drug concentrations (mg/l) were needed to inhibit 90% of the
strains tested: ciprofloxacin 0.25, norfloxacin 1, azlocillin 16,
piperacillin 16, thienamycin 2, ceftazidime 4, cefsulodin 8, cefoperazone 16, tobramycin 1, sisomicin 4. Thus, ciprofloxacin is the most
active antipseudomonal drug among the agents tested; its antibacterial
activity was identical against mucoid or non mucoid strains.

The production of extracellular proteases (elastase and alkaline protease)
was investigated using a radio immuno assay. Viable bacterial counts as
well as enzyme concentrations were determined daily for 5 days. Samples
were taken daily prior to the transfer of an aliquot of the cultures
into fresh media. Bacteria were exposed to drug concentrations being
achievable in the sputum of CF-patients. Following an incubation for 5 days
neither drug reduced the viable counts as compared to the drug free control.
However, ciprofloxacin reduced to a high extend the production of both
proteases whereas cefsulodin and sisomicin respectively were ineffective.
Because of the superiority of ciprofloxacin over the other agents tested,
its broad spectrum of activity and favourable pharmacokinetics, ciprofloxacin may be a promising drug for the treatment of cystic fibrosis.

**POSTER GROUP FOUR No. 4.24a**

PHARMACOKINETICS OF CIPROFLOXACIN IN PATIENTS WITH CYSTIC FIBROSIS

FRITZ SÖRGEL, ULLRICH STEPHAN, HANS GEORG WIESEMANN, BERNHARD BÖWING, DIETER DALHOFF
DEP. OF PEDIATRICS, UNIVERSITY OF ESSEN, FRG
DEP. OF PEDIATRICS, UNIVERSITY OF ERLANGEN, FRG
BAYER AG, WUPPERTAL, FRG

Ciprofloxacin (BAY 09867) which is chemically a 1-cyclopropyl-6-fluoro-1.4-dihydro -4-oxo-7(1-piperazinyl)-3-quinolone carboxylic acid has shown extremely promising antimicrobial activities which may make it an important drug for treatment of Pseudomonas aeruginosa infections in patients with cystic fibrosis.

Several reports on the pharmacokinetics of cephalosporines suggest that compounds with anionic properties have an increased renal clearance in the cystic fibrosis patients. Ciprofloxacin as a 3-quinolone carboxylic acid may therefore also undergo increased renal elimination which would then require higher doses than in patients without cystic fibrosis.

We therefore studied eight patients with cystic fibrosis on a 500 mg dose and compared the data with those of healthy volunteers. The results of this comparison will be presented.

**OSTER GROUP FOUR No. 4.24b**

# PHARMACOKINETICS OF CEFOTIAM IN PATIENTS WITH CYSTIC FIBROSIS

FRITZ SÖRGEL, ULLRICH STEPHAN, HANS GEORG WIESEMANN,
BERNHARD BÖWING, FRIEDER KEES, HORST GROBECKER
DEP. OF PEDIATRICS, UNIVERSITY OF ESSEN, FRG
DEP. OF PEDIATRICS, UNIVERSITY OF ERLANGEN, FRG
DEP. OF PHARMACOLOGY, UNIVERSITY OF REGENSBURG, FRG

Although several reports indicate that cephalosporines
are handled differently in patients with cystic fibrosis,
there is no clue yet as to what mechanism causes this
unique pharmacokinetic change. In an attempt to establish
a relationship between chemical structure and changes in
drug clearance, we tested cefotiam as a compound with high
water solubility, high molecular weight, low protein binding and high renal clearance.
We studied the distribution and elimination of cefotiam
in ten patients with cystic fibrosis following intravenous
injection of 1 gm of cefotiam.
The data from healthy volunteers and patients with cystic
fibrosis will be compared and discussed on the basis of
literature data with other antibiotics. An attempt will
be made to explain the pharmacokinetic changes seen in
cystic fibrosis.

**POSTER GROUP FOUR No. 4.24c**

PHARMACOKINETICS OF CEFADROXIL AND CEFACLOR IN PATIENTS
WITH CYSTIC FIBROSIS

FRITZ SÖRGEL, ULLRICH STEPHAN, HANS GEORG WIESEMANN,
BERNHARD BÖWING
DEP. OF PEDIATRICS, UNIVERSITY OF ESSEN, FRG
DEP. OF PEDIATRICS, UNIVERSITY OF ERLANGEN, FRG

It could be shown for several antibiotics that the elimination via the renal route is enhanced in patients with
cystic fibrosis when compared with normal volunteers. Mos
of those studies have been performed with antibiotics administered intravenously. Few data are available on antibiotics given orally.
In this investigation we were interested in the effect
of cystic fibrosis on the absorption, distribution and
elimination of two chemically very closely related cephalosporines. Both drugs were given at doses of 1 gm to
eight patients with cystic fibrosis and four healthy
volunteers in a cross over fashion.
The results as to the different absorption process and
renal elimination in cystic fibrosis will be discussed
and the consequences for drug therapy with these agents
are considered.

**POSTER GROUP FOUR No. 4.25**

ORAL CIPROFLOXACIN FOR PSEUDOMONAS BRONCHOPNEUMONIA IN CF
Bender,S.W., Posselt,H.-G., Wönne,R., Stöver,B., Strehl,R.,
Shah,P.M. Centers of Paediatrics and Internal Medicine,
J.W. Goethe-University, D-6000 Frankfurt/M., FRG.

Ciprofloxacin, a new substituted quinoline derivate with
inhibition of bacterial gyrase,is both highly active against
pseudomonas (minimal inhibitory concentration,MIC<1.0 µg/ml
in all strains from 20 CF patients tested) and well absorbed
from the intestinal tract. Ciprofloxacin was taken by 10 CF
patients (age >18, except one boy age 16 years), in an
open phase II therapeutic trial. A therapy course of 3 weeks
was planned but extended up to 8 weeks in seven patients.
Pharmacokinetic studies (5 patients on 0.5 and 5 patients
on 1.0 g every 12 hours) showed rapid absorption (t max
1-2 hours) with serum and sputum concentrations higher than
MIC after 12 hours. Good penetration of ciprofloxacin and
prolonged concentration in the sputum were registered in all
patients. Recruitment was restrictive and confined to
patients with acute infectious exacerbations only.

Clinical response, evaluated in weekly intervals, was good
to excellent in 8 and fair in 2 patients (the latter with
rises in MIC). In the responders, auscultatory findings
(reduction of lung fields with rhonchi), cough frequency and
amount of sputum improved markedly. Though subjective parameters of well-being, it is important to note an increased
appetite, weight gain and higher activity in all responders.
Extensive pulmonary function tests showed significant
(p<0.05) improvement for thoracic gas volume, specific airway resistance, peak exspiratory flow rate and flow at 50 %
forced exspiratory vital capacity after 3 weeks on ciprofloxacin. Trapped air changed insignificantly for the whole
group but decreased markedly in 4 patients. Due to extensive primary lung destruction, the x-ray scores according
to Chrispin and Norman did not improve after 3 weeks of
therapy.

With the exception of 2 patients, complaining of loose
stools, no further subjective and objective adverse reactions to major organ systems were noted.

Minimal inhibitory concentration, MIC (<1.0 µg/ml initially,
subsequently tested weekly) remained low in 4 and increase
slightly (2 µg/ml) in another 4 patients. The marked increase of MIC(4+8 µg/ml) observed in 2 patients after 1-2
weeks decreased 2-3 weeks after cessation of therapy thus
enabling two further treatment courses with ciprofloxacin.-
Selection with temporary overgrowth of pseudomonas wild
strains is likely to occur in the mixed flora of markedly
destructed lung tissue.

## POSTER GROUP FOUR No. 4.26

IS THE NEW ORAL QUINOLONE, PEFLOXACINE, USEFUL FOR THE MANAGEMENT OF CHRONIC PSEUDOMONAS AERUGINOSA INFECTIONS IN CHILDREN WITH CYSTIC FIBROSIS?

STERU D, CHERON G, PERIGNON F, FAUCHERE JC, LENOIR G.
Hôpital Necker-Enfants Malades - 149, rue de Sèvres, PARIS, FRANCE.

Twelve children with cystic fibrosis (C.F.) were treated with pefloxacine, a new oral quinolone, with antipseudomonas activity. Treatment was started after a three-week parenteral administration of antibiotics. A posology of 15 mg/kg/day was used. Serum and sputum concentrations of pefloxacine were measured with a bacteriological method 3 hours after administration. Dosage were done after one month of treatment. Clinical and bacteriological efficacy were evaluated.

Individual results are shown in table I

|  | 1 | 2 | 3 | 4 | 5 | 6 | 7 | 8 | 9 | IO | II | I2 |
|---|---|---|---|---|---|---|---|---|---|---|---|---|
| Serum concentrations µg/ml | 4,2 | 8,1 | 6,2 | 4,5 | 14,5 | 0,75 | I | 5 | 3,3 | 2 | 0,8 | - |
| Sputum concentrations µg/ml | 1,1 | 3,3 | 2,4 | 2,8 | 6,2 | 1 | 1 | 2 | 1 | 0,3 | 0,9 | - |
| B/S % | 26,2 | 40,7 | 38,1 | 68,2 | 42,7 | ND* | ND* | 40 | 30 | I5 | ND* | - |
| Clinical efficacy 1=good 2=bad | 1 | 2 | 2 | 1 | 2 | 1 | 2 | 1 | 1 | 2 | 2 | 1 |

* Not used for statistical interpretation.

- Clinical efficacy (reduction of expectoration, better feeling) was observed in 50 % of the patients. B/S in this group was high compared to the rest of the population ($41,7 \pm 18,9$ % VS $34,1 \pm 12,9$ %; $p < 0,05$).

When Pseudomonas Aeruginosa (P.A.) was sensitive to pefloxacine (n=7), an important reduction of colonies' number and one eradication were observed. However, 3 strains became resistant to the drug. B/S in this case was equal to $44,4 \pm 14,2$ %. In 5/12 cases, P.A. was resistant to pefloxacine before the beginning of the treatment, but could be eradicated in 2 cases. B/S ratio was $26,4 \pm 11,5$ % (N.S).

Tolerance to pefloxacine was good in 10/12 children. Vomiting, headache or joint pains were observed in 2 children.

Pefloxacine appeared to be useful in the treatment of cystic fibrosis patients in a stable state.

**OSTER GROUP FOUR No. 4.27**

PIPERACILLIN IN CYSTIC FIBROSIS

R.J. Stead., H.G. Kennedy., M.E. Hodson. and J.C. Batten,
Cardiothoracic Institute, Brompton Hospital, London SW3 6HP.

The majority of adult patients with cystic fibrosis (CF) have persistent bronchopulmonary infection with Pseudomonas aeruginosa. Piperacillin sodium is a semi-synthetic ureidopenicillin which has high in vitro activity against this organism. Thirty-eight patients (24 males; mean age 22·6 years) admitted with deterioration in their bronchopulmonary condition received 59 courses of piperacillin between 1981 and 1983. The 4 gram vials were mixed immediately prior to administration and given as an intravenous infusion 6 hourly. A mean dose of 0·36 g/kg/day piperacillin (range 0·29-0·64) was used in combination with an aminoglycoside.

Nine patients (24%) developed reactions considered to be due to piperacillin with fever of around $38·5^0C$ occurring at a mean of 13·5 days (range 5-28) after starting therapy. Two patients also developed rashes, in one maculopapular and in the other purpuric. Two patients complained of low back pain associated with piperacillin infusions, one of whom developed mild proteinuria. All these features resolved within 48 hours of discontinuing piperacillin. Two of the nine patients were each given a further course of piperacillin and had a second similar reaction.

For comparison the records of 35 patients given 47 courses of carbenicillin and 36 patients given 43 courses of azlocillin up to May 1983 were reviewed. No patients had similar reactions to carbenicillin although two patients who had received multiple previous carbenicillin courses had urticarial reactions. Four patients had reactions to azlocillin similar to the piperacillin reactions. Three of these had previously received piperacillin ($p<0·05$).

The aetiology of these reactions to piperacillin is not clear. However, the high incidence is of concern particularly as reactions to penicillins have not previously been a problem in this unit. The fact that piperacillin may sensitise patients to other pencillins is of further concern since these patients depend on future courses of antibiotics.

**POSTER GROUP FOUR No. 4.28a**

SULTAMICILLIN - A NEW ANTIBIOTIC IN THE TREATMENT OF LOWER RESPIRATORY TRACT INFECTIONS CAUSED BY HAEMOPHILUS INFLUENZAE

Tanja Pressler, Svend Stenvang Pedersen, Lene Christensen, Christian Koch and Niels Høiby.

Department of Paediatrics, Rigshospitalet, and Statens Seruminstitut, Department of Clinical Microbiology at Rigshospitalet, Copenhagen, Denmark.

H. influenzae frequently cause recurrent or chronic lower respiratory tract infections in CF and other patients suffering from chronic obstructive pulmonary diseases (COPD). Ampicillin and amoxycillin are the cornerstones of treatment, but resistant strains producing β-lactamase have necessitated the use of other antibiotics in our patients. Sultamicillin is an oral drug consisting of ampicillin in combination with sulbactam, which is a β-lactamase inhibitor. This combination is very efficient in vitro against many β-lactamase producing bacteria including ampicillin-resistant H. influenzae.

Eight CF children and ten children with other COPD, who suffered from chronic H. influenzae infection of the lower respiratory tract were treated with sultamicillin orally (25 mg/kg b.i.d.) for two weeks. Ten of the patients harboured ampicillin-resistant strains. At the end of the treatment 2/3 of the patients were free of H. influenzae, but half of these patients were reinfected within one month. The only adverse reaction was diarrhea which occurred in 14 patients, whereas haematology, blood chemistry and urinalysis remained normal.

In conclusion, sultamicillin is a promising new drug for the treatment of ampicillin-resistant respiratory infections in CF patients and other COPD patients.

**OSTER GROUP FOUR No. 4.28b**

TREATMENT OF H. INFLUENZAE INFECTION IN CHILDREN WITH
CYSTIC FIBROSIS AND CHRONIC AIRWAY DISEASE.

M Pedersen, S Størving, E Mørkassel, C Koch and N Høiby.
Cystic Fibrosis Centre, Dept. of Pediatrics and Statens
Seruminstitut, Dept. of Clinical Microbiology, Rigshospi-
talet, Blegdamsvej 9, 2100 Copenhagen, Denmark.

The efficacy of pivampicillin and amoxicillin against
H. influenzae cultured from the lower respiratory tract
was compaired in a double blind cross over study in 20
children with chronic airway disease (10 CF and 10 non CF)
and a history with high incidence of treatment failure
to pivampicillin.
Equivalent oral dosis of pivampicillin (80 mg/kg/day) and
amoxicillin (62 mg/kg/day) were prescribed for 2 weeks
courses. The average concentrations of antibiotics obtained 2 hours after medication was 9.7 $\mu$g/ml for pivampicillin and 19.1 $\mu$g/ml for amoxicillin ($p < 0.01$).
Both drugs were well tolerated, but a more pronounced nausea was associated with pivampicillin. No significant difference was found between the antibiotics with respect to
clinical and bacteriological efficacy, and in only 1/3 of
the patients H. influenzae was eradicated from sputum after treatment. Although sensitive strains in all cases
was cultured before treatments, a remarkable high frequency of ampicillin resistent strains was developed during
treatment with amoxicillin (57%), which was higher than
during pivampicillin treatment (17%) ($p < 0.001$).

**POSTER GROUP FOUR No. 4.29**

CEFOPERAZONE KINETICS IN CYSTIC FIBROSIS

J.C. Kramer, B.B. Sharma, M.L. Henley. Hillcrest Medical Center, 1120 S. Utica, Tulsa, Oklahoma 74104, USA. (Department of Pediatrics, University of Oklahoma, Tulsa Medical College, Tulsa, Oklahoma).

Cefoperazone (C) has good in vitro activity against Pseudomonas aeruginosa (PA), Staphylococcus aureus and Haemophilus influenzae. The therapeutic dose of C in Cystic Fibrosis (CF) patients with PA endobronchial and pulmonary infections is unknown. Our goal was to find a dose whose serum excretion curve most closely approximated the 4 gram single adult dose reported[1](mean serum conc 251 ug/ml. one hr. post dose). Six CF patients, ages 2 to 19 yrs, were treated with combination of C and azlocillin or piperacillin or colistin or tobramycin based on in vitro sensitivity data. C was infused over 1 hour. Doses ranged from 70 to 135 mg/kg and were given at 6 to 8 hr. intervals. Ten sets of kinetic data were obtained. Serum C conc was measured by HPLC.

| DOSE (mg/kg) | NUMBER of pts. | MEAN SERUM C CONC (ug/ml) | | |
|---|---|---|---|---|
| | | 1 Hr | 3 Hr | 5 Hr |
| 135 | 1 | 293 | 151 | 112 |
| 120 | 2 | 163 | 82 | 43 |
| 110 | 1 | 228 | - | 72 |
| 100 | 4 | 201 | 114 | 58 |
| 70 | 2 | 177 | 73 | 36 |

One patient died of overwhelming pulmonary infection after 30 days of therapy. One patient developed CNS depression and a pruritic skin rash, and C was stopped. The other patients improved after 2 to 4 weeks of antibiotic therapy. Two patients relapsed and were retreated. C in combination with other antipseudomonal antibiotics can be used in CF patients with PA pulmonary infection in a range of 70 to 135 mg/kg/dose, at 6 to 8 hr. intervals. Until this can be confirmed by a larger study serum C conc, where available, should be monitored to guide therapy.

Reference:
1. Cefobid (Cefoperazone sodium), "Reference Monograph". Roerig (Pfizer Pharmaceuticals), October 1982.
2. Danzer, L., "Liquid Chromatographic Determination of Cephalosporin and Chloramphenicol in Serums". Clinical Chemistry, Vol. 29: 856-858, 1983.

**POSTER GROUP FOUR No. 4.30**

ASPERGILLOSIS AND CYSTIC FIBROSIS - EFFICACY OF
COMBINED TREATMENT WITH INTRAVENOUS AMPHOTERICIN B AND
ORAL 5-FLUCYTOSINE

M. GUILLOT, A. PLUS, C. LEVEQUE and M. ALEXIS, LISIEUX
HOSPITAL, 1400 LISIUX (FRANCE)
E. DROUHET and G. TOURNIER, PASTEUR INSTITUTE,
TROUSSEAU HOSPITAL, 75 PARIS (FRANCE)

B.G., born in 1970, was referred in October 1983 for
sudden fever (39$^{\circ}$), shortness of breath and acute
wheezing.  Cystic fibrosis had been diagnosed in 1979
(sweat chloride, 129-136) with steady follow-up.  The
clinical data and admission chest radiograph were
consistent with acute respiratory infection.
Pseudomonas aeruginosa and Hemophilus influenzae were
found in sputum, and i.v. therapy (Tobramycin,
6 mg/Kg/day; Ceforaximen 140 mg/Kg/day) was initiated.
Nine days later dyspnoea increased, and a chest X-ray
revealed  diffuse mucoid infiltrates.  Aspergillus
fumigatus (A.f.)infection was confirmed by the presence
of organisms in sputum and bronchus aspirate, by
immunoprecipitins against the metabolic and somatic
antigen (4 bows), by hypereosinophilia (2185/mm3),
serum IgE (>1000 IU/ml), and by IgE antibody activity
against A.f. (RAST Class II).  Intravenous amphotericin
B, with increasing doses up to 1 mg/Kg/day to give a
total dose of 2 g, combined with oral 5-flucytosine
(140 mg/Kg/day) was administered for 60 days.  Marked
clinical improvement was immediately obtained with
later full recovery.

In conclusion, A.f. should be screened for routinely in
cystic fibrosis, and combined i.v. amphotericin B and
oral 5-flucytosine in combination is an effective
treatment.

**POSTER GROUP FOUR No. 4.31**

RIGHT ATRIAL ACCESS CATHETER PLACEMENT IN CYSTIC FIBROSIS PATIENTS
FOR HOME ANTIBIOTIC THERAPY

M. Alley, P. Wells, A. Spock, Department of Pediatrics, Duke University Medical Center, Durham, North Carolina 27710

Efforts have been made to decrease the frequency of hospitalization for intravenous antibiotic therapy in cystic fibrosis patients
by offering oral and inhaled medications. However, the central line
intravenous route of therapy at home has not been extensively pur-
sued. Such a route of medication delivery, along with continuous
routine care, should improve the quality, if not duration, of life
in these patients. Right Atrial Access Catheters have been placed
in four patients, age 11 through 31 years, who met the criteria of
having severe lung disease requiring hospitalizations every 6 to 8
weeks for at least a 3-week period each, sputum culture of Pseudomonas sensitive only to intravenous medications, a negative history
for renal or otologic disorders, strong family support and a desire
to be actively involved in their medical management. The complic-
tions of catheter placement, importance of its maintenance and drug
side effects were carefully explained to each patient and his or her
family prior to enrollment. Depending upon the sputum sensitivity,
either piperacillin (300 mg/kg/d) or an aminoglycoside (gentamicin
or tobramycin at 5 to 9 mg/kg/d to achieve optimal peak and trough
drug levels) were infused by the patient over thirty minutes three
times per day, with each infusion followed by heparin flush. Laboratory studies included baseline electrolyte and drug levels, urinalysis and otologic evaluations, with repeat otologic studies at two
month intervals or with any symptom of hearing loss, vertigo or
tinnitus. Physical examination and baseline studies were otherwise
repeated on a monthly basis. Thus far, the longest duration of
catheter usage has been eight months and no complications have
occurred from catheter insertion or maintenance. Cost effectiveness
of catheter placement is great, as 50% of the charge for a 3-week
hospitalization for antibiotic therapy is saved when compared to that
of the procedure and subsequent home therapy. Home therapy costs
alone are less than 10% of a comparable 3-week hospitalization. All
patients have reported an improvement in quality of life, in part due
to a notable decrease in hospitalization time. We conclude that this
method of therapy should be considered in patients with cystic
fibrosis who demonstrate chronic and severe pulmonary infection.

**OSTER GROUP FIVE No. 5.01**

GASTROESOPHAGEAL REFLUX (GER) IN CYSTIC FIBROSIS (CF)

R. Brent Scott, Edward .V. O'Loughlin, D. Grant Gall

Department of Pediatrics,
Alberta Children's Hospital and University of Calgary,
3330 Hospital Drive N.W.,
Calgary, Alberta, Canada.
T2N 4N1

GER is a recognized problem in CF.  The aim of this study was to define the frequency of GER in a clinic population of CF patients as compared to a group of asymptomatic siblings, and to assess the effect of supplemental nocturnal nasogastric (NG) feedings on the frequency of GER in patients with CF.

METHODS:  Children in the CF clinic and their asymptomatic siblings were surveyed to determine the incidence of symptomatic GER.  A subgroup of CF patients with poor nutritional status were studied with esophageal manometry and 24-hour esophageal pH recording before and after initiation of supplemental continuous night-time NG feeds.

RESULTS:  Of 68 CF patients $\geq$5 yr of age (13.1±7.1 yr, $\bar{x}$±SD) 20.6% experienced regurgitation and 26.5% heartburn.  In the control group of asymptomatic siblings $\geq$5 yr of age (13.8±5.07 yr) 0% experienced regurgitation and 5.6% heartburn.  Amongst the CF patients there was no significant association between symptoms of GER and bronchodilator therapy.  Eight CF patients studied with manometry and 24-hour pH recording (15.5±6.6 yr) had normal lower esophageal sphincter pressure of 24.8±8.8 mmHg and thoracoabdominal pressure gradient of 11.4±4.6 mmHg.   Peristalsis and upper esophageal sphincter function were normal.  There was a significant increase in reflux episodes,  episodes greater than 5 minutes duration, and percent time esophageal pH was less than 4 in CF patients compared to published control data for the entire 24-hour period or during sleep.  During sleep continuous NG feeding significantly increased episodes of reflux.

CONCLUSIONS:  Our findings indicate that symptoms of GER, heartburn and regurgitation, are more frequent in CF patients than in asymptomatic siblings, and when quantitated by 24-hour esophageal pH monitoring GER is significantly more common in CF compared to controls.  GER was not related to bronchodilator therapy but was aggravated by night-time NG feedings.

**POSTER GROUP FIVE No. 5.02**

DEFECTIVE GALLBLADDER FILLING AND EMPTYING IN PATIENTS WITH CYSTIC
FIBROSIS. E.A. Shaffer, D.G. Gall. GI Research Unit and CF Clinic,
University of Calgary, Calgary, Alberta, Canada. T2N 4N1
 Bile salt malabsorption has been linked to pancreatic insufficiency
and fat malabsorption in patients with cystic fibrosis (CF). The excess loss depletes the bile salt pool. This results in deficient
intraluminal bile salt concentration which aggrevates fat malabsorptio
and decreased bile salt secretion which leads to lithogenic bile and
cholesterol gallstone formation. Although gallbladder abnormalities
are considered common in CF, gallbladder function has only been defined radiologically. Gallbladder dysfunction, if it occurs, would
further contribute to the problems of malabsorption and gallstone
formation.
Methods: 16 CF patients (average age 18.7 yr) were compared to 41
healthy controls, using cholescintigraphy to quantitate gallbladder
filling and emptying in response to low dose cholecystokinin infusion
(.02 U/kg-min). The CF patients also had oral cholecystograms and abdominal ultrasounds. Parameters measured were: % partitioned, i.e.
percent hepatic bile entering the gallbladder rather than the duodenum
$T\frac{1}{2}$, time to empty half the contents; *emptying rate*, the linear decreas
in the square root of percent maximum activity, and % *ejected*, the
percent of GB bile ejected (Gastroent 79: 899, 1980).
Results ($\bar{X}\pm SE$; p<.05)

|  | n | GB Filling | | GB Emptying | |
|---|---|---|---|---|---|
|  |  | % Partitioned | $T\frac{1}{2}$(min) | Rate(min$^{-1}$) | % Ejected |
| CF Patients | 7 | 0 | - | - | - |
|  | 6 | 37.2±10.0* | 22.5±5.35* | -.14±.08* | 30.7±14.9* |
|  | 3 | 80.3±12.4 | 6.3±1.1 | -.34±.03 | 79.3± 6.4 |
| Control | 41 | 74.4± 2.5 | 10.3±0.7 | -.28±.01 | 81.5± 2.3 |

In 7/16 patients the gallbladder failed to accumulate the radionucleo-
tide and did not visualize on oral cholecystography. 6 patients had
reduced filling and/or emptying as defined by being 2 SD beyond the
means of cholescintigraphic values for the controls; 3 had normal
radiological function on oral cholecystography. Only 3 CF patients had
normal cholescintigrams.
All 13 patients with abnormal or absent GB function had significant
pulmonary disease and were malnourished: 2 had gallstones, 1 a micro-
gallbladder and 3 normal fat absorption. The 3 patients with normal
gallbladder function had minimal disease and were well nourished;2 had
normal fat absorption. There was no difference in age (10-23 yr vs 14-
23 yr) or duration of recognized illness (½-21 yr vs 1-15 yr) between
those with abnormal vs normal gallbladder function.
Conclusion: Abnormal gallbladder filling and emptying in CF patients i
best related to their general health. Gallbladder dysfunction occurred
in the absence of gallstones or gross morphological anomalies and was
not specifically related to fat malabsorption. The abnormalities of
gallbladder function most likely result from obstruction of the cystic
duct or an intrinsic **defect** in gallbladder motility.

**POSTER GROUP FIVE No. 5.03**

BILE ACID MALABSORPTION IN CYSTIC FIBROSIS: HOW AND WHY ?

F.W.M. de Rooij, J.W.O. van den Berg, E.P. Bosman-Jacobs,
A.C. Touw-Blommesteijn, M. Sinaasappel *.
Dept.of Internal Medicine II and Dept.of Pediatrics subdiv.Gastroente-
rology (*), Erasmus University, 3000 DR Rotterdam, The Netherlands.

In Cystic Fibrosis (CF) increased fecal bile acid loss is found (1),
furthermore a decreased bile acid pool is found in CF (2). This might
be due to bile acid malabsorption. Fondacaro et al.(3) suggested that
reduced bile acid absorption in the terminal ileum of CF patients may
cause bile acid loss in CF. Although bile acids are absorbed by passive
diffusion, most important is the $Na^+$-dependent active absorption
of conjugated bile acids (against a concentration gradient) in the terminal ileum. We have been able to characterize the ileal $Na^+$-dependent
taurocholate transport across the brush border membrane in vitro by
preparing brush border membrane vesicles (BBMV) from microquantities
(25-200 mg) of ileum, allowing the use of biopsy specimen (4). BBMV
were prepared according to an adaptation of the "$Ca^{++}$ precipitation"
method of Kessler et al.(5). The outer side of these membrane vesicles,
prepared in this way from the enterocyte brush border membrane, normally is exposed to the luminal content. No mucus layer is
present on these BBMV. The absorptive capacity of the ileal enterocytes
for specific components like bile acids can be studied in vitro at a
low bile acid concentration of 4 $\mu M$, measuring only the active absorption, isolated from the complex in vivo situation. In this study uptake
of 3H-taurocholate into the BBMV in the presence of a 100 mM NaCl gradient, is followed during 1 minute by sampling at 20, 40 and 60 seconds
after starting the incubation. In various patients with e.g. ileitis
(histologically diagnosed) and with increased fecal bile acid loss, a
decreased in vitro taurocholate uptake was found (see table).

TABLE:TAUROCHOLATE UPTAKE INTO BBMV FROM ENDOSCOPICAL BIOPSY SPECIMEN OF
CROHN PATIENTS AND CONTROLS AND FROM ILEAL SEGMENTS OF TWO CF PATIENTS.

| | uptake in 60 sec. pMoles/mg BBMV protein | | |
|---|---|---|---|
| controls | 284 | 143 (SD) | n=52 |
| crohns | 58 | 57 (SD) | n= 7 |
| cf pat. 1 | 105 | | |
| cf pat. 2 | 90 | | |

Preliminary results obtained with ileal specimen from 2 CF patients,
taken from the resection area during the closure of their ileostomy,
show that in vitro ("active") bile acid uptake is low but not abnormal.
The viscous mucus layer in vivo might cause decreased bile acid absorption.

Ref.:1)Weber, A.M.et al. N.Engl.J.Med. 1973;289:1001.2)Watkins, J.B. et
al. Gastroenterology 1977;73:1023.3)Fondacaro, J.D. et al. Pediatr.Res.
1982;16:494-498.4)de Rooij, F.W.M. et al. Gastroenterol.Clin.Biol.
1983;7:511.5)Kessler, M. et al. Biochim.Biophys.Acta 1978;506:136-154.

**POSTER GROUP FIVE No. 5.04**

CONJUGATED BILE ACIDS IN SERUM AND SECRETIONS OF CYSTIC FIBROSIS
PATIENTS.

G.P. Davidson, T.A. Robb, C. Kirubakaran.
Gastroenterology Unit, Adelaide Children's Hospital, South Australia,
Australia. 5006.

Eighty-five percent of patients with cystic fibrosis (CF) have poor
pancreatic function and have large, daily faecal bile acid (BA) loss,
a postulated cause of lowered intraluminal BA concentration and
altered fat absorption.  We studied quantitative duodenal conjugated
BA secretion after secretin - cholecystokinin infusion in 55 CF
patients and 6 controls (C) by use of a non-absorbable marker
technique.  Fasting serum conjugated BA's were also measured.  BA's
were measured by high performance thin layer chromatography (HPTLC)
and densitometry.  Post stimulation BA secretion was above the
critical micellar concentration in CF and C (13.7 + 8.9,
5.2 + 2.9 mmole/l), and total BA post stimulation secretion rate was
similar in both groups (CF 1.9 + 1.4, C 2.1 + 1.5).  The glycine/
taurine ratio (G/T) was significantly elevated in CF patients
pre (CF 5.5 + 4.0, C 1.5 + 1.1, P < 0.01) and post stimulation
(CF 5.6 + 4.7, C 1.3 + 0.9, P < 0.01).  Thirty-eight percent of CF
patients had elevated total fasting serum BA concentration and
a significantly decreased duodenal BA secretion rate.  The serum G/T
ratio was significantly elevated in CF (CF 4.4 + 4.8, C 1.6 + 0.6,
P < 0.01).  HPTLC is a simple, rapid and sensitive measure of
conjugated BA's in serum and secretions.  Total BA concentration and
secretion rates are normal in CF children but the G/T ratio is
markedly altered which may directly affect fat absorption and may
provide a clue to the aetiology of the liver disease in CF.

**POSTER GROUP FIVE No. 5.05**

FECAL BILE ACID EXCRETION IN PATIENTS WITH CYSTIC FIBROSIS : CORRELATION WITH
CLINICAL AND BIOCHEMICAL PARAMETERS.

C.Colombo,A.M.Morselli°,P.Rucci°,R.Maiavacca,M.Ronchi,A.Giunta.
CF Center,Department of Pediatrics,University of Milan,Italy
°Clinica Medica III,University of Bologna,Italy.

Seventysix patients with Cystic Fibrosis on enzymatic therapy (36 males,40 females,
ranging in age from 3 to 22 years) were studied;20 of them were on oral antibiotic
therapy.
Fecal bile acid (GLC) and fat excretion was simultaneously determined in the stool
collected throughout 72 hours;conventional liver function tests (alkaline phosphatase,
$\gamma$GT,transaminases,bilirubin,albuminemia and protrombin activity) were also performed.
Multifactorial analysis of variance was used to evaluate the influence of the following parameters on fecal bile acid (BA) loss:degree of pancreatic insufficiency,en-
zymatic therapy,antibiotic therapy and liver function tests.
For this purpose,each parameter has been firstly evaluated alone and then in association with the others,to determine a possible interrelation between factors.
Data have been evaluated by subdividing patients into 4 groups,according to the values
of coefficient of fat absorption,performed in basal condition at the time of the
diagnosis.
For statistical analysis we considered as significant a level of $P < 0.05$.
Results: 1) Fecal BA excretion was significantly correlated with the simultaneous
coefficient of fat absorption and with serum transaminases,total bilirubin and
albuminemia concentration,suggesting the possible physiopathological role of chronic
BA malabsorption in determining liver disease in Cystic Fibrosis.
No correlations were found between fecal BA and degree of pancreatic insufficiency,
enzymatic and antibiotic therapy and other liver function tests.
2) As far as the interrelation between parameters is concerned,we found that enzymatic
therapy has a different efficacy in reducing fecal BA excretion,depending on the degree of pancreatic insufficiency.
This finding confirms that endoluminal factors are mostly responsible of BA malabsorption in Cystic Fibrosis patients with severe pancreatic insufficiency.

**POSTER GROUP FIVE No. 5.06**

COMPOSITION AND DISTRIBUTION OF LIPIDS IN CF CHYME

D.R. Fine, C. Brown, P.L. Zentler-Munro, K. Bala, J.C. Batten and T.C. Northfield. St George's Hospital Medical School, London SW17, and The Brompton Hospital, London SW3, U.K.

It is generally believed that in CF a deficiency of pancreatic lipase prevents hydrolysis of dietary lipid to monoglyceride and fatty acid (MG and FA - the "solute"); this conversion of non-polar to polar lipid is considered essential for micellar solubilisation by bile acid (the "solvent"). We have previously shown that some lipolysis does occur in CF despite the absence of pancreatic lipase, but that uptake of the resultant FA into the micellar phase is reduced. Despite this, the concentration of all lipids in the micellar phase is normal, suggesting solubilisation of non-polar diglyceride (DG) and tri-glyceride (TG). We therefore set out to answer three questions: 1. What causes lipolysis in CF if there is no pancreatic lipase? 2. Where does the resulting FA go if not into the micellar phase? 3. What lipid is in the micellar phase if not FA? We aspirated postprandial jejunal chyme from 6 CF subjects and 6 healthy subjects (HS) and separated the physical phases by ultracentrifugation. In addition to the micellar (optically clear) phase conventionally described, we identified two novel aqueous phases in chyme from HS, one of which was consistently present in CF. In HS the micellar phase contained 44% of the FA mass at a concentration of 4.0 mM/l; the two new phases contained higher concentrations (20.3 and 11.5 mM/l) but accounted for only 10 and 12% of the FA mass because of their lower volumes. In CF, the micellar phase contained only 30% of the FA mass at a sub-normal concentration of 1.0 mM/l, whereas the new aqueous phase contained 44% of the FA at a concentration of 8.2 mM/l. This new phase seemed to be "filled in" in preference to the micellar phase. Micellar phase MG concentration was also lower in CF than in HS (0.05 vs 0.18 mM/l, $p < 0.05$) but DG and TG concentrations were similar (0.24 vs 0.45 mM/l, NS; and 0.15 vs 0.13 mM/l, NS). The preponderance of DG > MG in CF is consistent with the action of lingual lipase, and we are currently measuring lingual lipase concentrations. The presence of non-polar lipids in CF micellar phase contradicts the conventional requirement for hydrolysis before solubilisation. We conclude that: 1. Lipolysis in CF is probably due to lingual lipase; 2. The FA it produces may be trapped in a non-micellar phase whence it may not be absorbable; 3. The micellar phase itself contains non-polar lipids which also may be non-absorbable. These findings throw new light on the mechanism, and therefore possibly on the management, of steatorrhoea in CF.

HEPATIC COMPLICATIONS IN CYSTIC FIBROSIS (CF): CLINICAL AND PATHOLOGI-
CAL FEATURES. John D. Lloyd-Still, M.D., Frank Crussi, M.D.
Children's Memorial Hospital, Chicago, Illinois 60614, USA.
    The bile is lithogenic in CF, and hepatic involvement occurs in 2-
5% of patients. We have reviewed our experience of liver involvement
in our CF Center between 1975-1983; 180 pts. were followed, of whom
45% were below the age of 5 yrs. One had viral hepatitis during this
interval; 5% presented with hypoproteinemia in infancy. Clinically
significant hepatic involvement was seen in: 1) meconium ileus and
prolonged neonatal cholestasis (3 pts). Average duration of hyper-
bilirubinemia was 7.3 mos. Two have normal liver function 8 yrs.
later, but 1 died at 11 mos. 2) Massive fatty infiltration of the
liver 2° to malnutrition with hypoproteinemia and zinc deficiency (1
pt. age 3 mos.) and 2° to fever without malnutrition (1 pt. age 2
yrs.) which progressed to cirrhosis within 6 mos. 3) Macronodular
cirrhosis with portal hypertension in 3 older pts. (ages 8, 8 and 12
yrs.) all of whom had initially presented in infancy with hypoproteinemia. One pt. died from hepatic and respiratory failure; 1 pt. died
of post-shunt complications, and 1 is alive with hypersplenism. 4)
Gallstones. One pt. required cholecystectomy at 19 yrs. for abdominal
pain.
    Data on hepatic involvement was obtained from 23 CF Center Direc-
tors. 76 (2.2%) of 3520 pts. surveyed had either cirrhosis, portal
hypertension or hepatosplenomegaly. Information on albumin levels
was available in 31 of the 76; 14/31 (45%) had hypoproteinemia in infancy. Previous studies have demonstrated elevated levels of alkaline
phosphatase (38%) and serum bile acids (21-33%) in our CF pts. Clinical examination is as effective in demonstrating significant hepatic
involvement as any biochemical parameter. Although liver/spleen scans
and ultrasound detect abnormalities in a high proportion of pts.,
liver biopsy is the definitive procedure to document cirrhosis. Pathological changes included granular eosinophilic concretions, with
ductular dilatation, hyperplasia, proliferation, cholestasis and fibrosis in neonates, to massive fatty infiltration with eosinophil and
polymorph infiltration and hypertrophy of smooth endoplasmic reticulum on electron microscopy, to end stage findings of macronodular
cirrhosis. These findings suggest that in CF, unlike Kwashiorkor, the
presence of hypoproteinemia and fatty infiltration of the liver may be
complicated by cirrhosis. Conclusions: 1) Clinically significant
liver disease was present in 9/180 (5%) of our CF population. 2)
There was a direct association between meconium ileus and prolonged
neonatal cholestasis. 3) 45% of pts. with macronodular cirrhosis present with hypoproteinemia in infancy. 4) Massive fatty infiltration
of the liver in CF may be complicated by the rapid development of
cirrhosis. 5) Liver biopsy differentiates these hepatic complications. 6) Neonatal screening programs could prevent the development
of hypoproteinemia and lower the incidence of these hepatic complications.

**POSTER GROUP FIVE No. 5.08**

LIVER DISEASE:  PRELIMINARY RESULTS ON CORRELATION OF ULTRASOUND, LABORATORY AND CLINICAL FINDINGS.

J.M. McHugo, A.J. Day, C.M.E. McKeown, P.H. Weller & K.J. Shah

The Children's Hospital, Ladywood Middleway, Birmingham,B16 8ET, UK

As survival improves in cystic fibrosis (CF), liver disease becomes an increasingly important cause of morbidity and mortality.  A pilot study was undertaken to assess the value in CF of abdominal ultrasound (US) scanning to detect and monitor liver disease and to compare it with clinical and laboratory evidence of liver involvement Forty-three children with CF (22 male, 21 female), mean age 11 years (range 1-18), had a US examination of the abdomen.  The liver and spleen were scanned in all patients using an ATL real time scanner. The gall bladder, common bile duct and pancreas were also scanned whenever possible; although not all patients were starved.  In addition, in all cases, when technically possible, the vascular anatomy of the upper abdomen, in particular the portal venous system, was imaged.  Seven children were selected for scanning because of clinical splenomegaly, 4 because of hepatomegaly, 14 during admission to hospital for antibiotic therapy, and the remaining 18 at the time of their annual chest X-ray.  Standard liver function tests (LFT) were available in 41 patients.

The most consistent abnormality on US was of irregularity of the inferior border of the liver.  The earliest changes were also associated with liver enlargement.  The liver was small in those with more well established liver disease.

Seventeen of the 43 children had abnormalities on scan, of whom 14 had abnormal LFTs (raised transaminases ± abnormalities of bilirubin, alkaline phosphatase, albumin or coagulation).  Of the 26 with normal scans, 3 had abnormal LFTs (one had a hepatitic illness at the time), and in 2 the LFTs were not available.  The sex ratio of the 14 with abnormalities on both scan and LFTs was M/F 3.7:1 and their mean age was 10.8 years.  The 23 with normal scans had no abnormalities on LFTs and had a sex ratio of M/F 0.77:1 and mean age 11.9 years.

These preliminary results suggest that US examination is a quick, non-invasive method of detecting liver involvement in CF and following its evolution.

**POSTER GROUP FIVE No. 5.09**

LIGHT AND ELECTRONMICROSCOPY OF THE LIVER IN CHILDREN WITH
CYSTIC FIBROSIS

Rolf Hultcrantz and Birgitta Strandvik, Departments of Medicine,
Paediatrics and Research Center, Karolinska Institutet, Huddinge
University Hospital, Stockholm, Sweden.

The frequency of liver disease among patients with cystic fibrosis
is high and it seems to increase with age. The most common ethiolo-
gical hypothesis is that bile with high viscosity leads to obstruction of the bile ducts. This hypothesis is in line with the morphology of the liver disease in the terminal stage, which has been called
focal biliary cirrhosis.
In search for early alterations which could indicate the cause of
the liver disease, we have performed light and electron microscopical
studies on liver biopsy specimens from five patients with Cystic
Fibrosis. The patients aged 6-11 years had normal height and weight
for age and clinical score 58-90. At the time of the biopsy none
had clinical or laboratory evidence of liver insufficiency, but they
had slightly elevated levels of serum transferases and serum bile
acids. The serum gammaglutamyltransferase was normal. One has
later on developed liver cirrhosis.
The liver of three of the patients had fibrosis and all had moderate
fatty infiltration. None had inflammatory infiltrates and their
bile ducts were normal. An increase in Ito-cells were seen in the
glycogen. The Kupffer cells were sometimes hypertrophied. Electron
microscopical examination showed that the cytoplasm of the hepatocytes had a generally normal appearance although some abberations
were seen. In the peribiliary areas the smooth endoplasmic reticulum
was often hypertrophied and dilation of the Golgi Apparatus was seen.
The bile canaliculi were not dilated, no bile plugs were found and
intracellular bilepigment were absent. Other organelles such as
the rough endoplasmic reticulum, mitochondria and peroxisomes seemed
to be unaffected. Large heterophagic vacuoles were sometimes seen
in the Kupffer cells.
In summary very mild changes were seen in the ultrastructure of the
liver. Evident features of cholestasis were lacking. The unspecific
pathological findings which were noted cannot clearly explain the
basis of the cell damage, suggesting that metabolic disturbances
are probably more important than viscous bile in the pathogenesis
of the liver disease.

310

**POSTER GROUP FIVE No. 5.10**

NEOFORMATION OF ISLET TISSUE IN CYSTIC FIBROSIS

J. I. Kerr, A. O. B. Redmond and K. D. Buchanan, Department of
Medicine, The Queen's University of Belfast and The Royal Belfast
Hospital for Sick Children

The islets of Langerhans in cystic fibrosis (CF) have been described
as being either normal or enlarged due to coalescence of islet tissue
within the atrophying pancreas. The low incidence (1-2%) of diabetes
mellitus in CF confirms this apparent preservation of islet tissue.
However, in view of the destructive events occurring within the CF
pancreas, it is difficult to understand how the islets can remain
functionally intact. Indeed the reported deficiency of circulating
pancreatic polypeptide (PP) in CF suggests that the islets are not
functioning normally. The aim of this study was to assess the
morphology and degree of survival of islet tissue within the CF
pancreas using immunofluorescence techniques to visualise insulin,
glucagon and PP containing cells. Pancreatic tissue was obtained
post-mortem from 3 CF subjects (aged 0.5, 3 and 10 yr) and processed
routinely to wax sections (5μ). Immunofluorescence studies were
performed using primary antisera directed against insulin (GP11),
N-terminal glucagon (YY234), C-terminal glucagon (YY89) and PP (204),
and secondary antisera conjugated to fluoroscein. Haematoxylin and
eosin staining was also employed. Apart from extensive fibrous and
fatty replacement of acinar tissue, the most striking feature was
ductal hyperplasia. Numerous islets were seen, although many
displayed abnormal morphology including fibrous infiltration and core
acellularity. Immunofluorescence revealed further abnormalities of
islet architecture. Beta cells occupied the islet periphery rather
than their usual central location. Bizarre patterns of immunofluorescence were also seen in regions of ductal hyperplasia.
Glucagon containing cells were most abundant occurring in rows
(>50 cells) alongside the ductal epithelium. Insulin and PP
containing cells were also seen in these areas where islet-like
structures could be seen budding off from ducts. In conclusion, these
immunofluorescence studies suggest that the apparent preservation of
islet tissue in CF is in fact a continual process of islet destruction paralleled by islet regeneration. Presumably, this remarkable
regenerative capacity protects against the onset of diabetes mellitus
in CF. Furthermore, there was no direct evidence of selective loss
of PP cells. Consequently the aetiology of circulating PP deficiency
remains uncertain.

**POSTER GROUP FIVE No. 5.11**

CHYMOTRYPSIN EXCRETION IN THE NEWBORN

G A Brown, R B Halliday, C A Smalley.

Institute of Child Health, University of Birmingham and
Sorrento Maternity Hospital, Birmingham, England

Procedures for the direct assessment of exocrine
pancreatic function are complex, costly and invasive
and for the latter reason cannot be used for
developmental or sequential studies in the newborn.
In the adult, faecal chymotrypsin measurements have
been found a simple, useful, non-invasive and readily
repeatable alternative. This study defines faecal
chymotrypisn reference data for the healthy neonate.

Chymotrypsin was measured in random meconium and faecal
specimens (n=160) from 26 neonates. Mean values were
calculated for the whole group for each 24h period from
birth to 14 days. The mean rose from an initial value
of 290 $\pm$ 37 ug chymotrypsin/g stool (mean + SEM) to a
peak at the fourth 24 hour period (697 + 66); then
decreased again to 278 $\pm$ 36 ug/g stool (last 4 days
data pooled). The lowest individual values relating to
these 3 means were 120, 300 and 120 ug/g stool
respectively. Mean chymotrypsin concentrations
calculated for each baby showed a significant positive
correlation with birth-weight. (r=0.563; p = <0.01).

A peak has also been described for pancreatic enzyme
concentrations in the duodenum in the first week of
life. Faecal chymotrypsin measurements appear
sufficiently sensitive, therefore, to follow the
physiological changes in pancreatic function in the
neonate and may provide a simple non-invasive, readily
repeatable method of assessment.

In neonates presenting with meconium ileus and
subsequently shown by the sweat test to have cystic
fibrosis, faecal chymotrypsin is usually absent.

**POSTER GROUP FIVE No. 5.12**

UNSATURATED Cbl R BINDER IN CYSTIC FIBROSIS MECONIUM.

Vidailhet M, Guéant JL, Monin B, Pasquet C, Djalali M, Morali A, Nicolas JP. Laboratoire de Biochimie Médicale et Pédiatrique et Service des Maladies Infantiles 1, CHU Nancy-Brabois, Vandoeuvre-lès-Nancy 54500, France.

A malabsorption of crystalline vitamin B12 (Cbl) is observed in 100% of cystic fibrosis (CF) patients. Recently we have studied the faecal excretion of unsaturated cobalamin binders and the faecal and seric concentrations of cobalamin (Cbl) and Cbl analogues, before and after 4 days interruption of a pancreatic extract treatment in 9 CF and in 5 healthy children (1). We observed that interruption of the treatment lowered significantly the Cbl analogues concentration in CF sera and the level of degradation of Cbl R binders in the corresponding faeces. In the present study, we have completed our investigation with a determination of the unsaturated binding capacity and the physicochemical properties of Cbl binders in the meconium of CF (n=2) and healthy neonates (n=13). Meconium aqueous extracts were desalted. The unsaturated binding capacity was determined using the radioisotope dilution method of Gottlieb et al. and also Sephacryl S-300 radio-immuno-gel filtration. Molecular weights were estimated in gel filtration using standard labelled proteins as reference and the microheterogeneity and the mean isoelectric point were determined in liquid isoelectrofocusing chromatography. The unsaturated Cbl binding capacity corresponded mostly to R binder (unsaturated intrinsic factor $<$5%). It was of 122.0 ng/g and of 1.0 $\pm$ 1.5 ng/g in CF meconiums and control meconiums respectively. In CF meconiums, the estimated molecular weight of R binder was of about 127 500 ; the mean isoelectric point was 3.37, the microheterogeneity corresponded to 3 isoproteins. In control meconiums, R binder eluted in two positions corresponding to estimated molecular weights of 102 000 $\pm$ 3 400 (4 cases) and of 53 400 $\pm$ 13 900 (9 cases). The mean isoelectric point was 3.08 $\pm$ 0.33 and the microheterogeneity corresponded to 3 isoproteins. Unsaturated R binder was thus partially degraded in control meconiums but it was undegraded and in much greater amounts in CF meconiums. The results were compared to the trypsin seric concentration and they confirmed our previous hypothesis (1) that exocrine pancreatic dysfunction is responsible for a failure to degrade endogenous digestive R binder in CF. The malabsorption of crystalline Cbl may correspond to a sequestration of Cbl to undegraded R binder and this process could be increased by a low gastric pH. A further extensive study is necessary to investigate the diagnostic value of the unsaturated Cbl binding capacity of meconiums in CF.

(1) Guéant JL, Vidailhet M, Pasquet C, Djalali M, Nicolas JP, Clin. Chim. Acta, 1984, in press (n° 02751)

COMPARATIVE STUDY OF GLYCOPROTEINS FROM MECONIUM OF CYSTIC
FIBROSIS, NORMAL PRE-TERM AND FULL-TERM NEWBORNS.

I. GARCIA, M.C. BOISSON, G. FAVRE, E. BANNIER, A. REVOL
CENTRE HOSPITALIER LYON-SUD, Laboratoire de Biochimie,
Secteur Sainte-Eugénie, 69310 PIERRE-BENITE.

We studied the glycoprotein content of meconium from four cystic
fibrosis newborns compared to three healthy newborns and three
prematures. Meconium is shaken overnight in distilled water and
centrifuged and the supernatant is freeze-dried. Aliquots of the
lyophilisat are dissolved in Tris/HCl buffer and subjected to
chromatography on a column of Sepharose CL 2B (PHARMACIA FINE
CHEMICALS) using Tris/HCl buffer ph 8.00 as eluent. The protein
content of the eluates is determined by measuring the absorbance
at 260 nm, the hexose content by an orcinol technique and the
sialic acid content by the thiobarbituric acid method of Aminoff
after hydrolysis with 0,1M $H_2SO_4$ for 30 min at 80°C. Fractions are
pooled according to the profile obtained and subjected to electrophoresis. The carbohydrate content of Glycoprotein is determined
using gas chromatography by the method of LEHNARDT et WINZLER.

Meconium from cystic fibrosis newborns contain more protein and
less hexose and sialic acid (five to six fold) than meconium from
controls. Prematures are intermediate. The chromatographic and
electrophoretic patterns of proteins, hexoses and sialic acid of
meconium of cystic fibrosis newborns are different from meconium
of pre-term and full-term healthy newborns.

314

**POSTER GROUP FIVE No. 5.14**

ALTERATION IN THE PROPORTION OF THE MAJOR ISOELECTRIC FORMS OF SERUM ALBUMIN IN CYSTIC FIBROSIS.

Noa Alon and John R. Riordan
Research Institute, The Hospital for Sick Children
555 University Avenue, Toronto, Ont., Canada M5G 1X8

Albumin concentrations are sometimes reduced in advanced cystic fibrosis due to increased plasma volume, or in some cases with liver involvement due to a diminished synthetic rate (1). However, no qualitative changes have been reported. We have found that on isoelectric focusing of CF sera in the presence of urea, the amount of the more acidic form of the molecule (pI ∿4.8) is markedly reduced compared to control sera. It is known that bound fatty acids account for the bulk of this low pI form of the protein (2). Quantitative determination (GLC) of total and individual fatty acids in sera confirmed the reduced amount of linoleic acid in CF (1) and a mean reduction of total fatty acids presumably reflecting diminished lipase activity. Despite this, we have not been able to demonstrate a strict correlation between the reduced amount of the pI 4.8 band and pancreatic insufficiency. Furthermore, even though the differences in the intensities of this bands between normal and CF sera disappeared or were diminished on fatty acid removal (charcoal defatting), the CF albumin showed a band of greater than normal intensity after adding back excess exogenous fatty acid. After albumin purification by chromatography on either an immunoabsorbent column or a Cibicron-blue column, the differences were minimized. If in fact the observations reflect changes other than fatty acid levels, several possibilities must be considered. For example, $Ca^{++}$ ions are known to inhibit the removal of fatty acid from albumin and hence the diminution of the pI 4.8 form (2). Albumin also functions to regulate free $Ca^{++}$ concentrations (3). The characteristic CF change is not seen in sera from asthmatics.

(Supported by the Canadian Cystic Fibrosis Foundation and the Sellers Foundation)

1. Chase, H.P. (1978) Lancet. July 29, p. 236.
2. Evenson, M.A. and Deutsch, H.F. (1978) Clin. Chim. Acta 89, 341.
3. Lohse, J., Verine, H.J. and Moore, E.W. (1978)
   Arzneim. Forsch. 28, 881.

# MECHANISM OF DEFECTIVE PROTEOLYSIS IN CYSTIC FIBROSIS

Helen K. Berry and Monica C. Hsieh, Children's Hospital Medical Center and the Department of Pediatrics, University of Cincinnati College of Medicine, Cincinnati, Ohio U.S.A.

We carried out screening tests for cystic fibrosis (CF) based on measurement of albumin, other proteins (lactase, B-fucosidase), or proteolytic activity in meconium from newborn infants. To understand the mechanism for defective proteolysis which resulted in accumulation of protein in meconium, we measured immunoreactive trypsinogen (IRT), trypsin catalytic activity (CA) and trypsin inhibitory activity (IA) in meconium specimens with increased albumin from infants later shown to have CF by sweat chloride measurements, with increased albumin from low birth weight infants without CF (LBW), and albumin negative specimens from normal infants. IRT was normal in CF meconium based on total protein content but was elevated based on wet weight. IRT was increased in LBW specimens. Trypsin CA was decreased in CF meconium. Trypsin IA was pronounced in CF meconium, but barely detected in normal or LBW. Albumin and total protein were increased in CF and LBW compared to normal specimens:

| | Albumin Positive | | Albumin Negative |
| | CF | LBW | Normal |
| | n = 22 | n = 10 | n = 26 |
|---|---|---|---|
| IRT[a] | 7.1 ± 4.2*,≠ | 19.3 ± 6.2≠ | 3.1 ± 2.7 |
| IRT[b] | 38 ± 24≠ | 128 ± 49≠ | 54 ± 44 |
| Trypsin CA[c] | .25 ± .27*,≠ | 1.45 ± 1.18 | 1.03 ± .99 |
| Trypsin CA[d] | 1.48 ± 1.89*,≠ | 8.32 ± 5.18 | 17.7 ± 16.0 |
| Trypsin IA[e] | 33 ± 27*,≠ | 2 ± 3 | 1 ± 3 |
| Albumin[f] | 72 ± 40 | 54 ± 40 | <10 |
| Total prot.[f] | 205 ± 81* | 179 ± 58≠ | 57 ± 12 |

a = $\mu$g/g mec (wet wt); b = $\mu$g/g prot; c = $\mu$mol substrate hydrolyzed/g mec; d = $\mu$mol substrate hydrolyzed/g prot; e = $\mu$g porcine trypsin inactivated/g prot; f = mg/g mec; * CF - normal $p < .001$; ≠ CF - LBW $p < .001$; ≠ LBW-normal $p < .001$.

Trypsinogen, an inactive precursor of trypsin, is synthesized by pancreatic acinar cells and secreted into intestinal lumen. The results show this process is normal in CF and LBW infants. In CF infants presence of trypsin inhibitor(s) accounts for accumulation of protein in meconium, whereas in LBW infants failure of activation of trypsinogen either through defective bicarbonate secretion or decreased production of enterokinase may account for defective proteolysis.

**POSTER GROUP FIVE No. 5.16**

INTERRELATIONSHIP OF NUTRITIONAL STATUS AND PULMONARY DISEASE
SEVERITY IN CYSTIC FIBROSIS (CF)

Lucille A. Lester, M.D., Angelita Lopez, R.D., Zenaida Corpuz, R.N.,
Richard M. Rothberg, M.D. Department of Pediatrics, The University
of Chicago School of Medicine, Box 133, 5841 S. Maryland Ave.,
Chicago, Illinois 60637.

To further characterize the relationship between nutritional
status and course of pulmonary disease in CF, 33 children and young
adults with CF (ages 4-31 years) underwent serial assessment of their
nutritional status using anthropometric measurements (triceps skinfold thickness (TSF), and arm circumference (AC) in addition to
careful height and weight measurements. TSF and AC values were expressed as % predicted normal (%pn) for age using standard tables.[1]
Taussig - NIH clinical scores (CS) were calculated on all children
over age 6 yrs who could perform pulmonary function testing; Shwachman
scores were calculated for 6 pts under age 6 yrs. All pts had measurements made by the same observer (over a 1 to 5 year period) at the
time of outpatient visits or at the beginning of a hospitalization.
In a cross-sectional analysis of the data using the first set of
values for each pt, clinical scores correlated well with TSF, (r=0.69)
and with AC (r=0.71). TSF values were closely related to AC values
for the group as a whole (r=0.82). For individual pts, TSF measurements were more reduced than AC values. Twenty-five of 33 pts had TSF
6 to 46 percentage points lower than AC values, possibly indicating
a relative preservation of lean body mass as compared to fat stores
in these pts.

Detailed serial anthropometric measurements (over 2-3 yrs) and
pulmonary function test results were analyzed in 4 pts (age 14-17 yrs;
CS 52 to 80), and changes in TSF were examined as a function of %pn
for FVC, $FEV_1$, and $FEF_{25-75}$. Graphic displays of 5-10 paired data
points (TSF vs pulmonary function parameter) revealed a close parallel
in the decline of %pn TSF and %pn for FVC and $FEV_1$. The $FEF_{25-75}$
values were in the 10-30% range in all patients and did not vary as
significantly with changes in TSF. Improvements in pulmonary function
parameters after in-hospital treatment of pulmonary exacerbation and
the use of nutritional supplementation was associated with transient
improvement of %pn TSF in these pts.

Conclusion: These studies demonstrate a close association between
nutritional status and pulmonary disease, and suggest that serial
measurements of TSF and AC add to our ability to objectively monitor
the clinical course in CF pts.

Long term longitudinal studies are required to assess whether
decline in nutritional status preceeds and predicts the onset of a
decline in pulmonary status, or whether nutritional status worsens
as a result of progressive loss of pulmonary function.
(1) Frisancho, AR, Am J. Clin. Nutr. 27:1052, 1974.

**POSTER GROUP FIVE No. 5.17**

NUTRITION IN YOUNG ADULTS WITH CYSTIC FIBROSIS (CF):
EPIDEMIOLOGIC DATA AND EMERGING PROBLEMS.

C. Romano, G.F. Gargani, M. Cotellessa, R. Cerone, C. Micalizzi,
S. Scalisi, M. Nantron.
G. Gaslini Institute, Genoa, Italy: University Dept. of PediatricsR

Nutritional status has been evaluated (on clinical grounds; serum
Zinc values: in the normal range in a large series of CF pts) in 42
CF young adults (17 males, 25 females). The mean age is 20 yrs (range
16-28 yrs). CF was diagnosed after age 15 yrs in 7 pts. The NIH
clinical score ranges from 39 to 96: 29 pts (70%) are in the good
or excellent score (>71). Pancreatic insufficiency was absent in 8.
EPIDEMIOLOGIC DATA. Absolute (<3rd centile) or relative for height
underweight is present in 24/42 CF pts (57%). 11/24 pts have FVC
values below 70% pred. In the 18 CF pts with normal weight (43%),
only one has abnormal lung function. No significant correlation was
found between nutritional status and age at diagnosis. Underweight
is present in 4/8 CF young adults without pancreatic insufficiency.
8 CF pts followed a normal weight channel until the mean age of 14
yrs (range 12-15 yrs), when weight decline became the rule,
corresponding to an increased severity of lung disease.
NUTRITION AND DIABETES MELLITUS. Diabetes mellitus (DM), requiring
regular treatment with oral hypoglycaemics or insulin, is present
in 6/42 CF pts (14%). In all pts, DM onset was accompagned by
impairment of nutritional status and of clinical and respiratory
function scores. The diagnosis and proper treatment of DM lead to
a significant improvement of energy intake/nutrition and of pulmonary
status. Conclusively, in our experience, DM onset, particularly if
unexpected, determines in CF a significant impairment of pulmonary
status.
NUTRITION AND PORTO-SYSTEMIC SHUNTS. In the last 10 yrs, porto-
systemic shunts were performed in 3 CF pts. In all pts, hyperammoniaemia (occasional in 2 pts) was present. In the 3rd patient
(male, 17 yrs with pancreatic insufficiency) DM onset proposed complex
nutritional problems: DM, poorly controlled by oral therapy, determined a severe impairment of nutritional and pulmonary status, with
persistent hyperammoniaemia, not responsive to low-protein diet and
conventional therapy. Regular insulin treatment allowed a significant
improvement of clinical score with a better control of hyperammoniaemia.

318

**POSTER GROUP FIVE No. 5.18**

THE RELATIONSHIP OF CALORIC INTAKE AND DIETARY COMPOSITION TO SEVERITY OF CLINICAL STATUS IN CYSTIC FIBROSIS. Alice E. Smith, Hans U. Wessel, and John D. Lloyd-Still. Children's Memorial Hospital, 2300 Children's Plaza, Chicago, Illinois 60614, U.S.A.

Inadequate dietary intake is a significant factor in growth failure; however, the precise relationship of caloric intake and dietary composition to growth failure in CF is unclear. We analyzed caloric intake and specific nutrient composition in 64 CF patients (pt.), aged 0.3-18 years, to determine if such detailed knowledge could predict clinical status.

Source data were: 1) Anthropometrics (age, hgt, wgt, %ile of hgt and wgt), 3) dietary parameters (%RDA for calories, protein, Fe, $Ca^{++}$, % total calories as protein, fat, carbohydrate, fat/Kg), 3) Shwachman Score (SS), and 4) lung function data (% of Pred.: FEV, $MEF_{25-75}$, $\dot{V}max_{75}$) were available in 35 pts. Dietary data were derived from 72 hr dietary records supplied by parents. To estimate the accuracy of parent records, in 12 pts. we compared the outpatient parent records to inpatient records obtained by a dietician. To assess reproducibility we evaluated 11 records obtained in 2 hospitalized pts.

Results: Caloric intake averaged 95 ±31% RDA; range of 42-206%. Protein intake averaged 214 ±77% RDA, range 85-380%. Other constituents were ≥100% of RDA in all pts. SS ranged from 48-100, mean 69 ±13. %FEV, $\%MEF_{25-75}$, $\dot{V}max_{75}$ averaged 70 ±17, 75 ±38 and 74 ±48% respectively. Linear regressions and multiple stepwise regressions revealed no significant correlations between any individual dietary parameter and age, hgt, wgt, %ile of wgt or hgt, SS and pulmonary parameters. No dietary parameter predicted either SS, %ile of wgt, or lung function (minimum entering F value 2.5). Of all parameters SS correlated best with %ile of wgt (r .495), %FEV (r .451), $\%MEF_{25-75}$ (r .442), $\%\dot{V}max_{75}$ (r .377), age (r -.368), wgt (r -.333), and hgt (r -.305) in that order. All other correlation coefficients were <.230.

Comparison of parent- and dietician-derived data showed no significant differences except that parents estimated a significantly higher % of carbohydrate calories (p <.01) and % fat calories (p <.05).

Conclusions: Although detailed dietary intake analysis provides important information about dietary composition, it has no predictive value with regard to clinical status of CF pts. as determined by SS, lung function or %ile of wgt. Of all parameters directly related to diet, %ile of wgt is the best predictor of clinical status. Our data indicate that SS and %ile of wgt decrease progressively with age whereas dietary intake parameters do not change appreciably. This would suggest that dietary manipulations have in all probability only limited effects on deterioration of pulmonary status which ultimately determines outcome in CF.

**POSTER GROUP FIVE No. 5.19**

A STUDY OF THE RELATIONSHIP BETWEEN NEUROLOGICAL FUNCTION AND
SERUM VITAMIN E LEVELS IN PATIENTS WITH CYSTIC FIBROSIS.
HJ WILLISON (1), S JONES (2), A KRISS (2), RJ STEAD (1), S
MATTHEWS (3), DPR MULLER (3), ME HODSON (1) AND AE HARDING (2).
From the Brompton Hospital, Fulham Road, London SW3 (1), the
Institute of Neurology, Queen Square (2), and the Institute of
Child Health, Guilford Street, London WC1 (3).

A progressive spinocerebellar syndrome has been described in
a small number of patients with chronic fat malabsorptive states,
including cystic fibrosis (CF), which is thought to be caused by
severe vitamin E deficiency [1]. The most striking pathological
abnormality in such cases is degeneration of the posterior
columns in the spinal cord [2]; this can be demonstrated during
life by the use of somatosensory evoked potentials (SSEPs)[3].
Ten unselected patients with CF, who had no overt neurological disease, were assessed by means of clinical neurological
examination. In addition, SSEPs were recorded over the clavicle,
cervical spine, mastoid process and sensory cortex following
stimulation of the median nerve at the wrist and the tibial nerve
at the ankle and compared with age and sex matched control subjects. Visual evoked potentials (VEPs) were also performed in
some cases. The findings were correlated with serum vitamin E
concentrations which were unknown to the neurological investigators prior to completion of the study.
One patient, in whom serum vitamin E was virtually undetectable (less than 1 umol/l), had mild reflex and sensory
abnormalities but the other nine were clinically normal. Abnormal
VEPs were recorded from two patients. SSEPs were normal in all
10 cases. There was no correlation between latency or amplitude
of any of the SSEP components and serum vitamin E levels, which
ranged from undetectable to within the normal range.
This study suggests that, on detailed assessment, a small
proportion of patients with CF have evidence of neurological
dysfunction which is likely to be related to severe vitamin E
deficiency. We conclude that serum vitamin E concentrations
should be monitored in CF, and oral supplements given to maintain
normal levels.

REFERENCES
1. MULLER DRP, LLOYD JK, WOLFF OH. Vitamin E and neurological
function. Lancet i:225-228, 1983.
2. ROSENBLUM JL, KEATING JP, PRENSKY AL, NELSON JS. A progressive
neurologic syndrome in children with chronic liver disease. N
Engl J Med 304:503-508, 1981.
3. HARDING AE, MULLER DPR, THOMAS PK, WILLISON HJ. Spinocerebellar degeneration secondary to chronic intestinal malabsorption: a vitamin E deficiency syndrome. Ann Neurol 12:419-424,
1982.

**POSTER GROUP FIVE No. 5.20**

VITAMIN A AND ZINC STATUS IN CYSTIC FIBROSIS

DR. M.Z. MUGHAL, MISS L. CLEMENTS, DR. G. HAMBLETON & DR. M. SUPER
ROYAL MANCHESTER CHILDRENS HOSPITAL, MANCHESTER

DR. F.E. WELLS, DR. G.M. ADDISON,
BOOTH HALL CHILDRENS HOSPITAL, MANCHESTER

Low plasma Vitamin A (Vit. A) levels, despite supplementation have
been reported in patients with Cystic Fibrosis (C.F.).  It has been
suggested that zinc deficiency, which has been reported in growth
retarded patients with C.F., impairs mobilisation of Vit.A from the
liver due to impaired hepatic synthesis of retinol binding protein
(R.B.P.).  R.B.P. bound to Vit. A is complexed with prealbumin (P.A.)
a rapid turnover transport protein, in the circulation.

We have studied the interrelationship between Vit.A, R.B.P., P.A.and
zinc status in 37 children with C.F. and 25 healthy controls.  Zinc
status was assessed by estimation of serum and hair zinc
concentrations.

The mean serum Vit. A concentrations in C.F. and controls were
similar, $450 \pm 113$ µg/l and $462 \pm 106$ µg/l respectively.  2 out of
24 C.F. patients so far studied·and none out of 17 controls had
plasma Vit. A levels below the normal range (200-670 µg/l).  P.A.
was correlated with the following clinical, biochemical and
pulmonary function parameters:-

|  | C.F. | | Controls | |
|---|---|---|---|---|
|  | r | p | r | p |
| P.A. vs Vit. A | + 0.82 | <0.001 | + 0.48 | >0.05 (NS) |
| P.A. vs Schwachman Score | + 0.50 | <0.01 | | |
| P.A. vs Wt.velocity(kg/yr) | + 0.38 | <0.05 | | |
| P.A. vs Ht.velocity(cm/yr) | + 0.48 | < 0.01 | | |
| P.A. vs serum zinc | + 0.19 | NS | + 0.38 | >0.05 (NS) |
| P.A. vs hair zinc | + 0.08 | NS | | |
| P.A. vs FVC | + 0.55 | <0.01 | | |
| P.A. vs $FEV_1$ | + 0.61 | <0.001 | | |

There was no evidence of zinc deficiency in C.F. or the control
patients.  Results obtained so far suggest that in a fairly healthy
group of C.F. patients (mean Schwachman score 79), mean Vit. A
level was similar to the control value.  In C.F. patients, P.A.
concentration and not zinc status correlated with plasma Vit. A
levels.  Remaining results, including RBP levels will be presented
and discussed.

**POSTER GROUP FIVE No. 5.21**

FATTY ACID PATTERN OF PLATELET PHOSPHOLIPIDS IN C.F.,
HETEROZYGOTE, AND CONTROL SUBJECTS .

C. Galabert, J.P. Chazalette, M. Filliat and Ph. Delmas
Centre de soins pour mucoviscidoses . Hopital Renée Sabran
Giens - 83406 - Hyeres Cedex - FRANCE .

Altered essential fatty acid (EFA) composition of platelet lipids was
observed by G.B.Burns and J.A. Dodge (1) in both CF and heterozygote
subjects compared with controls.
The aim of the present study was to further examine EFA in blood platelet from CF, heterozygote, and control subjects, with an assessment
of the dietary fat consumed .

The fatty acid pattern of platelet phosphatidylcholine (PC) and phosphatidylethanolamine (PE) was determined in 15 CF, 17 heterozygote,
and 19 control subjects .
Platelets were separated according to the procedure of M. Lagarde and
al. (2). Lipids werw extracted according to the method of Bligh and
Dyer (3). Phospholipids were separated by HPTLC on silica gel . The
fatty acid pattern of PC and PE was determined by gas chromatography.
In CF patients, we observed modifications of the fatty acid pattern
in both PC and PE: the main features were a decrease of essential fatty acids linoleic and arachidonic in PC, together with an increase of
palmitic and oleic acids in PC and PE .
In heterozygote subjects, we did not observe a decrease of the arachidonic content of PC and PE .

References :

(1) - G.B. Burns and J.A. Dodge . Elevated levels of 13,14 dihydro-15
keto prostaglandin metabolites and essential fatty acid deficiency in
CF and heterozygote subjects . in: Proceedings 11th annual meeting
EWGCF, Brussel, 1982, pp 76 .

(2) - M. Lagarde, P.A. Brion, M. Guichardant and M. Dechavanne .
A simple and efficient method for platelet isolation from their plasma . Thrombosis Research, 1980, 17, 581-588 .

(3) - E.G. Bligh and W.J. Dyer . A rapid method of total lipid extrac-
tion and purification . Can. J. Biochem. Physiol., 1969, 57, 911-917 .

322

**POSTER GROUP FIVE No. 5.22**

PROLONGED SMALL INTESTINAL TRANSIT TIME IN CYSTIC FIBROSIS

Ambika Bali, David Stableforth, Peter Asquith. Alastair Frazer and
John Squire Metabolic and Clinical Investigation Unit, East
Birmingham Hospital, Bordesley Green East, Birmingham. B9 5ST

Measurement of breath hydrogen concentration after ingestion of
lactulose can be used to estimate small-intestinal transit time.
The test is based on the fact that lactulose is not absorbed in the
small intestine in man. On reaching the colon it is fermented by
bacteria and hydrogen is released, which is then absorbed and
exhaled.

We have performed the lactulose hydrogen breath test on 10
patients with cystic fibrosis and 15 control subjects (matched for
age and sex) using a Hoek Loos unit. All normal subjects had a
fasting breath hydrogen concentration of less than 20 ppm. In
contrast, seven of the patients with cystic fibrosis had high
concentrations (25-170 ppm), which fell to 20 ppm or below on
prolonged fasting (14-23 hours). Seven of the patients had prolonged small bowel transit times (160-390 minutes) compared with
those in the control group (50-150 minutes).

Delayed small intestinal transit in cystic fibrosis might be
related to viscid intestinal mucus slowing propulsion of food along
the intestine. An intrinsic defect in contraction of intestinal
smooth muscle or altered gastrointestinal hormone concentrations in
the disease may also effect motility. Finally, apparent delay in
small bowel transit time might be due to delayed gastric emptying,
but this has not been studied in adults with cystic fibrosis.

Prolonged small intestinal transit time in cystic fibrosis could
have clinical implications. It might be relevent to the 10%
incidence of small intestinal obstruction (meconium ileus equivalent).
Moreover, intestinal motility is one of the important factors in
controlling bacterial colonisation in the intestine, and therefore
delayed small bowel transit time in cystic fibrosis may encourage
bacterial overgrowth of the small bowel. This in turn could increase
existing malabsorption and further impair nutritional status.

**POSTER GROUP FIVE No. 5.23**

EVIDENCE FOR BACTERIAL CONTAMINATION OF THE SMALL INTESTINE IN
ADULTS WITH CYSTIC FIBROSIS

Ambika Bali, David Stableforth, Peter Asquith. Alastair Frazer and
John Squire Metabolic and Clinical Investigation Unit, East
Birmingham Hospital, Bordesley Green East, Birmingham. B9 5ST

Many patients with cystic fibrosis (C.F.) now reach adult life,
and while respiratory disease still dominates the clinical picture,
gastrointestinal symptoms and malnutrition are common. A major
cause for the poor nutrition is malabsorption, which may be only
partially corrected by pancreatic enzymes and Cimetidine. Persistent steatorrhoea could be due to small intestinal bacterial overgrowth already described in children with C.F.

Twelve patients with C.F. were admitted to a Metabolic Unit;
antibiotics were stopped at least four weeks earlier whilst the dose
of pancreatic enzyme were kept constant throughout the study period.
The nutritional status was assessed and a measured fat diet (60-100
gm) was started. After a 48 hour equilibration period, baseline
determination of nitrogen and fat balance was made. Investigations
for small intestinal bacterial overgrowth included $H_2$ breath test,
[14]C-Glycocholic acid breath test and jejunal aspiration for microbiology. Treatment with antibiotics (Metronidazole and Co-trimoxaz-
ole) was then started. After 4-6 weeks, fat balance studies were
repeated and nutritional status reassessed. Control groups consisted
of 25 normal subjects (healthy staff) and 24 patients with diarrhoea
(10 with small intestinal bacterial overgrowth (SIBD), 4 Crohn's
disease and 10 irritable bowel syndrome).

Bacterial colonisation of the upper jejunum with faecal microorganisms (Streptococcus fecalis, Coliforms) was detected in 4
patients with C.F., 10 diarrhoea controls and none of the normal
subjects. The $H_2$ breath test was abnormal in 1 and [14]C-GCA breath
test in 2 of the C.F. patients. One other patient with C.F. had
abnormal breath tests suggestive of small intestinal bacterial overgrowth. Repeat fat balance studies after antibiotics showed
improved fat absorption (between 12.6% and 29.3%).

Amongst diarrhoea controls, 6 patients with bacterial overgrowth
had an abnormal $H_2$ breath test and [14]C-Glycocholic acid breath test
was abnormal in 10 (6 with SIBD and 4 Crohn's disease).

Evidence of bacterial contamination of upper small bowel has thus
been detected in 4 of 12 adult patients with C.F. (2 of whom had
previously received Cimetidine). It is suggested that cyclical
antibiotics could improve the nutritional status of these patients
and hence improve their quality of life.

324

ELECTROPHORETIC ANALYSIS OF SALIVARY PROTEINS IN CF AND IN AN ANIMAL
MODEL OF THIS DISEASE

Frank M. Hallinan, M. Rose, J.R. Martinez* and E. Tempany: Children's
Research Centre, Our Lady's Hospital for Sick Children, Crumlin,
Dublin 12, Ireland and *Department of Child Health, University of
Missouri–Columbia, School of Medicine, Columbia, Missouri 65201, USA.

CF primarily affects exocrine glands and the CF defect, at least in
the sweat glands, appears to be a result of breakdown of post
secretory ductal processes, mediated by factors in the secretion.
Similar events have also been envisaged in other exocrine glands
(1,2). Hence, the products of these glands may be altered. We have,
therefore, undertaken a study of human parotid saliva (as an easily
obtainable abundant exocrine secretion) from CF patients, their
parents, and a control group. The protein composition of saliva from
these individuals was examined in a number of polyacrylamide gel
electrophoresis (PAGE) systems and by isoelectric focusing in
polyacrylamide gels. Lectin binding proteins were also analysed by
sodium dodecyl sulphate (SDS)/PAGE of salivary proteins bound to
lectin affinity colums. No differences were seen between the three
groups although an inherently large extent of individual variation in
salivary protein patterns may obscure subtle differences.

In an attempt to overcome the problems of individual variation and to
enable subtle variations in individual proteins to be detected we
are at present raising antisera against certain salivary proteins.
Thus to date we have compared by crossed immuno isoelectric focusing
the patterns of CF and control parotid saliva amylase but no
differences were apparent.

Adult rats, after repeated injections of reserpine, exhibit several
morphologic and secretory alterations resembling those observed in CF
patients. We have, therefore, compared the protein composition of
parotid and submandibular saliva samples from control and reserpinised
rats secreted in response to $\alpha$ adrenergic and $\beta$ adrenergic agonists.
Saliva samples were analysed by SDS/PAGE and by native PAGE for both
anionic and cationic proteins. No alterations in protein pattern
were evident in either type of saliva after reserpine treatment.
Hence, although reserpine treatment causes a variety of alterations in
secretory gland function, including the development of ciliary
dyskinesia and sodium reabsorbtion factor(s) the final saliva is
largely unchanged at the protein level. However, the possibility of
more subtle changes e.g. at the enzymatic level remains an interesting
alternative both for the animal model and the human disease.

**POSTER GROUP SIX No. 6.02**

ANIMAL MODEL: PANCREAS AND SUBMANDIBULAR GLAND OF
PILOCARPINE TREATED RATS STUDIED BY X-RAY MICROANALYSIS

R.M. Müller and G.M. Roomans
Wenner Gren. Institute, University of Stockholm, Sweden

Among the various animal models proposed for the study
of cystic fibrosis (CF) we have earlier carried out
elemental analysis of submandibular glands in the chronically reserpine treated rat and in the chronically isoproterenol treated rat (Müller and Roomans, 1984, Exp.
Mol. Pathol. in press). In the present study, we have
investigated submandibular gland and pancreas of the
chronically pilocarpine treated rat by X-ray microanalysis
in the electron microscope. In this animal model it
has been demonstrated that the exocrine glands show
hyperreactivity. Rats were treated with the cholinergic
agonist pilocarpine for a period of 7 days (50 mg/kg/day).
After 24h of starvation, the animals were anaesthesized,
the glands were excized, cut into small pieces and rapidly
frozen. Sections of 16 μm were cut in a cryostat and
freeze-dried. The submandibular gland and pancreas were
then studied in the electron microscope with X-ray microanalytical techniques. The preparation of the tissue
by this method exacts rapid immobilization of the metabolism of the cells and conservation of their content.
The results can be summarized as follows:

|     | Submandibular gland | | Pancreas | |
|-----|---------|------------|---------|------------|
|     | control | pilocarpine | control | pilocarpine |
| Na  | 122± 8  | 71± 5      | 130±15  | 76± 6      |
| Mg  | 72± 6   | 60± 3      | 54± 3   | 47± 2      |
| P   | 506±35  | 529±21     | 816±24  | 748±23     |
| S   | 190±12  | 200±13     | 234±11  | 270± 7     |
| Cl  | 134± 9  | 145± 9     | 152± 7  | 138± 6     |
| K   | 497±19  | 481±19     | 528±20  | 568±24     |
| Ca  | 43± 5   | 77± 7      | 11± 2   | 19± 4      |

(data in mmol/kg dry wt. mean and SE of 10 animals)

Chronic pilocarpine treatment induced changes in elemental
concentrations in the submandibular gland that are similar
to those induced by chronic isoproterenol treatment
but different from chronic reserpine treatment (Müller
and Roomans, 1984). The increase in Ca levels in both
exocrine glands studied in this animal model parallels
the increased Ca levels found in cells of CF patients.

**POSTER GROUP SIX No. 6.03**

EFFECT OF CF FIBROBLAST MEDIUM ON RAT SUBMANDIBULAR
GLAND ACINAR CELLS

Anne M. von Euler (1), Ove Ceder (2), Hans Kollberg
(2,3) and Godfried M. Roomans (1)
(1) Wenner-Gren Inst., Univ. Stockholm, Sweden, (2)
Dept. Pediatrics, Univ. Umeå, Sweden, (3) Dept.
Pediatrics, Univ. Kuwait.

Body fluids from CF patients, as well as conditioned medium from cultured CF skin fibroblasts, have been
reported to contain a factor (or factors) that cause
diverse biological effects in various tissues. Among
these effects is an increase in mucus secretion from
rabbit tracheobronchial epithelium (Czegledy-Nagy &
Sturgess (1976) Lab. Invest. 35: 588-595), increased
$K^+$ efflux from rat submandibular gland (Bogart et al.
(1980) Pediatr. Res. 16: 223-226), and influx of Ca
into normal human fibroblasts (Ceder & Roomans (1983)
Ultrastruct. Pathol. 4: 305-309). Chronic treatment
with CF serum causes atrophy of rat parotid gland
(Schneyer & Wilborn (1976) Cell Tiss. Res. 169: 111-121).
In a previous X-ray microanalytical study we showed
that incubation of submandibular gland acinar cells
with CF serum or fibroblast medium causes a significant
decrease of the K and the Ca levels (von Euler et al.
(1983) Ultrastruct. Pathol. 5: 38-44), which parallels
the action of secretagogues.
In the present study, the effect of chronic treatment with CF fibroblast medium on rat submandibular
gland acinar cells was investigated. Rats were injected
for 7 days with conditioned medium from normal or CF
fibroblasts. The elemental content of the acinar cells
was analyzed by X-ray microanalysis on semi-thick (4-6
µM) cryosections.
A significant increase (p<0.01) in cellular Ca
was found after treatment with CF medium, compared to
normal medium. No differences in Na or K content could
be detected. The ultrastructure of the submandibular
gland acinar cells was not affected by the conditioned
medium. No evidence for atrophy was observed.
Apparently, a factor in conditioned medium from
cultured CF fibroblasts induces an influx of Ca into
rat submandibular acinar cells. Possibly, this factor
acts in a similar way in CF patients and causes the
elevated Ca levels found in CF cells.

**POSTER GROUP SIX No. 6.04**

EFFECTS OF RESERPINE AND ISOPROTERENOL ON CELLULAR
CALCIUM LEVELS IN RAT SUBMANDIBULAR GLAND

R.M. Müller, T. Grundin, and G.M. Roomans
Wenner Gren Institute, University of Stockholm, Sweden

It has been shown that Ca levels in the saliva and in
the secretory cells of the parotid gland in CF patients
are abnormally high. Since the role of Ca in the secretory
process in the exocrine glands is not completely understood, further elucidation of the regulation of Ca secretion would be of great importance in the exploration
of CF ethiology. Hence, in this study we focused on
the changes in cellular Ca levels in the acinar cells
of the rat submandibular glands after stimulation with
reserpine, a noradrenaline depleter, and the adrenergic
agonist isoproterenol. Rats (female Sprague-Dawley,
200g) were injected with reserpine (0.5 mg/kg b.w.)
and isoproterenol (160 mg/kg b.w.) respectively. Glands
were removed 1, 2, 3, 4, 7, 9 and 24 hours after injection
with reserpine and 1, 4, 8, 12, 16, 20 and 24 hours
after injection with isoproterenol. X-ray microanalysis
was performed on 16 $\mu$m sections, cut at 20°C. The sections
were freeze-dried, viewed in the electron microscope
in the scanning mode and analyzed at 20kV.
Reserpine caused a small increase in cellular Ca levels
after 4h. After 7-9h the Ca levels are doubled and 24h
after injection cellular Ca levels are even higher.
Isoproterenol causes depletion of the mucous granules
from the acinar cells and a parallel extrusion of cellular
Ca. From 8h after injection on the Ca level increases
and it reaches at 16h the initial level. At 24h the
Ca concentration is doubled.
This study clearly shows that reserpine and isoproterenol
influence the regulation of total cellular Ca concentrations. The Ca levels measured after chronic treatment
with these drugs, 24h after last injection, are about
the same as after one single injection. This may mean
that in order to obtain increased Ca levels in exocrine
glands in animal models of CF, chronic treatment is
not required.

**POSTER GROUP SIX No. 6.05**

SUBSTANCE P AND EXOCRINE SECRETION IN THE RAT SUBMANDIBULAR GLAND

N. Fleming, P.T. Bilan and K.W. Graham
Dept. of Oral Biology, University of Manitoba, 780 Bannatyne Avenue,
Winnipeg, Manitoba, Canada   R3E OW3

The active peptide, substance P (SP), is present in neurons innervating the rat submandibular gland, and may play a role in controlling exocrine secretion.  Its effect on the release of mucin and peptide hydrolases from enzymatically-dispersed cells of the gland was studied. Mucin was quantitated by radioimmunoassay, enzymes (arginine esterases) by the rate of hydrolysis of $\alpha$-N-benzoyl arginine ethyl ester.

In 40 min, SP ($1 \times 10^{-7}$M) stimulated the secretion of $31.9\pm3.0\%$ (mean$\pm$SEM) of intracellular mucin, compared with values of $12.5\pm1.5$ in unstimulated controls; $66.8\pm3.0$ in cells exposed to $1 \times 10^{-6}$M isoproterenol (IPR); and $48.8\pm5.9$ in cells treated with $1 \times 10^{-6}$M norepinephrine (NE) ($p<0.01$).  The SP effect was not inhibited by the antagonists propranolol or phentolamine and was therefore independent of adrenergic receptor stimulation.  The intracellular levels of cyclic nucleotides were measured at 5 and 10 min after SP stimulation in the presence or absence of a phosphodiesterase inhibitor.  The peptide did not enhance cyclic AMP or cyclic GMP concentration, indicating that these nucleotides are not involved in the SP stimulus-secretion coupling sequence.  Potential modulation of adrenergic responses by SP was examined by treating cells with SP for 30 sec followed by IPR or NE for 40 min.  Preincubation with SP reduced the IPR mucosecretory response to 75% of its normal value ($p<0.01$), probably via intracellular mechanisms rather than by cell receptor inhibition.  SP followed by NE produced a value of 161% of the NE figure and may reflect an additive response to independent stimulation of SP and NE receptors.

In the enzyme secretion studies, control cells released $9.9\pm0.6\%$ of their arginine esterase in 40 min.  Secretion was not stimulated above this level by SP ($9.9\pm0.8\%$).  Isoproterenol provoked a release of $16.3\pm1.5\%$ and NE of $37.3\pm4.2\%$ of enzyme.

It is concluded that substance P can act both as a secretagogue and as a modulator of adrenergic stimulation in the secretion of mucin from rat submandibular acinar cells.  Its failure to initiate enzyme secretion suggests that serous cells of the granular convoluted tubule may lack appropriate peptide receptors.

Supported by the Canadian Cystic Fibrosis Foundation

**POSTER GROUP SIX No. 6.06**

ABNORMAL CARRIER-MEDIATED ANION TRANSPORT IN REDUCED FLUID SECRETION FROM THE SUBMANDIBULAR GLAND OF THE RESERPINE-INDUCED MODEL FOR CF

M. Baldwin and J. R. Martinez, University of Missouri School of Medicine, Columbia, MO 65212

Fluid secretion from the isolated, perfused rat submandibular gland is significantly inhibited by replacement of either $Na^+$ or $Cl^-$ or by the presence of furosemide in the perfusate (1, 2). Furosemide is a "loop" diuretic, which inhibits $Na^+$-coupled $Cl^-$ transport in several epithelial tissues. Chronic reserpine administration to rats causes morphological and functional changes in the salivary and other exocrine glands which resemble those of cystic fibrosis (3). A major secretory abnormality is reduced fluid secretion (3). In view of the demonstrated importance of NaCl cotransport for fluid secretion by the submandibular gland, the function of this system in reserpine treated rats was studied in these experiments.

Male Sprague-Dawley rats were used. Some rats received seven daily i.p. injections of reserpine (0.5 mg/kg body weight). Both control and treated rats were anesthetized with sodium pentobarbital and the trachea, the arterial supply to the gland and the excretory duct were cannulated as previously described (1, 2). The gland was excised, placed in a bath at 37°C and perfused with an oxygenated, enriched Krebs Ringer bicarbonate medium at 3 ml/min. Secretion was stimulated with acetylcholine ($10^{-6}$M). Saliva samples were collected at timed intervals in microsample tubes and their volume and composition determined as described (1, 2). In some experiments the perfusate contained either $10^{-3}$M furosemide or its $Cl^-$ was replaced with $SO_4^=$.

In control glands, furosemide or replacement of perfusate Cl caused a 74% reduction in the volume of saliva secreted in 60 minutes and a significant reduction in salivary $Cl^-$ concentrations, but no change in $Na^+$ or $K^+$. In glands from reserpine treated animals, acetylcholine-induced fluid secretion was reduced 72% and addition of furosemide or Cl replacement reduced the response 53-56% and caused similar changes in salivary electrolytes. The results suggest that the reduced fluid secretion in the gland of the animal model is likely to result from abnormalities in $Na^+$-coupled $Cl^-$ transport. This may represent quantitative or qualitative changes in the carrier protein involved in the cotransport. The possibility is raised that a similar defect in cation-coupled $Cl^-$ transport may underlie the disturbances in fluid secretion reported in the salivary and other exocrine glands of CF patients.

(1) Arch. Oral Biol. 28:1101, 1983.
(2) Am. J. Physiol. 245:G711, 1983.
(3) Ped. Res. 9:470, 1975.

**POSTER GROUP SIX No. 6.07**

LACATE CONCENTRATION IN THERMAL SWEAT FROM CHILDREN WITH CYSTIC
FIBROSIS

Labbe, A.,* Fellmann, N.,*** Gachon, A.M.** and Coudert, J.***.
* Departement de Pediatrie, ** Laboratoire de Biochimie, Hotel
Dieu; et *** Laboratoire de Physiologie, Faculte de Medecine 63001
CLERMONT-FERRAND Cedex - France.

The sweat of children with cystic fibrosis (CF) exhibits greater
concentration of sodium ($[Na^+]$), potassium ($[K^+]$) and chloride
($[Cl^-]$) than found in healthy subjects. It has been shown that the
sweat gland energy metabolism is linked to cation transport. Accordingly we attempt to determine whether electrolyte sweat excretion in
such patients was associated with change in glandular anaerobic
metabolism evaluated by sweat lactate concentration ($[L]Sw$).

Five subjects with CF and 11 control children (C), 5 months to 14
years old were exposed to external thermal load (infrared radiation,
IR=5,000 W). After 20 min. heat exposure, the sweat was collected
from the frontal area on a 17.5 cm filter paper during 4 minutes.
When possible, 2 or 3 serial collections were performed. The amount
of sweat collected was determined by weighing the paper in an air-
tight tube immediately before and after each sweat collection and
sweat rated (QSw) was calculated in $ul.min^{-1}. cm^{-2}$ filter paper.
On each sweat sample, $[Na^+]$ and $[K^+]$ were measured by flame photo-
meter $[Cl^-]$ by amperometric titration and $[L]$ by enzymatic method.
The same measures were made on capillary blood drawn during IR
exposure.

After the tests, the mean increase of rectal temperature was $0.4^\circ C$
for both groups. In blood, the electrolytes and $[L]$ in CF did not
differ from C. In sweat, CF had significantly ($p < 0.001$) higher
$[Na^+]$ (156.3+12.4 mM), $[K^+]$ (33.0+7.1 mM) and $[Cl^-]$ (163.7+14.0)
than C ($[Na^+]$ = 48.6+4.8 mM; $[K^+]$ = 11.4+0.9 mM; $[Cl^-]$ = 53.7+5.8 mM);
but they had the same $[L]Sw$ (15.2+7.8 mM) and QSw 2.8+0.4 $ul.min^{-1}$
$cm^{-2}$) as C ($[L]Sw$ = 16.3+1.1 mM; $\bar{QSw}$ = 3.6+0.5 ul. $min^{-1}.cm^{-2}$)
(mean+SEM).

In both groups, the sweat output of sodium ($Na^+$) and potassium ($K^+$)
increased linearly with that of lactate (L), but the slopes in CF
were significantly higher than in C.

In conclusion, the same QSw and $[L]Sw$ in both groups suggests that
the glandular anaerobic metabolism is not modified in CF. This
metabolism is known to be linked mainly to cation transport by the
secretory coils. Therefore, the higher electrolyte excretion in CF
with the same LSw could be due to some defect of primitive sweat
reabsorption by ducts.

**POSTER GROUP SIX No. 6.08**

METABOLIC STUDIES ON ISOLATED HUMAN ECCRINE SWEAT GLANDS

C. Lee*, T. Kealey* and C. Jones**
*Department of Clinical Biochemistry, University of Newcastle,
Royal Victoria Infirmary, Newcastle upon Tyne NE1 4LP and
**Department of Zoology, Durham University Science Laboratories,
South Road, Durham, DH1 3LE.

We have developed a new method for the isolation of human eccrine sweat glands based upon the shearing of skin biopsies by the repeated use of scissors which supersedes our previous one based upon the collagenase digestion of skin biopsies [Kealey,T. (1983) Biochem. J. $\underline{212}$ 143–148]. This yields 20–50 glands per biopsy which are viable by the criteria of light and electron microscopy and adenine nucleotide contents; $81.0\pm12.7$ pmol ATP/gland, $13.8\pm3.3$ pmol ADP/gland, $3.8\pm1.0$ pmol AMP/gland. Glands can be maintained for 7 days on RPMI 1640 and retain viability as judged by electron micrographic appearance and adenine nucleotide contents of $63.2\pm7.3$ pmol ATP/gland, $8.5\pm2.2$ pmol ADP/gland and $3.5\pm0.8$ pmol AMP/gland.

Following 7 days' maintenance the rate of $[^{3}H]$ –leucine uptake into glands rises from $25.9\pm4.6$ fmol/fresh gland/h to $72.2\pm15.3$ fmol/maintained gland/h and autoradiographs of polyacrylamide gels of protein from $[^{3}H]$ – leucine exposed glands will be shown.

Following exposure to $10^{-5}$M acetylcholine and isoprenaline respectively the cyclic GMP content of freshly isolated glands rose from $5.4\pm0.8$ to $80.3\pm20.3$ fmol/gland and the cyclic AMP content from $39.5\pm4.4$ to $351.6\pm63.7$ fmol/gland (maintained glands show a hypersensitivity to isoprenaline which induces a cyclic AMP content of $1225.7\pm235.6$ fmol/gland) and autoradiographs of gels of $^{32}P$ incorporated into sweat gland proteins following exposure to secretagogues will be shown.

**POSTER GROUP SIX No. 6.09**

THE RHEOLOGICAL PROPERTIES OF CYSTIC FIBROSIS SPUTUM

M.I. Lethem, S.L. James and C. Marriott
Department of Pharmacy, Brighton Polytechnic, Moulsecoomb, Brighton
BN2 4GJ, U.K.

Cystic fibrosis (CF) is characterised by chronic obstructive airway disease, which accounts for much of the morbidity and mortality associated with this condition. Clinical workers have reported that the respiratory complications of CF are associated with the hypersecretion of an abnormally 'sticky' tracheobronchial mucus. Despite these reports a number of studies of the rheological properties of sputum from various respiratory diseases failed to find a significant difference between the purulent sputum of CF patients and other respiratory diseases. In this study we have analysed the rheological properties of purulent sputa from patients with CF and chronic bronchitis (CB) and correlated these properties to the DNA content of the sputum.

Samples of sputum from 12 patients with CF and CB were frozen immediately after collection. After thawing the sputum was blotted to remove saliva and loaded into a creep compliance rheometer where it was allowed to equilibrate at 25°C, 100% relative humidity, for 30 minutes. The sample was exposed to a constant stress in the linear viscoelastic region for approximately 1 hour, and the resulting trace analysed to yield values for the elastic and viscous components of the flow. The dry weight and DNA content of the sputum were also determined.

The results of the rheological analyses of the sputa indicated that samples from patients with CF comprised a group which had greater elasticity and viscosity than samples from CB patients ($p < 0.01$ for both parameters). Dry weight values and DNA content were also significantly higher for CF samples when compared to CB sputum ($p < 0.05$ and $p < 0.01$ respectively).

Linear regression analysis of the data shows a good correlation between dry weight and DNA content ($r = 0.877$) suggesting that a majority of the increase in dry weight in CF samples is due to DNA, which is presumably bacterial in origin. A good correlation between DNA content and elasticity ($r = 0.882$) and between dry weight and both elasticity ($r = 0.877$) and viscosity ($r = 0.810$) suggests that the major factor responsible for the unusually viscid sputum in CF is the severe degree of infection leading to high DNA levels.

**POSTER GROUP SIX No. 6.10**

COMPARISON OF PHYSICO-CHEMICAL PROPERTIES OF NATIVE MUCINS FROM
RESPIRATORY SECRETIONS OF CYSTIC FIBROSIS AND ASTHMATIC PATIENTS.
Kenneth V. Chace,* Marinus Flux+ and Goverdhan P. Sachdev*.
*Biomembrane Research Program, Oklahoma Medical Research Foundation
and +Cystic Fibrosis Pediatric Pulmonary Clinic, University of
Oklahoma Health Sciences Center, Oklahoma City, Oklahoma 73104.

The presence of excessive amounts of viscous secretions in the respiratory tract is the most widely known feature of cystic fibrosis
(CF). The viscoelastic and gelation properties of these secretions
are determined, to a large extent, by the presence of mucous glycoproteins (mucins) in the secretions. Thus, abnormalities in the viscoelastic properties of CF secretions, may be caused, at least in
part, by changes in the chemical and/or physical properties of the
mucins. In order to examine this possibility, the mucins were isolated and purified from the sputum specimens of CF and asthmatic patients. The purified mucins were characterized for their physico-
chemical properties.
Native (non-reduced) mucins were purified as follows: The sputum
specimens were solubilized in 0.22 M potassium thiocyanate and subsequently chromatographed on a Bio-Gel A 5m column. The excluded
fraction which contained mucin and DNA, were digested with D'Nase and
subject to another gel filtration step using the same column. The
excluded fraction from the second column was further purified by hy-
droxylapetite column chromatography. The mucins isolated using this
procedure were found to be electrophoretically homogeneous. The purified mucins were studied for their chemical and physical properties.
The native CF mucin contained 11.9% protein, 88.1% carbohydrate (i.e.,
fucose, galactose, N-acetylgalactosamine, N-acetylglucosamine, sialic
acid and sulfate) while native asthmatic mucin contained 18.2% protein, and 81.8% carbohydrate. The molar ratios of carbohydrate components with respect to N-acetylgalactosamine were similar for both
the CF and asthmatic mucins. A comparison of the amino acid content
of the two mucins indicated that CF mucin contained 412 residues of
serine + threonine/1000 amino acid residues while asthmatic mucin had
289 residues of serine + threonine/1000 amino acid residues. In contrast, asthmatic mucin contained significantly more aspartate and
glutamate residues than CF mucin. The native CF mucin had a considerably higher molecular weight (11.3 x $10^6$ daltons), as determined by
Rayleigh light scattering, as compared to that observed for asthmatic
mucin (7.2 x $10^6$ daltons).
The observed higher molecular weight of the CF mucin than the
asthmatic mucin suggests that the CF mucin may be present in a higher
state of aggregation which may influence the viscoelastic properties
of CF secretions.
This study was supported in part by a grant from National Cystic
Fibrosis Foundation.

334

**POSTER GROUP SIX No. 6.11**

ISOLATION AND PURIFICATION OF THE NATIVE GLYCOPROTEIN FROM THE SPUTUM
OF PATIENTS WITH CYSTIC FIBROSIS

A.E. Bell, M.I. Lethem, S.L. James and C. Marriott
Department of Pharmacy, Brighton Polytechnic, Moulsecoomb, Brighton
BN2 4GJ, U.K.

Cystic fibrosis (CF) patients hypersecrete an abnormal
tracheobronchial mucus. Rheological studies using creep compliance
techniques have shown this material to be viscoelastic (i.e. having
both fluid and elastic characteristics). It has been demonstrated
for other mucus secretions that this behaviour is predominantly a
function of the constituent glycoprotein. This work investigates
methods of separating such glycoproteins.

Fresh sputum from CF patients was collected, pooled and deep frozen
until required. The secretion was solubilised by gentle stirring at
4° for 24 hours in 200 mM NaCl solution. This soluble preparation
was then centrifuged (10,000 g for 1 hour, 4°C) to remove undissolved
material, loaded onto a gel filtration column (Sepharose cross-linked
4B, 10 x 30 cm) and eluted using 200 mM NaCl. This separated the
bulk of the glycoprotein ( 90% of the total glycoprotein as assayed
by the periodic acid-Schiff method) from the included non-covalently
bound protein ( 80% of total protein assaayed by coomassie brilliant
blue method). This excluded material was further purified by caesium
chloride density gradient ultra-centrifugation (1.42 g dl$^{-1}$ starting
density, 150,000 g for 48 hours). This gave a glycoprotein fraction
free from all detectable non-covalently bound protein as evidenced by
SDS polyacrylamide gel electrophoresis.

Previous workers have suggested that enzyme inhibitor 'cocktails' may
cause aggregation of mucus glycoprotein. However the addition of a
mixture of 1 mM phenylmethyl sulphonyl fluoride, 0.02% w/v $NaN_3$ and 5
mM ethylene diamine tetra acetic acid to solutions of the purified
glycoprotein in 200 mM NaCl produced no changes in either the
solution viscosities or their turbidity (600 nm) indicating no change
in the shape or degree of association of the glycoprotein in
solution. It would therefore appear essential to use such mixtures
in the isolation of glycoproteins from CF sputum so that spurious
results will not be caused by sample deterioration.

**POSTER GROUP SIX No. 6.12**

IDENTIFICATION OF TWO DIFFERENT MUCIN COMPONENTS IN CF SPUTUM

Ingemar Carlstedt[1] & John K. Sheehan[2]
[1]Department of Physiological Chemistry 2, University of Lund, Sweden
and [2]Department of Biological Sciences, University of Lancaster, U.K.

The secretory cells of the air-way mucosa, e.g. the serous and mucous cells of the submucosal glands and the goblet cells of the surface epithelium, are likely to contribute structurally different glycoproteins (mucins) to respiratory mucus. The isolation of mucins from sputum should therefore aim at separating the macromolecules into their individual secretory entities. The likely presence of degradative enzymes in infected samples must also be considered. We have devised a protocol for the isolation and purification of cervical mucins (Carlstedt et al., 1983, Biochem. J. 211, 13-22) with stringent control of proteinase activity and adapted this method to CF sputum.

Sputum collected at sessions of physiotherapy was stored frozen. After thawing, the samples were mixed with an equal volume of ice-cold 0.2M-NaCl supplemented with proteinase inhibitors (DFP, EDTA and N-ethylmaleimide), and centrifuged at 45000 rev./min to separate the mucus gel from the sol phase. The sol was mixed with 6M-guanidinium chloride/proteinase inhibitors whereas the gel was solubilized with gentle stirring in this solvent. Subsequent purification from non-mucin proteins was achieved by using isopycnic density-gradient centrifugation in CsCl/4M-guanidinium chloride (repeated once). Nucleic acids were finally removed in a gradient containing CsCl/0.2M-guanidinium chloride.

The mucins from the gel banded at 1.44-1.56 g/ml (CsCl/0.2M-guanidinium chloride) with the major peak (´light´ fraction) close to 1.47 g/ml. A pronounced shoulder (´heavy´ fraction) was noted at approx. 1.52 g/ml in some samples. The major part of the ´light´ fraction chromatographed with the void volume of a Sepharose CL-2B column (component A) whereas a large proportion of the ´heavy´ one was included. Mucins from the sol phase banded at 1.42-1.58 g/ml (CsCl/0.2M-guanidinium chloride) with the peak at 1.50 g/ml and were all included on Sepharose CL-2B. Reduction of disulphide bonds followed by trypsin digestion of component A afforded glycopeptides which were of approx. the same size as the major mucin population of the sol phase. Ion exchange chromatography showed, however, that the latter macromolecules are much more ´acidic´ than the glycopeptides derived from component A. The mucins from the sol phase are thus not likely to be proteinase-derived fragments of the much larger species from the gel phase but appear to represent a separate population.

**POSTER GROUP SIX No. 6.13**

PARTIAL CHARACTERISATION OF SPUTUM FROM CYSTIC FIBROSIS PATIENTS

M.I. Lethem, A.E. Bell, S.L. James and C. Marriott
Department of Pharmacy, Brighton Polytechnic, Moulsecoomb, Brighton
BN2 4GJ, U.K.

It has been suggested that the mucus secretions in cystic fibrosis
(CF) exhibit abnormal biophysical behaviour. Mucus glycoproteins
from a variety of sources have been shown to have the same general
structure, consisting of a protein core surrounded by a sheath of
carbohydrate side chains. Several of these glycoproteins have been
shown to be oligomers of subunits linked together by disulphide
bonds, which can be reduced using mercaptans. The rheological
properties of these secretions have been shown to be dependent upon
these interactions.

Samples of CF sputum were solubilised in 200 mM sodium chloride
containing 0.02% w/v sodium azide, 5 mM ethylene diamine tetra acetic
acid and 1 mM phenylmethyl sulphonyl fluoride, by homogenisation.
The insoluble cell debris was removed by centrifugation and the
soluble mucus fractionated by gel filtration at 4°C on cross-linked
Sepharose 4B (CL4B) using the same buffer as eluant. This separated
the bulk of the non-covalently bound protein (included) from the
constituent (excluded) glycoprotein.

Samples of the excluded glycoprotein were reduced using 200 mM
2-mercaptoethanol, and subsequently carboxymethylated using 220 mM
iodoacetamide. Samples of the non-reduced and reduced glycoprotein
were subsequently rechromatographed at 4°C on cross-linked Sepharose
2B (CL2B), using both the original buffer and the buffer containing
8.0 M urea. Glycoprotein was measured using a modified periodic
acid-Schiff method and protein by the coomassie brilliant blue assay.

The material excluded from the Sepharose CL4B gel (92% w/w
glycoprotein) was found to be only partially included on a Sepharose
CL2B column, both in dissociating and non-dissociating conditions
(22% and 27% with and without urea respectively). The reduced
glycoprotein when examined on Sepharose CL2B under non-dissociating
conditions gave essentially the same profile as the non-reduced
material (32% included). However if the same reduced glycoprotein
was chromatographed in 8.0 M urea a large proportion of the
glycoprotein was found to be within the included volume of the column
(68% included).

These studies suggest that the glycoprotein isolated from the sputum
of CF patients can form thiol independent, high molecular weight
aggregates, and the 'sticky' nature of CF sputum may be a reflection
of these apparently strong non-covalent interactions.

**POSTER GROUP SIX No. 6.14**

ACTIVE LIPID : A POTENTIAL FLUIDIFIZER OF CYSTIC FIBROSIS MUCUS

C. MOTTA[*], A.M. TOUILLON[*], G. SIMON[**] and B. DASTUGUE[*]
[*]Laboratoire de Biochimie Hôtel-Dieu - 63 000 CLERMONT-FERRAND France
[**]Centre Hélio-marin - 17 370 ST TROJAN LES BAINS France

Actin lipid (A.L.) is a lipid mixture which has been recently demonstrated to be a potent fluidifizer for rigidified natural membranes (1). This lipid mixture, extracted from egg yolk, contains 70 % of neutral lipids, 20 % phosphatidylethanolamin and 10 % phosphatidylcholine. Incorporation of this mixture in mucus from children with cystic-fibrosis has been investigated. The apparent effects have been analyzed by a physical method : the fluorescence polarization, using the fluorescent probe 1,6 Diphenyl 1,3,5 Hexatriène. The fluorescence polarization measurements are related to the movements of the probe embedded in the phospholipid domains of mucus and hence to the microviscosity of these domains. Aniso-tropy (r) measurements indicated a progressive incorporation of active lipid into the phospholipids structure contained in mucus, leading to a progressive decrease of r. This decrease is associated with a macroscopic mucus fluidification and a loss of adhesivity of mucus to plastic and glass tubes. Optimum macroscopic effects were obtained after 45 minutes of contact between A.L. and mucus. The most drastic results were obtained on mucus exhibiting the highest initial microviscosity values. If this initial value was relatively low, no fluidity improvement was recorded. It is suggested from these in vitro studies a possibility of therapeutic use of A.L. in cystic-fibrosis.

(1). - HERSHKOWITZ M HERON D, SAMUEL D, SHINITZKY M.
Modulation of protein phosphorylation and receptor binding in synaptic membranes by changes in lipid fluidity : implication for ageing. Progress in Brain Rescarch. Vol X. (In Press)

**POSTER GROUP SIX No. 6.15**

CYSTIC FIBROSIS MUCUS : PHOSPHOLIPIDS-PROTEINS INTERACTIONS

C. MOTTA, A.M. TOUILLON and B. DASTUGUE

Laboratoire de Biochimie Hôtel-Dieu - 63 000 CLERMONT-FERRAND France

The analysis of phospholipids dynamics and phospholipids-proteins interactions is essential to understand the molecular organization of mucus in cystic-fibrosis. Polarization fluorescence is a classic method to perform such investigations. Fluidity data and related parameters such as Activation Energy depend of molecular interactions. Previous studies on natural membranes and biological fluids have proved the validity of the method. Using two different fluorescent probes (1,6 Diphenyl 1,3,5 Hexatriène and Perylène) on 180 samples of mucus from 22 children, microviscosity $\eta$ and Energy Activation $\Delta E$ were measured either directly on mucus or on phospholipids vesicles from mucus extracts. The differences observed on $\eta$ values can be related to phospholipids-proteins type interactions, and could be related to the severity of the disease or to the lung bacterial infection. Arrhenius plots of $\eta$ versus the temperature exhibited in some cases residual phase transitions, this corresponding to noticeable amounts of saturated phospholipids in mucus. Fluidity measurements and related parameters correspond to a submacroscopic level of investigation which is physiologically relevant. These measurements can provide a convenient mean to follow the evolution of the disease. Precise knowledge of the molecular mucus organization in cystic-fibrosis could lead to the design of therapeutics aiming the disorganization of the mucus.

**POSTER GROUP SIX No. 6.16**

THE COMPOSITION OF MUCIN OF JEJUNUM AND ILEUM.  A.W. Wesley,
D. Manning, J. Wong, A.M. Roberton.  Depts. of Paediatrics and
Biochemistry, University of Auckland, Auckland, New Zealand.

Mucins have been isolated and purified from human autopsy small
intestine in order to determine the variation in composition of mucin
of jejunum and ileum.

Intestine was obtained from two adult subjects who died as a
result of accidents (H & M).  Purification of mucin was undertaken
by a sequence of homogenisation of mucosal scrapings, centrifugation,
Sepharose 4B chromatography and preparative CsCl density gradient
ultracentrifugation.  The purified mucins were analysed using
cellulose acetate electrophoresis (CAE), carbohydrate analysis by
gas liquid chromatography and sulfate analysis by the Ba chloranilate
method.

Mucin from both subjects separated into 3 species by CAE. Species
1 was the least mobile, and differed from species 2 and 3 by
staining with PAS only, while species 2 and 3 stained with Alcian
Blue (AB).  All three species were present in the upper jejunum,
but species 1 was dominant.  Species 1 and 3 decrease markedly in
mucin of distal small intestine.  Major differences in sulfate and
sialic acid content were seen between the two subjects as well as
different regions of the intestine.

|  | Sialic Acid | | Sulphate % by Wt. | |
| --- | --- | --- | --- | --- |
|  | H | M | H | M |
| Upper jejunum | 4.1 | 11.3 | 1.06 | 2.96 |
| Jejunum-ileum | 2.2 | 9.7 | 1.53 | 6.65 |
| Lower ileum | 5.8 | 15.3 | 1.17 | 5.24 |

Purified mucins from one subject with cystic fibrosis has also
been subjected to CAE.  PAS staining mucin was seen as in the
previous specimens but virtually no soluable AB staining material
was present.  However sulphate analysis of the CF mucin showed a
high content - similar to Subject M.

Mucin of the small intestine contains 3 mucin species with
differing PAS and AB staining and probable different sialic acid
and sulfate content properties.  This observation may be
important when interpreting studies of CF versus normal small
intestinal mucins.

**POSTER GROUP SIX No. 6.17**

QUANTITATION OF LEUKOTRIENES AND PROSTANOIDS IN THE SPUTUM OF PATIENTS WITH CYSTIC FIBROSIS

J T Zakrzewski, N C Barnes, P J Piper[1] & J F Costello, Chest Unit, King's College Hospital Medical School, London SE5 and [1]Department of Pharmacology, Royal College of Surgeons of England, London WC2.

Leukotrienes (LTs) and prostanoids (Ps) formed from the common precursor - arachidonic acid - are biologically active substances which may be mediators of inflammation and bronchoconstriction in cystic fibrosis (CF). Sputum samples from CF patients (n = 11) were collected in ethanol (80%) on ice and immediately homogenized. After centrifugation (12,000g for 20 min at $4^{\circ}C$), the supernatant was removed and evaporated to dryness under vacuum. Using synthetic LTs $B_4$, $C_4$, $D_4$ as standard markers initial analysis of extracts by reverse phase HPLC (5 $\mu$m $C_{18}$ column in methanol, water, glacial acetic acid 69:31: 0.01, pH 5.4)[18] and bioassay of corresponding fractions, indicated the presence of LT-like material. Sputum extracts containing $LTB_4$ and peptidolipid LTs $C_4$ and $D_4$ were then directly quantitated by bioassay on a combination of guinea-pig lung parenchyma (GPP) and ileum smooth muscle (GPISM). The use of these two tissues discriminates between $LTB_4$ and peptidolipid LTs (see Ford-Hutchinson et al, 1982); furthermore only the peptidolipid LTs are antagonised by FPL-55712. $LTC_4$ was quantitated by radioimmunoassay (RIA) using an antiserum which also cross-reacts with $LTD_4$ (Hayes et al, 1983). Prostaglandin $F_{2\alpha}$, $E_2$ (PGF$_{2\alpha}$, PGE$_2$), thromboxane $B_2$ (T x $B_2$) and 6-oxo-prostaglandin $F_{1\alpha}$ (6-oxo-PGF$_{1\alpha}$) were also measured by RIA. The average amount of sputum produced in CF patients was 5.3 g $\pm$ 1.3. Bioassay of extracts showed a contraction of GPP (26.5 $\pm$ 4.9 pmol equivalents LTD$_4$/g) which was partially inhibited by FPL 55712 1 ug/ml (29.0 $\pm$ 6.0% n = 7) Activity on GPISM could only be detected in one patient. These results suggest a major $LTB_4$ component in addition to low levels of peptidolipid LTs. Measurement of $LTC_4$/$LTD_4$ by RIA (5.7 $\pm$ 1.5 pmol/g) confirmed the presence of peptidolipid LTs which were antagonised by FPL 55712. PGF$_{2\alpha}$ (8.6 pmol/g $\pm$ 1.6), PGE$_2$ (37.7 pmol/g $\pm$ 9.2), T x $B_2$ (8.7 pmol/g $\pm$ 2.2) and 6-oxo-PGF$_{1\alpha}$ (14.9 pmol/g $\pm$ 4.4) were also formed. Initial experiments with BW 755c (25 ug/ml) suggest that although these substances may be formed during homogenization, the majority of activity is not produced by this procedure. Our results show that LTs and Ps are present in sputum of patients with CF at levels likely to contribute to inflammation and bronchoconstriction.

We thank the Asthma Research Council for financial support and Dr J Rokach, Merck-Frosst for LTs and antiserum to $LTC_4$.

Ford-Hutchinson A W et al (1982) Br J Pharmac 76; 215-220.

Hayes E C et al (1983) J Immunol 131, 429-433.

MACROMOLECULAR PROPERTIES OF THE MAJOR MUCIN COMPONENT FROM THE GEL
PHASE OF CF SPUTUM

John K. Sheehan[1] and Ingemar Carlstedt[2]
[1]Department of Biological Sciences, University of Lancaster, U.K. and
[2]Department of Physiological Chemistry 2, University of Lund, Sweden

Morbidity and mortality in CF are intimately associated with a
deterioration of the lung function with infection and the secretion of
a viscid mucus being prominent features of the pathological process.
The macromolecules responsible for the properties of mucus are high-$M_r$
glycoproteins referred to as the mucus glycoproteins or the mucins. In
order to understand how mucus is formed and how its properties are
regulated physiologically or deranged as a consequence of disease,
macromolecular features such as size, shape and ´architecture´ of
mucins representative of those present in situ must be studied. We have
extracted mucins from the gel phase of CF sputum into 6M-guanidinium
chloride supplemented with proteinase inhibitors. Subsequent purification was achieved by using isopycnic density-gradient centrifugations
followed by preparative gel chromatography. A major population which
chromatographed with the void volume of Sepharose CL-2B was studied
further. The macromolecules appeared as a single unimodal peak in
sedimentation-velocity as well as analytical isopycnic density-gradient
centrifugation. The hydrodynamic properties were studied with laser
light-sacttering performed as total intensity measurements ($M_r$ and $R_G$)
as well as photon correlation spectroscopy ($D_T$). The results are
summarized in Table 1:

TABLE 1

| $s^o_{20,w}$ (S) | $10^{-6}$ x $M_w$ | $R_G$ (nm) | $10^8$ x $D^o_{20,w}$ (cm$^2$/sec) |
|---|---|---|---|
| 47 | 15 - 20 | 260 | 1.8 |

The size of the fragments obtained after reduction of disulphide
bonds (´subunits´) and of the glycopeptides isolated after subsequent
trypsin digestion of ´subunits´ were of approx. the same size as the
corresponding fragments from cervical mucins (Carlstedt et al., 1983,
Biochem. J., 213, 427-435). The relationship between log$R_G$ and log$M_r$
also conform with the cervical mucins. We suggest that the major mucin
component from the gel phase of CF sputum is a linear flexible chain
within a spheroidal solvent domain.

**POSTER GROUP SIX No. 6.19**

---

LIPID BOUND SIALIC ACID IN CYSTIC FIBROSIS

Occari C., Giurioli R., Panin G., Giunta A.M.*, Amoretti M.*, Chiandetti L., Zacchello F.
Dept.of Pediatrics, University of Padua, Via Giustiniani, 3, 35128
Padua, Italy; *II Pediatric Clinic, University of Milan, Via Commenda, 9, 20122 Milan, Italy.

Plasma and fibroblasts of patients with cystic fibrosis (CF) appear
to have normal activities of the enzymes: sialic acid-glycoprotein
sialyltransferases. Less knowledge is available concerning sialyltransferases involved in the biosynthesis of gangliosides. Since these
enzymes are different in specificity, and gangliosides play an important role in membrane associated functions, we studied lipid bound
sialic acid in sera from CF patients and obligate heterozygotes to find
out if a defect of sialo-glycolipid biosynthesis in involved in CF.
MATERIALS AND METHODS. Serum samples were obtained from 6 CF homozygotes, 16 obligate heterozygotes, 10 control children and 12 healthy
adults. All the samples were kept frozen at -70°C and analyzed at the
same time interval from the collection (8 days). Total sialic acid
was assayed according to Warren (1959). Lipid bound sialic acid was
measured according to the procedure described by Katopodis and Stock
(1980).

RESULTS:

| | N | TOTAL SIALIC ACID ($\mu$g/ml) $\bar{x} \pm$ S.D. | LIPID BOUND SIALIC ACID ($\mu$g/ml) $\bar{x} \pm$ S.D. |
|---|---|---|---|
| CF (2-14yrs) | 6 | 867.0 $\pm$ 118.9 | 173.2 $\pm$ 25.5 |
| CONTROLS (2m-11yrs) | 10 | 823.1 $\pm$ 108.4 | 241.4 $\pm$ 33.9 |
| HETEROZYGOTES (23-45yrs) | 16 | 684 $\pm$ 110.1 | 202.2 $\pm$ 37.6 |
| CONTROLS (24-40yrs) | 12 | 702.4 $\pm$ 44.1 | 186.2 $\pm$ 14.2 |

DISCUSSION

Lipid bound sialic acid concentration is lower ($p < 0.001$) in CF homozygotes than in age matched control children. Obligate heterozygotes
do not differ significantly from healthy adults subjects. Further
work is in progress to elucidate the pathophysiological relevance of
these findings.

**POSTER GROUP SIX No. 6.20**

ISOPROTEIN PATTERN OF COBALAMIN R BINDER AND INTRINSIC FACTOR IN CYSTIC FIBROSIS.

Guéant JL, Vidailhet M, Djalali M, Michalski JC, Naimi D, Hambaba.L, Nicolas JP. Laboratoire de Biochimie Médicale et Pédiatrique et Service des Maladies Infantiles 1, CHU Nancy-Brabois, Vandoeuvre-lès-Nancy 54500, France.

R binder and intrinsic factor are 2 glycoproteic binders of vitamin B12 (Cbl). In the present work, we studied physicochemical properties of R binder in saliva and sera from 8 cystic fibrosis (CF) patients and 5 healthy children, R binder was labelled with CN $^{57}$Co Cbl and was semi-purified by Sephacryl S-300 gel filtration and by ultrafiltration. The molecular mass was estimated in gel filtration using $^{125}$I labelled reference proteins. Isoelectrofocusing chromatography was carried out in LKB 110 ml columns using carrier ampholines of pH 2.5-4.0 and 3.5-5.0 in a final concentration of 1% and in 0-50% sucrose gradient. The estimated molecular mass of R binder from CF saliva was similar to that from control saliva (95 300 ± 13 200 and 103 600 ± 4 900 respectively) but the mean isoelectric point was increased significantly (4.3 ± 0.20 and 3.78 ± 0.08 respectively) and the microheterogeneity was reduced (1-5 isoproteins and 10 isoproteins respectively).This physicochemical modifications were not observed with R binder from CF sera. The augmentation of the mean isoelectric point of CF salivary R binder correspond in part to a decrease of its sialic acid content. The activity of β -galactosidase, α-mannosidase, α-L-fucosidase and neuraminidase was thus determined in saliva and sera. Only β-galactosidase and α-mannosidase activities were significantly increased in CF saliva (p < 0.05). The isoelectric change of CF salivary R binder could be explained by this increased glucosidase activities but 1) no correlation was found between glycosidase activities and the mean isoelectric points 2) no neuraminidase activity was detected in CF saliva. It could be also explained by a modified composition or structure of the carbohydrate chains of the molecule. The molecular mass, the mean isoelectric point and the microheterogeneity of intrinsic factor from CF gastric juice were normal (53 800 ± 2 300, 5.05 ± 0.22, 3 isoproteins respectively) compared to control values. In conclusion, R binder could be a good model molecule to study the glycoprotein metabolism in CF since it contains 30-40% carbohydrates and it is present in most tissues and fluids of the organism.

**POSTER GROUP SIX No. 6.21**

SYNTHESIS OF PROTEOGLYCANS AND GLYCOPROTEINS IN SKIN FIBROBLASTS CULTURED FROM PATIENTS WITH CYSTIC FIBROSIS (CF).

M.F. Harmand, M. Colle*, R. Duphil, D. Ducassou, J. Battin*

INSERM-SC 31 - Université de Bordeaux II, 146, rue Léo Saignat, 33076 Bordeaux-Cédex (France)
*Hôpital des Enfants, Clinique des Maladies des Enfants, 168 Cours de l'Argonne, 33077 Bordeaux-Cédex (France).

Fibroblasts were cultured from forearm skin biopsies of CF patients and age matched controls in medium (NCTC 109/RPMI 1640, 50/50) supplemented with 10 % foetal calf serum, in 25 cm$^2$ culture flasks. Confluent cultures ($6 \times 10^4$ cells/cm$^2$) were labelled for 1, 3, 6, 12 and 24 hours with $[1-^{14}C]$-Sodium acetate. Media and cell layer $^{14}C$-glycoproteins were characterized by gel filtration chromatography on Sephadex G-200 columns (0.9 x 150 cm). Proteoglycans and hyaluronic acid from both compartments were assayed for hexuronic acid (per μg DNA).

Firstly, after 1 hour of incubation the content of hexuronic acid is already 50 % ($P < 0.01$) higher than control values, and after 24 hours the values are 3 times that of the normal ones ($P < 0.001$).

Secondly, the elution profiles of $^{14}C$-labelled components exhibit the same peaks in normal and CF cultures. However, there is a higher proportion of the largest molecules migrating in (or near) the void volume in CF cultures. For example, 35 $^{14}C$-dpm/μg DNA and 145 $^{14}C$-dpm/μg DNA are incorporated respectively in normal and CF void volume macromolecules ($P < 0.001$).

In conclusion : fibroblasts arising from CF patients exhibit higher synthesis rate of proteoglycans and glycoproteins. Larger molecular species synthesis seem to be favourised. These alterations could be related to the hypersecretion of abnormally viscous mucus observed in cystic fibrosis.

# ALTERED FUCOSYLATION OF GLYCOPEPTIDES FROM CYSTIC FIBROSIS (CF) FIBROBLASTS

Thomas F. Scanlin, Yu-Mei Wang and Mary Catherine Glick. Department of Pediatrics, University of Pennsylvania School of Medicine, The Children's Hospital of Philadelphia, Philadelphia, PA 19104, USA.

Previously we have demonstrated differences in the monosaccharide composition of the glycopeptides from the trypsin-sensitive glycoproteins from skin fibroblast membranes when CF was compared to matched controls. Similar differences were also found in high molecular weight glycoproteins purified from the growth media of CF skin fibroblasts (Biochemistry, 21, 491, 1982). However, the glycopeptides from the surface of the fibroblast membranes were obtained from a heterogeneous population of glycoproteins. Therefore we have further purified these glycopeptides to obtain a more detailed characterization of the differences in glycosylation in CF.

CF and matched control skin fibroblasts were metabolically labelled with L-[$^3$H]fucose. Trypsin-sensitive surface glycopeptides were purified using Sephadex G-50 column chromatography. The glycopeptides were further purified using lentil lectin affinity chromatography. Immobilized lentil lectin binds bi- and tri-antennary glycopeptides which are fucosylated at the asparagine-linked N-acetylglucosamine and which contain $\alpha$-mannosyl residues.

The glycopeptides obtained were analyzed for radioactivity and the carbohydrate composition was determined by gas liquid chromatography of the alditol acetate derivatives. The glycopeptides from the CF material which were eluted from the lentil lectin column with $\alpha$-methyl mannoside had an increased content of fucose, an increased ratio of fucose to the other monosaccharides and a much lower specific activity of incorporated L-[$^3$H]fucose. The mean values for duplicate experiments on three matched sets of CF and control fractions showed a specific activity of 355 ± 183 cpm per nmol fucose for the CF fractions compared to a value of 2707 ± 839 for the controls. This striking, seven-fold difference in the specific activity of the incorporated fucose suggests a different turnover for the fucose moiety in these CF glycoproteins. Supported by USPHS AM16859.

346

THE EFFECT OF CYTOSKELETAL DISRUPTION ON THE CARBOHYDRATE COMPOSITION OF GLYCOPROTEINS SECRETED BY NORMAL AND CYSTIC FIBROSIS FIBROBLASTS

V Gavrias and CJ Danpure
Division of Inherited Metabolic Diseases, Clinical Research Centre, Watford Road, Harrow, Middlesex HA1 3UJ.

There have been many reports that the carbohydrate composition of both O- and N-linked secretory glycoproteins is abnormal in cystic fibrosis. The reason for this is unknown but does not seem to be directly related to any known enzymic abnormality. It has also been shown that certain aspects of cytoskeletal, especially microtubular, function is altered in cystic fibrosis. The object of the present study is to investigate the possibility that cytoskeletal malfunction in cystic fibrosis cells may be responsible for some of the carbohydrate abnormalities observed in cystic fibrosis glycoproteins.

Confluent monolayers of normal and cystic fibrosis skin fibroblasts were labelled with $^3$H-fucose and $^{14}$C-mannose for 24 h. The radioactive medium was then removed and replaced with non-radioactive medium containing various combinations of the microtubule poison colchicine (10 $\mu$M) and the microfilament poison cytochalasin B (20 $\mu$M) for 1 – 24 h. The intracellular, trypsin-soluble and secreted glycoproteins were then assayed for $^3$H and $^{14}$C.

In both normal and cystic fibrosis cells, much more mannose was taken up than fucose, but a greater proportion of the latter was incorporated into glycoproteins. Most of the $^3$H-fucose-labelled glycoproteins were secreted over 24 h, whereas most of the $^{14}$C-mannose-labelled glycoproteins remained intracellular. The relative secretion of $^{14}$C-mannose-labelled glycoproteins was increased by both drugs, individually and in combination, to levels approaching those of the $^3$H-fucose-labelled glycoproteins, the latter remaining unaltered. The total secreted glycoprotein-bound $^3$H-fucose: $^{14}$C-mannose ratio was decreased by the presence of both drugs. In this system no overall difference was found between normal and cystic fibrosis cells.

Currently the effect of cytoskeletal disruption on the carbohydrate composition of specific glycoproteins, such as fibronectin, is being investigated in an attempt to distinguish between generalised changes in the rate of secretion of high mannose containing glycoproteins and specific changes in fucose: mannose ratios in specific glycoproteins.

**POSTER GROUP SIX No. 6.24**

IDENTIFICATION OF DEGRADED PROTEOGLYCANS IN THE SPUTUM OF
PATIENTS SUFFERING FROM CHRONIC BRONCHIAL HYPERSECRETIONS.

André Le Treut[1], Geneviève Lamblin[2], Geneviève Leray[1], Lucienne
Guenet[1] Monique Filliat[3] and Philippe Roussel[2].
Laboratoire de Biochimie Médicale B, Faculté de Médecine, 35403
Rennes[1] ; Unité INSERM N°16, Place de Verdun, 59045 Lille[2] and
Hopital Renée Sabran, 83406 Giens-Hyères, France[3].

The soluble phases of the sputum from 19 patients
suffering from bronchial hypersecretion (6 patients with cystic
fibrosis, 4 with bronchiectasis, 5 with chronic bronchitis and 4
with bronchoalveolar carcinoma) were analyzed for proteoglycans
by agarose electrophoresis before and after specific enzymatic
treatments.

Proteoglycans sensitive to chondroitinases but not to
Streptomyces hyaluronidase were characterized in six cases (5
patients with CF and 1 patient with bronchiectasis).

Proteoglycans were isolated from the sputum of one of the
patients with CF and were treated by pronase. The liberated
glycosaminoglycans (GAG) were subsequently purified by gel
chromatography on Sephacryl S-300 and by preparative agarose
electrophoresis. The chemical analysis of these GAG revealed
that they contained short chains of chondroitin sulfate probably
belonging to degraded proteoglycans.

The origin and significance of proteoglycans in tracheobronchial secretions are unknown ; however they might reflect
alterations of the basal lamina of the tracheobronchial
epithelium in relation with the severity of the bronchial
disease.

This work is supported by a grant from the Association
Française de Lutte contre la Mucoviscidose.

**POSTER GROUP SIX No. 6.25**

QUANTITATION OF MUCUS SECRETION FROM THE FERRET TRACHEA

Kyle, H., Robinson, N. and Widdicombe, J.G.  Department
of Physiology, St. George's Hospital Medical School,
Cranmer Terrace, London SW17 ORE.

Most methods used for the study of tracheal mucus
secretion involve either washing out secretions or the
collection of respiratory tract fluid which may be
contaminated with lung fluid and modified by the collection method.  Collections of 'pure' secretions from a
defined area have been made by micropipette collection
from a single submucosal gland, but the volumes collected
prohibit extensive chemical analysis.

Our method is to mount a whole ferret trachea (7cm
long, laryngeal end down) in an organ bath, with its
serosal surface bathed with Krebs-Henseleit solution, and
its lumen air-filled.  The lower laryngeal end is cannulated with a special perspex cannula which allows the
insertion of a fine polyethylene catheter for sample
collection.  The upper end is attached to a pressure
transducer to register changes in smooth muscle tone.
Drugs are given into the bathing solution and secretion
is collected at intervals of 10-30 min.  The secretions
are weighed to determine their volume, and their total
solute, sodium and potassium concentrations are measured.

The cholinergic agonist, methacholine (0.05mM) and the
adrenoceptor agonists adrenaline, phenylephrine and
salbutamol (0.1mM), all significantly increased secretion
rate compared to control ($p < 0.05$), with a range of 3.82µl/
min for methacholine to 0.23µl/min for salbutamol.  The
adrenoceptor agonists dobutamine and prenalterol (0.1mM)
did not increase the secretion rate.  Total solute concentration appeared to be inversely proportional to secretion
rate with a range of 1.78% (methacholine) to 3.8% (salbutamol).  Sodium but not potassium concentration also
appeared to be inversely proportional to secretion rate
with all mean ion concentrations being hypertonic to
Krebs-Henseleit solution.  Methacholine, adrenaline and
phenylephrine all caused a large smooth muscle contraction, while dobutamine and prenalterol had no effect, and
salbutamol caused a slight smooth muscle relaxation.

**POSTER GROUP SIX No. 6.26**

COMPLEXES WITH HUMAN TRACHEAL GLYCOPROTEINS

Thomas P. Mawhinney and Giulio J. Barbero
University of Missouri Medical Center, Departments of
Child Health and Biochemistry, Columbia, Missouri, 65212,
U.S.A.

One of the most prominent features associated with cystic fibrosis (CF), and other forms of chronic obstructive pulmonary disease (COPD), is the accumulation of pulmonary secretion within the respiratory tree. Through the course of our studies we have observed that many plasma and lung derived components, typically found in these secretions (e.g., albumin, transferrin, IgG, IgA, phospholipids, etc), showed expressed affinities for the large anionic tracheobronchial glycoproteins (TBG) which are the primary macromolecular constituent in these secretions. In an effort to better define these affinities we covalently bound well characterized TBG to CNBr-Sepharose, activated Thiol-Sepharose 4B/Thiopropyl-Sepharose 6B, and CNBr-Sepharose 6MB (for cell chromatography). We then employed these TBG-Sepharose columns as affinity columns and tested the ability of many plasma and lung derived compounds to bind to them under varying ionic strengths and varying concentrations of divalent cations. Our preliminary studies demonstrated that at low ionic strength (0.01M NaCl) albumin, transferrin, alpha$_1$-antitrypsin, IgA (7 and 11S) and P. aeruginosa outer membrane did bind, and that IgG, DNA, haptoglobin, alginate, P. aeruginosa mucoid slime and lipopolysaccharide did not. With the exception of haptoglobin, all compounds tested showed significant increases in their binding to these TBG-Sepharose columns in the presence of calcium (1-4 mmol/L in 0.15 M NaCl). Notably, at the higher concentration of calcium (4 mmol/L) DNA binding increased 87.2% and P. aeruginosa mucoid slime increased 98% over the amount bound in the absence of a divalent cation. Additionally, by using TBG-Sepharose 6MB for affinity cell chromatography, low ionic and strong lectin affinities were noted for smooth type P. aeruginosa and only ionic affinities for the mucoid strains (CF sputum isolates). These early studies suggest that TBG form ionic and non-ionic complexes with many plasma and lung derived protein, glycoprotein and phospholipid components found in sputum, and that these complexes, including those with bacteria and bacterial products, may play a prominent role in CF and COPD where many of these sputum components are significantly increased.

350

**POSTER GROUP SIX No. 6.27**

STRUCTURE DETERMINATION OF THE CARBOHYDRATE CHAINS OF CYSTIC
FIBROSIS BRONCHIAL MUCINS BY 500-MHz [1]H-NMR SPECTROSCOPY

H. van Halbeek*, J.N. Breg*, J.F.G. Vliegenthart*, G. Lamblin'
and P. Roussel'.  * Department of Bio-Organic Chemistry, University
of Utrecht, NL-3522 Utrecht (The Netherlands); ' INSERM No 16,
Biochimie des Proteines, Place de Verdun, F-59045 Lille Cedex
(France).

In cystic fibrosis (CF), bronchial hypersecretion leads to obstruction of the airways, thereby increasing the gravity of the disease
i.e. by inducing infections.  To determine whether these phenomena
are correlated with aberrant mucous glycoprotein structure, we
investigated the carbohydrate chains of bronchial mucins obtained
from 6 patients (bloodgroup O) suffering from CF.

The carbohydrates were released from the mucins by alkaline boro-
hydride treatment; the resulting oligosaccharide-alditols were
separated by ion-exchange chromatography and high-performance
liquid-chromatography.  The structures of the neutral and sialylated di- to hexasaccharide-alditols were characterized by
employing high-resolution [1]H-NMR spectrosocpy at 500 MHz.  This
approach allows the primary structure determination of carbohydrates at the level of nanomole amounts, even if present in
mixtures of related components, in a rapid and non-destructive
way (1,2).  It provided a unique means to gain insight into the
(micro) heterogeneity displayed by these carbohydrate chains.
Moreover, a determinant sequence was found to occur which had not
been observed before in mucins, namely,

$$\text{NeuAc } \alpha(2{\rightarrow}3)\text{Gal} \beta (1{\rightarrow}4) \left[\text{Fuc} \alpha (1{\rightarrow}3)\right] \text{GlcNac} \beta (1{\rightarrow}3/6).$$

The possible specificity of this determinant for CF mucins and its
role in bacterial infection promotion are currently under
investigation.

This study was supported by the Netherlands Foundation for Chemical
Research (SON/ZWO), the Netherlands Cystic Fibrosis Foundation,
the Department of Cell Biology and Genetics, Erasmus University
Rotterdam and the Association Francaise de Lutte contre la
Mucovisidose.

(1) J.F.G. Vliegenthart, L. Dorland and H. van Halbeek (1983)
Adv. Carbohyd. Chem. Biochem. 41, 209-374;
(2) H. van Halbeek, L. Dorland, J.F.G. Vliegenthart, W.E. Hull,
G. Lamblin, M. Lhermitte, A. Boersma and P. Roussel (1982)
Eur. J. Biochem. 127, 7-20.

**POSTER GROUP SIX No. 6.28**

COMPARISON OF CYSTIC FIBROSIS AIRWAY SUBMUCOSAL GLANDS
WITH AND WITHOUT OBSTRUCTED SECRETORY LUMENS.

R.L. Boyd[1], D. Njus[1], A. Spock[2], S.S. Spicer[3]. [1]Department of
Pediatrics, University of Texas, San Antonio, Texas 78284; [2]Department
of Pediatrics, Duke University Medical Center, Durham, North Carolina
27101;
[3]Department of Pathology, Medical College of South Carolina,
Charleston, South Carolina 29425.

Accumulation of mucus in airway submucosal gland lumens is
characteristic of cystic fibrosis. The present morphometric investigation
of the relationship between serous and mucous gland densities suggests a
possible mechanism for the accumulation of viscous mucus in gland
lumens.

The fractional volume (Vv) of submucosal mucous (M) and serous (S)
glandular cells and tubular lumens were measured in intrapulmonary
airways from cystic fibrosis patients. Using a 64 point ocular grid,
microscopic morphometric analysis of tissues stained with alcian blue and
high iron diamine enabled characterization of the proportion of M and/or
S cells containing sialyldated (sial), sulfated (sulf) or mixed (sial-sulf)
glycoproteins. Within the same airway section measurements were made
in glands with and without mucous cast obstruction of secretory lumens.
In the areas with obstruction compared to areas without obstruction the
following significant differences ($p < 0.05$) in Vv were observed: 1) the
sulf and sial-sulf were decreased in M tubules; 2) the sulf was decreased in
S tubules; 3) the proportion of cells containing neither sulf nor sial was
increased in M tubules; 4) the M, S, and total gland cell density (G=M+S)
were decreased; 5) the S/G ratio was decreased, whereas the M/G ratio
and mucous lumen/G ratio were increased.

These preliminary data indicate an attenuation of secretory function
of the submucosal glands associated with the presence of mucous casts in
the tubular lumen. This finding suggests that insufficient serous tubular
secretions may result in inadequate hydration of downstream mucous
tubular secretions, accumulation of the viscous mucus in the ductal lumen
and formation of casts in the lumen.

**POSTER GROUP SIX No. 6.29**

EFFECTS OF ION TRANSPORT INHIBITORS ON LABELED GLYCOPROTEIN RELEASE
BY THE TRACHEA OF CONTROL AND RESERPINE TREATED RATS

T. Mawhinney and J. Ricardo Martinez, University of Missouri School
of Medicine, Columbia, MO 65212

Release of $^3$H or $^{35}$S labeled glycoproteins is significantly
increased in isolated, perfused tracheas of rats treated with
reserpine (1), a drug which causes exocrine gland abnormalities in
rats resembling those of cystic fibrosis (2). In control tracheas,
release of this material is inhibited by replacing Na$^+$ or Cl$^-$ in the
bathing solution (3), which suggests that release depends on fluid
and ion secretion into the lumen. We compared, therefore, the
effects of inhibitors of ion transport on the release of $^3$H-labeled
glycoproteins by isolated tracheas of control and reserpine treated
rats.

Tracheas were excised from anesthetized rats and equilibrated
in oxygenated Hank's balanced salt solution for 30 min prior to a 3
hour pre-incubation in M199 medium and to a final transfer to fresh
medium containing 1 μCi/ml of N-acetyl-D-(6-$^3$H)-glucosamine.
Twenty-four hours later the tissues were washed 3 times in
isotope-free medium and placed in a perfusion chamber containing
oxygenated solution at 37°C. The lumen was perfused with a similar
solution (28 μl min$^{-1}$). Samples were collected every 10 min,
dialyzed against 0.15M NaCl and counted. Release was measured with
and without 10$^{-5}$M acetylcholine, furosemide (10$^{-4}$M), ouabain (10$^{-3}$M)
or amiloride (10$^{-4}$M).

The results indicated: 1) tracheas from reserpine treated
animals released more labeled material than control tissues in the
absence (32%) or presence (47%) of acetylcholine; 2) furosemide in
the bathing solution caused a significant reduction in the basal
(68% and 80%) and stimulated (58% and 79%) release from tracheas of
control and reserpine treated rats. Luminal furosemide had no
effect on labeled glycoprotein release in tracheas of control or
treated rats; 3) long incubations with ouabain were required in both
tissues for a reduction in release; 4) luminally, amiloride
significantly reduced basal secretion of labeled glycoproteins in
tracheas from reserpine treated, but not control, animals.
Glycoprotein release by the rat trachea is dependent on fluid and
electrolyte secretion, which involves a furosemide-sensitive NaCl
cotransport and an ouabain-sensitive Na$^+$, K$^+$ ATPase. Release is
enhanced in reserpine treated rats and is more sensitive to
furosemide, which suggests possible abnormalities in the cotransport
system.

(1) CF Club Abstracts 20:14, 1979.
(2) Ped. Res. 14:872, 1980.
(3) CF Club Abstracts 21:48, 1980.

**POSTER GROUP SIX No. 6.30**

Ca$^{2+}$-TRANSPORT AND Mg$^{2+}$ AND Ca$^{2+}$-ATPase ACTIVITY IN THE EXOCRINE PANCREAS

Twum Ansah,[*] Ph.D., Sidney Katz, Ph.D. Faculty of Pharmaceutical Sciences, The University of British Columbia, Vancouver, B.C. Canada V6T 1W5

A defect in Ca$^{2+}$-transport in tissues obtained from Cystic Fibrosis (C.F.) patients coupled to the increased levels of calcium in many glycoprotein-rich secretions in C.F. underscores the importance of Ca$^{2+}$ in the pathophysiology of exocrine tissues. The role of calcium in the rat pancreatic acinar cell was studied using isolated intact acinar cells and plasma membrane-enriched preparations obtained from these cells. The viability of the isolated cells was greater than 95% as evaluated by the exclusion of trypan blue dye. Secretin, pancreozymin and carbachol produced a dose-dependent release of amylase by the acinar cells. Trifluoperazine (TFP) inhibited carbachol-stimulated amylase release in a dose dependent manner (IC$_{50}$ of 10 µM). Chlorpromazine (CPZ) at a concentration of 10 µM inhibited carbachol- and pancreozymin-stimulated amylase release without affecting secretin-stimulated (non-calcium mediated) release. Propranolol did not show this selective inhibition. These studies indicate the possibility that phenothiazines inhibit calcium-mediated amylase release by acting on a calmodulin-regulated step in the stimulus-secretion coupling process. A Ca$^{2+}$-dependent ATP hydrolytic activity was present in plasma membranes of pancreatic acinar cells. This activity was stimulated almost equally by Ca$^{2+}$ or Mg$^{2+}$. Kinetic analysis though, revealed that the enzyme had a higher affinity for Ca$^{2+}$. Investigation of the partial reactions of the ATPase activity revealed two phosphoprotein intermediates (M.W. of 115,000 and 130,000) in the presence of Ca$^{2+}$ and Mg$^{2+}$. The Ca$^{2+}$-ATPase activity was stimulated by calmodulin (K$_d$ of 0.7 µM) and acidic phospholipids. The calmodulin-stimulated activity was inhibited by TFP and CPZ in the µmolar range Using an [125]I-labeled calmodulin gel overlay technique, it was shown that calmodulin binds in a Ca$^{2+}$-dependent fashion to a 133,000 and a 230,000 dalton protein present in the plasma membrane-enriched fraction. Under conditions that favour Ca$^{2+}$-dependent kinase activity, calmodulin enhanced the phosphorylation of a 30,000 and a 19,000 dalton protein. Ca$^{2+}$-flux measurements in plasma membrane vesicles indicated the presence of both ATP-dependent Ca$^{2+}$ extrusion and uptake processes. The major ATP hydrolytic activity in pancreatic acinar plasma membranes was present as an ecto-enzyme. The role of this system in the acinar cell remains to be elucidated.

Supported by grants from the Canadian Cystic Fibrosis Foundation.

* Present address: Dept. Physiology, University, Manchester, UK.

**POSTER GROUP SIX No. 6.31**

ISOLATION OF DUCTS FROM THE RAT PANCREAS

S. Arkle and B.E. Argent, Department of Physiological Sciences, The University Medical School, Newcastle upon Tyne, NE1 7RU, England

Duct cells comprise approximately 4% of the mass of the normal pancreas and are generally considered to be the site of pancreatic $HCO_3^-$ secretion. Micropuncture experiments indicate that interlobular ducts are a major site of secretin-stimulated $HCO_3^-$ transport in the rat (for review see Schulz, 1981).

Although in vitro (e.g. perfusion/micropuncture)experiments have provided some information about duct cell secretory mechanisms and their control by secretin, rigorous electrophysiological studies have not proved possible using the intact gland because of the inaccessibility of the duct cells. Clearly, the availability of an isolated duct preparation in which transmembrane and transepithelial potentials could be recorded, and which might be perfused, would greatly facilitate our understanding of transport processes in this epithelium.

Previously, a technique for the isolation of ducts from the rat pancreas has been reported (Githens, Holmquist, Whelan & Ruby, 1980) but the epithelium shows poor morphological preservation. We began with glands taken from rats which have been fed a copper-deficient diet containing a copper chelating agent. This dietary regime leads to a non-inflammatory atrophy of acinar cells (80% of the gland) but leaves the ducts structurally and functionally intact (Folsch & Creutzfeldt, 1977). As a starting point this preparation offers two major advantages (1) the relative proportion of duct cells in the gland is increased (2) potentially injurious digestive enzymes are virtually absent. Our isolation procedure, which involves dissociation of the gland with collagenase and hyaluronidase followed by microdissection of ducts under transmitted light, allows the separation of interlobular ducts up to 2-3mm in length. Frequently, the smaller intralobular ducts, can be observed as branches. The poster will describe the isolation technique in detail and present data on the morphological and functional integrity of the preparation.

REFERENCES

Folsch,U.R. & Creutzfeldt, W. (1977). Gastroenterology 20,554-577.
Schulz, I. (1981). In Physiology of the Gastrointestinal Tract, ed.
  Johnson,L.R. vol. 2, pp.795-819.NY: Raven Press.
Githens,S., Holmquist, D.R.G., Whelan, J.F. & Ruby, J.R. (1980).
  J. Cell. Biol. 85, 122-135.

**POSTER GROUP SEVEN No. 7.01**

IgA-IgG CIRCULATING IMMUNE COMPLEXES (CIC) AND PSEUDOMONAS SPECIFIC ANTIBODIES IN CYSTIC FIBROSIS (CF): PROGNOSTIC IMPLICATIONS. M.K. Dasgupta[1], F.L. Harley[1], J. Lam[2], G.Döring[3], M. Larabie[1], K. Lam[2], J. Costerton[2] and J.B. Dossetor[1]. From the Universities of Edmonton[1], Calgary[2], Alberta, Canada and Tübingen[3], West Germany.

Infection and persistent colonization of the lung with Pseudomonas aeruginosa (PA) is associated with poor prognosis in cystic fibrosis (CF). Immune response to PA occurs in these patients and immune complex (IC) formation may lead to additional lung injury. However, the role of circulating immune complexes (CIC) remains controversial. We have re-examined this question in 16 severely affected CF patients (aged 8-18) having persistent specific precipitins to PA in the serum by measuring serial CIC containing IgG, IgA and IgM IC.

CIC are detected by $^{125}$I C1q-BA (IgG + IgM-IC) and Raji RIA (IgG-IC). A modification of Raji RIA and anti-C3 solid phase RIA (by the use of goat anti-human IgA) are used to detect IgA-IC. Specific precipitins to PA are detected with PAO-1 antigen by crossed immunoelectrophoresis (XIE) (Inf. Immun. p. 88, Oct. 1983). Also, antibodies to alkaline protease (AP), elastase (EL) and exotoxin-A (EA) of PA are detected by ELISA technique (Inf. Immun. 42: 197, 1983).

Patients are divided into two groups according to CIC results: eight have positive results most of the time (Group A) and another 8 patients are rarely positive (Group B) for CIC. Average follow-up period in Group A is 22 months and 26 months in Group B. CIC and precipitin results are as given below:

| | | CIC POSITIVES | | | | No. of |
| --- | --- | --- | --- | --- | --- | --- |
| | Samples (n) | Total +ves | C1q | IgG-Raji | IgA-IC | PAO-1 precipitins ($\bar{X}$) |
| Group A (8 patients) | 91 | 62 | 26 | 47 | 36 | 13.3 (5-23) |
| Group B (8 patients) | 118 | 29 | 23 | 5 | 13 | 9.2 (8-15) |

In Group A, CIC mostly consist of IgG (76%) and IgA (58%), whereas in Group B C1q binding IC (79%) and IgA-IC (45%) are more prevalent than IgG-IC (17%). Four children died during the follow-up period in Group A and one in Group B. Number of precipitins to PAO-1 are equally high in both groups. Antibodies to AP, EL, and EA of PA are also similar in both groups.

Our data based on 16 cases indicate that presence of CIC in association with specific antibody response to PA heralds a poor prognosis in CF. (This project is supported by grants from AHFMR, MRC (Canada) and CCFF.)

**POSTER GROUP SEVEN No. 7.02**

IMMUNE COMPLEXES (IC) AND LEUKOCYTE ELASTASE ACTIVITY
IN THE SPUTUM OF CYSTIC FIBROSIS (CF) PATIENTS

G. Döring, W. Goldstein, N. Høiby, P.-O. Schiøtz, M. Dasgupta and F.L. Harley.

Hygiene-Institut, Universität Tübingen, Tübingen, West Ger-
many, Statens Seruminstitut, Rigshospitalet, Copenhagen,
Denmark, Department of Medicine, University of Alberta
Hospitals, Edmonton, Alberta, Canada.

Sputum samples from 16 CF patients were investigated for
IC, proteolytic activity due to P. aeruginosa proteases
and leukocyte elastase. P. aeruginosa lung infection was
demonstrated by detection of specific antibodies to P.
aeruginosa proteases or exotoxin A in sera of all patients
using radioimmunoassays. In 75% of the sputa IC of IgG or
IgA type were detected using the Raji cell assay; 6 sputa
were highly positive, and 6 were low positive. Detection
of P. aeruginosa proteases in patients' sputa was negative
in all cases. When leukocyte elastase activity was measured using $Suc(Ala)_3pNA$ as substrate high activity was
found in 8 patients, low in 7 and no activity in 1 patient
High proteolytic activity was correlated to low or negative IC values and low or negative activity was correlated
to high IC values. The study shows that a) the free proteolytic activity in the majority of sputa from CF patients, suffering from P. aeruginosa lung infections, is not
due to proteases of this pathogen when specific antibodies
are present, but is host derived, b) IC are found in the
sputa of most CF patients and c) high leukocyte elastase
activity is correlated to low or negative IC values; this
negative correlation suggests a probable influence of the
elastase on IC in the CF lung.

**POSTER GROUP SEVEN No. 7.03**

PROGNOSTIC VALUE OF CIRCULATING IMMUNE COMPLEXES, PLASMA COMPLEMENT ACTIVATION, AND PSEUDOMONAS ANTIBODIES IN CYSTIC FIBROSIS. RB Moss, H Milgrom, YP Hsu, J Curd, NJ Lewiston. Children's Hospital-Stanford, Palo Alto, CA, and Scripps Institute, La Jolla, CA, USA.

Circulating immune complexes (CIC) containing airway pathogen antigen and antibody have been detected frequently in CF patients, but their clinical significance remains unclear(1). To further investigate the relationship of infection, immune response, and clinical syndromes we obtained immunologic profiles in 51 patients: CIC were measured by C1q binding, CIC-induced classical pathway plasma complement activation by quantitative rocket immunoelectrophoresis for C4d/C4 ratio, Pseudomonas aeruginosa (PA) IgG1-4 subclass antibodies by immunoenzymatic assay, and sputum culture for presence of PA. Clinical parameters were also monitored. A comparison of factors by 2x2 contingency tables follows:

| Factors | P |
|---|---|
| PA vs mortality | $< 0.001$ |
| CIC vs mortality | $< 0.001$ |
| C4d vs mortality | $< 0.001$ |
| CIC vs C4d | $< 0.001$ |
| CIC vs PA IgG4 | $< 0.01$ |
| CIC vs PA IgG1 | NS |
| CIC vs PA presence | NS |

Longitudinal studies indicate a closer relationship between persistent CIC and/or C4d in a subgroup of older, sicker patients colonized with PA and development of extrapulmonary syndromes such as arthritis, vasculitis, and serum sickness-like illness, than between episodic CIC or C4d and acute exacerbations of lung disease. Conventional measures such as leukocytosis and acute phase serum reactants appear better markers in the latter case. Persistent CIC and/or C4d indicate a subpopulation of patients with poor prognosis and at risk for extrapulmonary immunopathology for whom more aggressive or unconventional therapy may be indicated(2). Our data agree with those of Naff et al(3); the relation of classical to alternate complement pathway activation and the role of poorly opsonic IgG4 antibody in particular require further study.

References
1. Moss RB. Immunology of cystic fibrosis. In Lloyd-Still JD, ed. Textbook of Cystic Fibrosis. John Wright/PSG Inc, Boston,1983, ch 10.
2. Lewiston NJ, Moss RB. Circulating immune complexes decrease during corticosteroid therapy in cystic fibrosis. Pediatr Res 16:354, 1982.
3. Naff GB, Wisnieski JJ, Dearborn DG, Boat TF. Increased mortality associated with deficient alternative complement pathway activity and/or circulating immune complexes in patients with cystic fibrosis. CF Club Abstracts 24:57, 1983.

358

**POSTER GROUP SEVEN No. 7.04**

PSEUDOMONAS CEPACIA AS A PATHOGEN IN CYSTIC FIBROSIS.

Jeffrey D. Klinger, Cystic Fibrosis Center, Department of Pediatrics, Case Western Reserve University, Rainbow Babies & Childrens Hospital, Cleveland, Ohio 44106, U.S.A.

Smooth and mucoid colonial forms of Pseudomonas aeruginosa, Staphylococcus aureus, and Hemophilus influenzae remain the most frequent bacterial isolates from CF sputum cultures. Appropriate antimicrobial chemotherapy increases the duration and quality of life of infected CF patients. Recently, investigators at a number of CF treatment centers in North America and Europe have noted increased isolation of non-aeruginosa gram-negative non-fermentative bacilli. Prominent species include Pseudomonas cepacia, P. maltophilia, other pseudomonads, Achromobacter spp., and Acinetobacter spp. Significant disease has been most often associated with P. cepacia. The spectrum of P. cepacia colonization/infection in CF patients ranges from long-term colonization (i.e., years) with no apparent untoward clinical effects, to a virulent process of infection, fever, possible bacteremia, and death over a period of several weeks. The extent to which such differences reflect variations in patient immune responses, status at initial colonization, and characteristics of infecting strains is under investigation. Strains of P. cepacia from CF patients are resistant to aminoglycosides, most antipseudomonas penicillins, and many disinfectants. With the possible exception of ceftazidime, most newer cephalosporins are also ineffective. We have biotyped 228 strains, and serotyped 277 strains of P. cepacia from CF patients, non-CF infections, and environmental sources and find a predominance of biotype "C" (system of Esanu & Schubert) and serotype "I" (system of Jonsson) strains in CF. This distribution is different than in the other two sources. Additionally we have begun characterization of potential virulence factors including a 30,000 dalton proteinase. Though highly resistant to many agents, P. cepacia strains often have a slow rate of growth, and do not survive well on ordinary bacteriologic media; hence they may be overlooked in some routine lab settings. The occurence of such organisms may have broad implications for how patients are seen and grouped in hospital settings, and calls attention to potential profound effects of selection on microbial populations as more effective anti-Pseudomonas aeruginosa agents are employed.

Supported in part by the C.H. Ivey Foundation, the Cystic Fibrosis Foundation, and the National Institutes of Health.

**POSTER GROUP SEVEN No. 7.05**

TECHNIQUE FOR BACTERIOCIN TYPING OF PSEUDOMONAS CEPACIA.

J.R.W. Govan and G.S. Harris
Medical School, University of Edinburgh.

Pseudomonas cepacia is recognised as probably the most adaptable of
the pseudomonads in its ability to utilise a wide range of carbon
sources.  Clinical isolation from the hospital environment, particularly from pharmaceutical solutions and instruments, has become increasingly common leading to colonisation and/or infection in compromised patients.
    In recent years a number of CF clinics in North America have
noted an increased incidence of P. cepacia in respiratory tract
cultures from patients with cystic fibrosis;  incidence was highest
either at post-mortem examination or immediately before death.
Epidemiological studies to find reasons for the increased incidence
of P. cepacia in CF patients and to assess its clinical significance
for the future management of CF are hampered by a lack of typing
methods.   We have attempted to develop a typing scheme based on
bacteriocin production and sensitivity.   The technique is based on
our revised pyocin typing scheme for the typing of P. aeruginosa.
Indicator strains to detect bacteriocin production by P. cepacia
strains were isolated following a study of over 130 pseudomonads
belonging to a variety of pseudomonas species.   For bacteriocin
production, test isolates of P. cepacia are rapidly applied to the
surface of agar plates using a multiple inoculator.   After incubation for 6h and exposure to chloroform, indicator strains are applied
in agar overlays without prior removal of test strain growth.   After
further incubation for 18h, inhibition zones due to bacteriocin
activity can be recognised.   The bacteriocin type of the test strain
can then be defined on the basis of bacteriocin production as judged
by the presence and size  of inhibition zones against standard indicator strains and by the sensitivity or resistance of the test
strains to bacteriocins produced by standard producer strains.
    In a small preliminary study carried out with 16 strains of
P. cepacia, including strains from two CF patients, all isolates
either produced or were sensitive to bacteriocin.   On the basis of
bacteriocin production and sensitivity 5 'cepaciacin' types were
recognised.
    The results of a larger trial to be carried out and the use of
the technique in other laboratories will assess the value of this
scheme for epidemiological studies of P. cepacia.

360

PSEUDOMONAS CEPACIA AND CYSTIC FIBROSIS: EVIDENCE FOR LACK OF PERSON TO PERSON TRANSMISSION. Richard Honicky, Glenn Seagren, Patricia Peek Isabel Leader, John Malnor, and Dennis Murray. Department of Pediatrics/Human Development, Michigan State University, East Lansing, MI and Ingham Medical Center, Lansing, MI.

Pseudomonas cepacia (Pc) is a lesser known, but important bacterium colonizing patients with cystic fibrosis (CF). Pc is resistant to many antibiotics commonly used to treat pulmonary infections in CF, including aminoglycosides. Concern had been expressed by several CF specialists about possible transmission of Pc from person to person while attending a summer camp. We evaluated the period prevalence and transmissibility of Pc during a 1 week CF camp in the Summer of 1983. Campers (cp) and camp staff (c-s) had cultures of sputum or deep throat swabs obtained on days 1 and 7 of camp. All Pseudomonas isolates were subjected to species identification. Antibiotic sensitivity testing was performed on all Pc isolates. Records of recent antibiotic therapy and hospitalizations were obtained from all participants. Camp activities and procedures (sleeping arrangements, etc.) were not changed.

At camp entry 5/98 (5.1%) cp and c-s with CF had Pc identified; only 2/5 had Pc identified prior to camp. At exit only 1/95 (1.1%) cp and c-s with CF had Pc identified; this individual was also positive for Pc on entry. At neither time did non-CF c-s have Pc isolated. The number of isolations of other Pseudomonas, including Pseudomonas aeruginosa, did not significantly change from day 1 to day 7. All Pc tested were resistant to carbenicillin and gentamicin. Compared with a quality control, patients' isolates of Pc required 4-8 fold higher concentrations of trimethoprim-sulfamethoxazole (TMP-SMX) to inhibit growth. Of patients from whom Pc was isolated, 3/5 were known to be taking TMP-SMX at time of camp entry.

Our data suggests Pc is not transmitted from person to person during a CF summer camp. In addition, TMP-SMX may not be effective antimicrobial therapy in controlling Pc colonization.

References:
1. Speert D., Layton D., Damm S: Communicability of Pseudomonas aeruginosa in a cystic fibrosis summer camp. J Pediatr 101:227-229, 1982.
2. Blessing J., Walker J., Maybury B., Yeager A., Lewiston N: Pseudomonas cepacia and maltophillia in the cystic fibrosis patient, abstracted. Amer Rev Resp Dis 119:262, 1979.
3. Isles A: Bacteriology of cystic fibrosis. In Pulmonary Infection In Cystic Fibrosis "GAP" Conference Report. pp 1-3, 1983.

The authors wish to gratefully acknowledge support from Roche Laboratories for this project.

**POSTER GROUP SEVEN No. 7.07**

QUANTATIVE SPUTUM ANALYSIS IN CYSTIC FIBROSIS (CF) PATIENTS:   SIGNIFI-
CANCE OF PSEUDOMONAS AERUGINOSA (PA) COLONY DENSITY
Bonnie W. Ramsey, M.D. and Arnold L. Smith, M.D.
Children's Orthopedic Hospital and Medical Center, University of
Washington, Seattle, Washington 98105

Qualitative changes in sputum bacterial isolates from CF patients
seldom reflect significant changes in clinical symptoms.  It is
difficult, therefore, to determine the efficacy of antibiotic therapy.
For this reason, use of quantitative sputum culture techniques have
been advocated in patients with CF and other chronic lung diseases.  As
part of a two year prospective study evaluating the role of viral infections in CF lung disease, we have obtained 77 sputums for quantitative analysis[1] as well as DNA[2] and albumin content on 17 patients.  At
the time of sputum collection, pulmonary function tests, Pseudomonas
aeruginosa antibody titers and antibody inhibition of exotoxin A, were
obtained.  We also gave each study member an objective numerical score[3]
for clinical symptoms.

These patients ranged in age from 6 to 21 years with Shwachman-
Kulczycki scores ranging from 90 to 38.  A scatter plot of the Pa
colony density against Staphylococcus aureus (Sa) colony density showed
a strong negative correlation ($p < .001$).  A density of $Pa > 10^6$ was
always associated with $< 10^6$ Sa and vice versa.  In 11 patients Sa was
the predominant organism and in 6 patients Pa.  Over the first 15
months of the study no patient has changed predominant organism,
although other bacterium is usually present at a lower density, i.e.,
$< 10^6$.  Those patients with $> 10^6$ Pa had significantly lower FVC
($p < .001$), $FEV_{1.0}$ ($p < .001$), and Shwachman-Kulczycki scores ($p < .001$)
as well as higher sputum DNA ($p < .001$) and albumin ($p < .05$) content.
At the same time the antibody inhibition of exotoxin A was higher
($p < .05$).  There was no difference in respiratory rate.  Two patients
with $> 10^6$ Pa  and high inhibition of exotoxin A died.  There was a
positive correlation ($p < .05$) between clinical exacerbation scores
and log Pa.

These results show the prognostic importance of determining sputum
bacterial colony densities by quantitative culture techniques.
Although both Pa and Sa may be isolated together, one always has a
greater colony density.  When Pa is the predominant organism, there is
a greater inflammatory response associated with increased airway
resistance and clinical symptoms.  It is possible that an increased
density of Sa is protective, which would have important therapeutic
implications.

References:  1.  Louria, DB, et al.  JAMA  1962  182:1082
             2.  Kissane, JM, et al  J Biol Chem  1958  233:184
             3.  Ramsey, BW, et al.  CF Club Abstracts  1983  24:43
Supported by Grant GO49-3 from the Cystic Fibrosis Foundation

362

THE ORIENTATION OF GLUCONATE DEHYDROGENASE ON THE
CYTOPLASMIC MEMBRANE OF <u>PSEUDOMONAS AERUGINOSA</u>

James G. Johnson, Dept. of Biology, Univ. of Calgary,
Calgary, Alberta, Canada   T2N 1N4

<u>P</u>. <u>aeruginosa</u> carries out the following reactions:

$$\text{glucose} \xrightarrow[\substack{\text{dehydrogenase} \\ \text{(GD)}}]{\text{glucose}} \text{gluconate} \xrightarrow[\substack{\text{dehydrogenase} \\ \text{(GAD)}}]{\text{gluconate}} \substack{\text{2-keto} \\ \text{gluconate}}$$

The enzymes GD and GAD are thought to be located on
the cytoplasmic membrane (CM) and to operate upon
substrate located outside the CM in the periplasmic
space (K. Matsushita, et al., Agric. Biol. Chem.,
44, 1505 (1980);  B.K. Roberts, et al., J. Gen.
Micro., 78, 319 (1973)).  This external orientation
is unusual, in that other bacterial enzymes linked to
the electron-transport chain (such as succinate
dehydrogenase) are located on the inner face of the CM.

The enzymes GD and GAD have been purified from the
same bacterial strain, and antibodies to the whole
enzymes and to the component subunits have been
raised.  Immunoelectron microscopy has been used
to prove the external orientation of the enzymes
on the CM.

**POSTER GROUP SEVEN No. 7.09**

The Structure and Properties of Extracellular Alginate
Produced by Mucoid  Pseudomonas aeruginosa Isolated from
Cystic Fibrosis Patients

P.Gacesa, V.Sherbrock-Cox & N.J.Russell,
Department of Biochemistry, University College, P.O.Box 78,
Cardiff CF1 1XL

It has been assumed previously that the extracellular
material produced by mucoid strains of Pseudomonas
aeruginosa isolated from the lungs of CF patients consisted
entirely of alginate - a linear co-polymer of the uronic
acids, $\alpha$-L-guluronic acid (G) and $\beta$-D-mannuronic acid (M).
We show that in addition to alginate the extracellular
material contains both protein and non-uronic acid based
polysaccharide(s).
To permit a proper investigation of the chemical and
physical properties of the alginate, we have developed an
ion-exchange method to purify it free of protein and other
polysaccharides. We have investigated the M/G ratio and
poly-G (or M) block structure and degree of acetylation
(which all affect the polymer viscosity) of purified
alginate from a number of clinical isolates of P.aeruginosa
using a combination of chemical, GLC and $^{1}$H-NMR analysis.
We show that P.aeruginosa alginate contains predominantly
random or poly-M block structures, and that the polymer is
highly acetylated. The absence of poly-G blocks and lack
of a correlation between M/G ratio and degree of
acetylation with viscosity will be discussed in terms of
the gelling (by $Ca^{2+}$) of P.aeruginosa alginate from CF
patients in the context of abnormal lung ionic composition.

**POSTER GROUP SEVEN No. 7.10**

Chemical Analysis of the Exopolysaccharides Synthesized by Mucoid
Strains of Pseudomonas aeruginosa Isolated from Patients with
Cystic Fibrosis

W. Bautsch[1], R. Kownatzki[1], B. Tümmler[1], R. Chan[2], J.W. Costerton[2]
1. Zentrum Biochemie II, Org.Nr. 4351, Medizinische Hochschule
Hannover, D-3000 Hannover 61, W. Germany
2. Department of Biology, University of Calgary, Calgary, Alberta,
Canada T2N 1N4

The chronic colonization of the lung by mucoid strains of Pseudomonas aeruginosa is a common finding in patients with cystic
fibrosis. The occurrence of mucoid strains correlates with age and
severity of the disease (Ref. 1). The exopolysaccharide synthesized
by these bacteria induces the formation of microcolonies and impairs
host defense mechanisms and diffusion of antibiotics.

We investigated the structure and the chemical composition of the
exopolysaccharide by TLC, GLC/MS, IR, and NMR techniques. Bacteria
were grown in liquid culture using a modified Vogel-Bronner medium.
The conditions for culturing and processing were optimized for
maximum purity of the exopolysaccharide. The purified polymer contained no detectable contaminations of lipid, protein, nucleic acid,
and monomeric sugar. The polymer was subjected to complete and
partial acid hydrolysis. Sugar monomers were identified by $R_f$-values
in TLC using several solvents of different polarity, differential
staining of spots by sugar sensitive dyes, and the combined GLC/MS
analysis of the permethylated partially deuterated alditols. The
glycosidic linkage was determined in NMR experiments. The analyses
revealed that mucoid strains of P. aeruginosa can synthesize at
least two different types of exopolysaccharides, an alginate-like
heteropolymer with varying relative amounts of mannuronic and
guluronic acid, and a homopolymer made up by hexonic acids. The
implication of these findings for the development of adjuvant antibiotic drugs which inhibit the biosynthesis of the exopolysaccharide
will be discussed in detail.

We would like to thank Drs. M. Slack and W.W. Nichols, John Radcliffe
Hospital, Oxford, U.K., for the supply of several mucoid P. aeruginosa strains.

Ref. 1: Thomassen, M.J.; Demko, C.A.; Boxerbaum, B.; Stern, R.C.;
Kuchenbrod, P.J. (1979) J. Infect. Dis. 140, 873 - 889.

**POSTER GROUP SEVEN No. 7.11**

Pseudomonas Isolation Agar (Difco) and Pseudomonas Selective Agar
(Oxoid) inhibit the growth of some strains of Pseudomonas aeruginosa
from cystic fibrosis.

Kevin Fonseca[1] and Tyrone. L. Pitt[2] [1]Department of
Microbiology, Wexham Park Hospital, Slough, Berks, UK. [2]Central Public
Health Laboratory, 175 Colindale Avenue, London, NW9 5HT, UK.

During the course of routine bacteriological examination of sputa from
cystic fibrosis patients attending an out-patients clinic, we observed
that some strains of P. aeruginosa were inhibited by the selective
agars- Pseudomonas Isolation Agar - (PIA Difco) - and Pseudomonas
Selective Agar (PSA - Oxoid). The active selective agent in PIA is
Irgasan (R) (2.4-4-trichloro-2-hydroxydiphenyl ether) at a concentration of 25 mg/1, and in PSA are sodium nalidixate (15 mg/1) and
cetrimide (cetyltrimethyl ammonium bromide) 220 mg/1.

The MIC of these compounds was determined by agar dilution on 200
cultures of P. aeruginosa from 70 patients. 18 isolates were
inhibited by 16 mg/1 Irgasan, 36 by 16 mg/1 nalidixic acid and 11 by
125 mg/1 cetrimide. There was no association between colonial
morphology and failure to grow on the selective media. Furthermore
the growth of some isolates was considerably reduced on the selective
media and in general these strains gave MIC values marginally above
the 'in use' concentration of the selective agents.

We recommend that sputum from CF patients be cultured on both
selective and non-selective media to maximise the isolation of
P. aeruginosa.

**POSTER GROUP SEVEN No. 7.12**

The effect of oleic acid and oxygen on respiration and slime production by Staphylococcus aureus and Pseudomonas aeruginosa in nutrient broth.

I.M. Campbell, D.N. Crozier, A.B. Pawagi, A.L. Symonds, F.C. Zagdanski and D.R. Houpt. Division of Life Sciences, Scarborough College, University of Toronto, CANADA.

The etiology of pulmonary bacterial infections in CF patients is not understood. Using an in vitro system, we investigated the possibility that the bacteria may be responding to abnormal changes in the fatty acid composition of the respiratory tract lipids (elevated oleic and diminished linoleic acid content) and to a decrease in the supply of oxygen. Whereas linoleic was found to be bacteriostatic to S. aureus, oleic acid induced the bacteria to drastically decrease their uptake of oxygen and to produce a slime (exopolysaccharide)in which they became encapsulated. This effect of oleic acid occurred only in broths at equilibrium with 100 mm (13.3 kPa) or less of oxygen. Increasing the oxygen pressure above 150 mm, after the interaction with oleic acid had occurred, completely reversed the effect. Normal oxygen uptake was restored and the slime capsule disappeared. Kinetic studies on the oxidation and reduction of the cytochromes and NAD in intact cells revealed that oleic acid decreases the demand for oxygen by interfering with the flow of electrons both to and from the coenzyme. Similar studies on the effect of oleic acid and oxygen on both mucoid and non-mucoid strains of the obligate aerobe, P. aeruginosa, gave similar results.
Since Williamson et al (Proc. N.A.S. (U.S.A.) 56:247,1966) found that oleic acid had the same effect on NAD activity in rat-liver mitochondria and, in so doing, stops glycolysis and intiates gluconeogenesis in the cells, it seems possible that slime (exopolysaccharide)production by the bacteria may well be the result of the fatty acid interfering with electron transport.
If, as several authors have suggested, the production of a slime capsule by bacteria can afford them protection against the defense mechanisms of the host and antibiotics, our results suggest that hyperbaric oxygen therapy may be useful in the treatment of pulmonary infections.

**POSTER GROUP SEVEN No. 7.13**

Hypersensitivity to antibiotics, surfactants and cell lytic agents of Pseudomonas aeruginosa from cystic fibrosis.

Kevin Fonseca[1], Tyrone. L. Pitt[2] and Andrea Penketh[3]
[1] Department of Microbiology Wexham Park Hospital, Slough, Berks, UK.
[2] Central Public Health Laboratory, 175 Colindale Avenue, London NW9 5HT and [3] Brompton Hospital, Fulham Road, London, UK.

The MIC of several antibiotics, surfactants and chelating agents for 200 cultures of P. aeruginosa from 70 cystic fibrosis patients was determined and correlated with colonial morphology, serotype and sensitivity to serum. 'Hypersensitive' cultures (1) were defined as those which gave an MIC value for an antibiotic or agent of 8-fold or less than the median for that compound.

Approximately 10% of the cultures were resistant to the aminoglycosides and 2.5% were hypersensitive. In contrast 33% of cultures were resistant to carbencillin although 21% were hypersensitive to this antibiotic. 14% of cultures showed increased sensitivity to the other antipseudomonal penicillins. Most penicllin hypersensitive cultures were mucoid and serum sensitive and a significant proportion of these reacted with antisera to defective lipopolysaccharides (LPS).

Hypersensitivity to other antibiotics and agents was varied; nalidixic acid (18%), trimethoprim (9%) rifampicin, colistin and tetracycline (3-7%). Of the nalidixic acid - hypersensitive cultures, 3.5% were also extremely sensitive to the aminoglycosides, carbenicillin and trimethoprim. 18% of cultures were inhibited by 500 mg/l of EDTA (median MIC = >4000 mg/l). EDTA-hypersensitive cultures were rarely hypersensitive to antibiotics. Chlorhexidine and cetrimide respectively inhibited 2% and 15% of cultures at concentrations markedly below the median MIC.

A variety of phenotypes of resistance were found within single specimens and the results of tests on repeated isolates from the same patient at different times suggested that there was continuous variation in these markers although strains which were hypersensitive remained so.

1. Irvin, R. T., Govan, J. R., Fyfe, J. A. M. & Costerton, J. W. (1981). Antimicrob. Agents & Chemother., 19, 1056

**POSTER GROUP SEVEN No. 7.14**

O-antigen defective strains of Pseudomonas aeruginosa in cystic fibrosis.

Tyrone. L. Pitt[1], Jane Ullmer[1], E. Mary Cooke[1], Andrea Penketh[2], Margaret Hodson[2] and J. C. Batten[2]. Central Public Health Laboratory, 175 Colindale Avenue, London NW9 5HT, UK. [2]Brompton Hospital, Fulham Road, London SW7, UK.

Many reports in the literature have commented on the difficulty of O-serological grouping of strains of P. aeruginosa from the sputum of CF patients. Recently in a study of 49 patients attending an out-patient department Penketh et al.(1) found that only 32.1% of strains reacted with a single O-antiserum, 50.5% were polyagglutinable (PA) and the remainder were not typable (NT). The emergence of these serologically aberrant forms was correlated with the clinical severity of respiratory infection in these patients. Furthermore both PA and NT strains were most often sensitive to the bactericidal action of freash normal human serum. Independently, Hancock et al.(2) confirmed that the majority of 26 isolates of P. aeruginosa from CF were serologically PA or NT and showed that these strains were deficient in lipopolysaccharide (LPS) O-antigen specific side chains.

We have constructed two variant strains defective in O-antigen specific side chains. One of these variants is polyagglutinable and is similar to those found in CF and the other is a non-typable variety derived from a wild-type 'O-typical' strain. The defective nature of their LPS was confirmed by SDS-PAGE electrophoresis. We prepared antisera towards these strains in rabbits and used the sera in conjunction with the standard O-typing serum set to classify 402 cultures of P. aeruginosa from 115 patients. In addition we determined the sensitivity of the cultures to fresh human serum by the method of Penketh et al.(1).

Of the 402 cultures, 324 (80.6%) were fully sensitive to serum, 29 (7.2%) were slightly sensitive and 49 (12.2%) were resistant. Approximately half (51.2%) of the serum-sensitive cultures reacted with one or both sera to defective LPS and 27 cultures (6.7%) only were O-typable. In contrast of the 78 resistant or partially resistant cultures only 4 gave a reaction with the LPS-defect antisera and 52 (66.6%) were O-typable. This study describes the serologically aberrant forms of P. aeruginosa found in CF and provides evidence suggesting that antigenic variation of bacteria within the lung may facilitate the continued colonisation of the host.

1. Penketh, A., Pitt, T., Roberts, D., Hodson, M. E., & Batten, J. C. (1983). Am. Rev. Resp. Dis. 127, 605

2. Hancock, R. E. W., Mutharia, L. M., Chan, Ł., Darveau, R. P., Speert, D. P., & Pier, G. B. (1983). Infect. and Immun. 42, 170

**POSTER GROUP SEVEN No. 7.15**

---

ANTIGENICITY OF OUTER MEMBRANE COMPONENTS OF MUCOID PSEUDOMONAS
AERUGINOSA ISOLATED DIRECTLY FROM THE LUNGS OF A CYSTIC FIBROSIS
PATIENT:  INFLUENCE OF ANTIBIOTICS

Hosmin Anwar[1], Michael R W Brown[1], Peter A Lambert[1], Peter Weller[2]
and Alan Day[2]
1.  Microbiology Research Group, Department of Pharmacy, University
of Aston in Birmingham, Gosta Green, Birmingham B4 7ET
2.  The Children's Hospital in Birmingham, Ladywood Middleway,
Birmingham B16

Mucoid Pseudomonas aeruginosa has been isolated from the sputum
of a cystic fibrosis patient without further subculture in laboratory
media.  The outer membrane (OM) was prepared by using sodium lauryl
sarcosinate  (Sarkosyl) and the OM protein profile was revealed by
electrophoresis in polyacrylamide gels containing sodium dodecyl
sulphate (SDS).  The results indicated that three OM proteins of
$M_r$ 80,000, 86,000 and 90,000 were induced.  The induction of these
proteins can be simulated by growing the same isolate under iron
restricted conditions in laboratory media.  A 21K $M_r$ protein (H1)
was also present.  The patient was treated with piperacillin and
tobramycin.  The isolate was also grown in the chemically defined
medium under iron restricted conditions in the presence of piperacillin or tobramycin alone or in combination at one tenth of their
minimum inhibitory concentrations.  The presence of antibiotics at
this concentration did not appear to alter the OM protein profiles
of the cells.

The antigenic profiles of the OM components of cells grown in vivo
and in vitro were revealed by blotting the antigens from polyacrylamide gels onto nitrocellulose sheets.  They were then probed
with sera from two patients.  The results indicated that the OM
proteins induced in vivo and in vitro under iron restriction were
antigenic.  The present study gives direct biochemical evidence that
mucoid Pseudomonas aeruginosa grows under iron restricted conditions
in the lungs of the cystic fibrosis patients and that the OM proteins
induced in vivo were also detected by the immune system of the
patients.

370

**POSTER GROUP SEVEN No. 7.16**

ANALYSIS OF PSEUDOMONAS AERUGINOSA SLIME BY CAESIUM CHLORIDE
ISOPYCNIC DENSITY CENTRIFUGATION

Yvonne Smedley, S.L. James, N.A. Hodges and C. Marriott
Department of Pharmacy, Brighton Polytechnic, Moulsecoomb, Brighton,
U.K.

The clinical condition of cystic fibrotics is reported to deteriorate
rapidly after opportunist infection of the lungs by mucoid
Ps.aeruginosa. The possibility exists that the disease state is
exacerbated by interaction of the bronchial mucus with the
exopolysaccharide 'slime' produced by Ps.aeruginosa, thereby altering
the rheological properties of the mucus. In order to investigate
this possible interaction it is first necessary to elucidate the
nature of the total 'slime' produced. The major component of the
slime has been variously identified as alginate and polysaccharide
and protein. Isopycnic density centrifugation of the slime will
fractionate it with respect to the bouyant density of its components,
thus yielding an alternative method to alcohol coacervation.

Mucoid strains of Ps.aeruginosa were isolated from fresh cystic
sputum and cultured in tryptone-soya broth for two days with aeration
followed by two days of static culture. The slime produced was
disaggregated in tetrasodiuim edetate and centrifuged at 36000 g for
1 hour to remove bacteria. After exhaustive dialysis against
distilled water the dialysate was centrifuged at 150000 g on a 42%
CsCl density gradient for 48 hours to achieve equilibrium. Each 1 ml
fraction was dialysed to remove CsCl and assayed for total hexose,
protein and DNA. The total hexose:protein:DNA ratio of the 'slime'
using this technique is typically 35:14:1. A single protein peak is
found at the tube meniscus with little or no protein being associated
with other fractions (Figure). Similarly little DNA was found in any

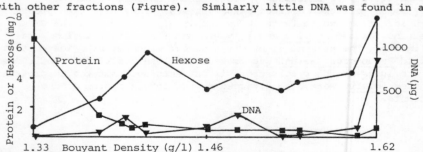

fraction other than the most dense. Hexose appeared throughout the
tube with two peaks occurring, one in the most dense fraction and the
other at a density of approximately 1.4 g/l. Thus the major
component of these slimes is a hexose polysaccharide and the protein
which is present is not covalently bound to the sugar.

**POSTER GROUP SEVEN No. 7.17**

THE DIFFUSION OF ANTIBIOTIC MOLECULES THROUGH MUCUS LAYERS

M.S. Cheema, C. Marriott and M.F. Beeson
Department of Pharmacy, Brighton Polytechnic, Moulsecoomb,
Brighton, U.K. and Beecham Pharmaceuticals Research Division,
Biosciences Research Centre, Great Burgh, Epsom, U.K.

The transfer of antibiotic molecules from the systemic circulation
to the mucus layer in the bronchial tree is known to be difficult.
If the barrier to this transfer is the mucus layer then it would be
predicted that it would be similarly affected in the
gastrointestinal tract particularly when this is occluded with
mucus as in cystic fibrosis. In this work the diffusion of benzyl
penicillin through mucus gels has been studied. The effect of
mucus concentration and contamination with plasma proteins such as
those found in the mucus secretions of cystic fibrotics has been
investigated. The experimental technique involves the dialysis of
the $^{14}$C benzyl penicillin into a capillary tube containing the
mucus and the subsequent diffusion from the mucus is measured as a
function of time.

The presence of a small concentration of purified mucus
glycoprotein decreased the diffusion of benzyl penicillin but
further increase up to 0.15 mg dl$^{-1}$ produced no further significant
change. However, above this concentration a precipitate and
significant fall ($p < 0.01$) occurred and this may be associated
with the concentration range over which a change occurs from an
aqueous solution of glycoprotein molecules to a gel: this change
occurs at a glycoprotein concentration between 0.15 and 0.24 mg
dl$^{-1}$. Unpurified mucus gels allowed a higher diffusion of benzyl
penicillin and this can be explained by the fact that soluble
proteins such as albumin will contribute to the dry weight but will
not present the same barrier to diffusion as glycoproteins because
of their lower molecular mass.

Thus the mucus gel lining the gut and the lung does present a
barrier to the diffusion of drug molecules and does not act merely
as an unstirred layer. When the ionic strength of the mucus gel is
increased above 0.1M then the barrier to diffusion is decreased.
However, this was with respect to monovalent ions and the effect of
the divalent ion calcium, which is known to be elevated in the
mucus secretions of cystic fibrotics, has yet to be evaluated.

**POSTER GROUP SEVEN No. 7.18**

CHARACTERIZATION OF THE ADHERENCE OF MUCOID PSEUDOMONAS AERUGINOSA TO THE RESPIRATORY TRACT EPITHELIUM.

Hilda Marcus and Neil R. Baker, Department of Microbiology, College of Biological Sciences, The Ohio State University, Columbus, Ohio 43210.

The interaction of mucoid Pseudomonas aeruginosa isolates from cystic fibrosis patients with tracheal epithelial cells was studied in order to characterize the colonization of the lower respiratory tract by these organisms. The effects of various agents on the adherence of mucoid P. aeruginosa to the tracheal epithelium were examined using the perfused tracheal explant model. Excised hamster trachea were mounted in a perfusion chamber and infected with $10^7$ CFU/ml of the bacterial suspension in the presence of D(-)mannose, N-acetylglucosamine, N-acetylgalactosamine, D(+)galactose, L(-)fucose, N-acetylneuraminic acid, or bovine submaxillary mucin. Control explants were infected in the absence of sugars or mucin. The infected explants were incubated for 2 hr at $37^\circ$C, rinsed, homogenized, and plated for quantitation of adherent bacteria. Each of the agents tested inhibited adherence but dose response curves indicate that N-acetylglucosamine and galactosamine were the best inhibitors. Mucin was a particularly potent inhibitor of adherence. These results indicate that interaction of the mucoid variants of P. aeruginosa with host mucus is an important factor in the colonization of the lower respiratory tract of cystic fibrosis patients.

**POSTER GROUP SEVEN No. 7.19**

PSEUDOMONAS AERUGINOSA AND CYSTIC FIBROSIS: IS THE ISOLATION OF NON-MUCOID PSEUDOMONAS AERUGINOSA REALLY OF NO CLINICAL SIGNIFICANCE?

J.R.W. Govan, J.A.M. Fyfe, C. Doherty and W.M. McCrae
Medical School, University of Edinburgh and Royal Hospital for Sick Children, Edinburgh.

Debilitating and intractable respiratory infection due to mucoid, alginate-producing Pseudomonas aeruginosa is now a major cause of morbidity and mortality in patients with cystic fibrosis. We have attempted to improve the management of pseudomonas infection by intensive bacteriological monitoring of CF patients and by basic studies of the genetics and pathogenicity of P. aeruginosa in relation to infection in CF patients. Our results help to explain some contradictions regarding the role of P. aeruginosa in cystic fibrosis and emphasise the co-operation assocation of bacterial and CF factors which ultimately result in chronic infection and pulmonary damage. The importance of asymptomatic colonisation with non-mucoid P. aeruginosa to the ultimate outcome of infection is indicated by the mutational basis of alginate biosynthesis. Our results indicate that the clinical signification of alginate lies in the adhesive and gelling properties of this unusual bacterial polysaccharide; in animal studies mucoid P. aeruginosa have been shown to be cleared less rapdily from the respiratory tract than isogenic non-mucoid strains. Microscopy of CF sputa and of mucoid P. aeruginosa grown inthe presence of suitable electrolytes suggests that, in CF lung, mucoid P. aeruginosa do not grow as individual cells but as micro-colonies imbedded in an alginate gel. We suggest that the micro-colony mode of growth would exacerbate pulmonary damage by localising the relatively weak pseudomonas toxins and by presenting the patients immune defences with an indigestable target leading to a "frustrated macrophage syndrome" and immunemediated tissues damage. Protected by a ionised alginate gel, the microcolony mode also helps to explain the intractibility of mucoid P. aeruginosa despite aggressive antibiotic therapy and the paradoxical emergence in CF patients of P. aeruginosa hyper-sensitive to certain antibiotics.

Although early colonisation with classic non-mucoid P. aeruginosa may appear to be of no clinical significance, it forms an essential microbial reservoir to allow expression of bacterial mutations which contribute to the survival of P. aeruginosa in the lower airways to pulmonary damage.

374

ANTIBODY RESPONSE TO PROTEASES AND EXOTOXIN A OF PSEUDO-
MONAS AERUGINOSA IN A RAT LUNG MODEL

G. Döring, K. Lam and J.W. Costerton

Hygiene-Institut, Universität Tübingen, Tübingen, West
Germany and Department of Biology, University of Calgary,
Calgary, Alberta, Canada.

The rat model of chronic pulmonary infection, developed
by Cash, was used to study the serum antibody response to
alkaline protease (AP), elastase (Ela) and exotoxin A
(ExoA) of Pseudomonas aeruginosa. Groups of rats were in-
oculated transtracheally with agar beads in which different P. aeruginosa strains were embedded. Animals from
each group were sacrified in weekly intervals up to 7
weeks after challenge; rat lungs were examined for bacterial numbers and sera for antibody titers to AP, Ela
and ExoA using radioimmunoassays. 7 to 14 days after
challenge specific antibody titers to the enzymes were
detected. Titers increased with time. No delay in detection of antibody titers to the proteases relative to
titers to ExoA was observed. Antibody titers did not
correlate with the in vitro enzyme production of the
strains. The study shows that nonspecific protease inhibitors cannot complex the proteases sufficiently thereby
preventing or delaying immune stimulation. The course
of the antibody titers to the enzymes seems to be similar
to human pulmonary P. aeruginosa infection in cystic
fibrosis and thus emphasizes the usefullness of this
animal model in the study of human pulmonary P. aeruginosa
infection.

**POSTER GROUP SEVEN No. 7.23**

ASPERGILLOSIS AND CYSTIC FIBROSIS

Diagnosis and therapeutic approach

J. FEIGELSON (1), M. GUILLOT (2), R. GIRAUD (3)
Y. PECAU (4) C. COMBIER (4), J. de BLIC (3) P. SCHEINMANN (3)

(1) 153, rue de Saussure 75017 Paris, (2) Hôpital de LISIEUX 14
(3) Hôpital des Enfants Malades 149, rue de Sèvres 75015 Paris
(4) Laboratoire d'analyses 41, rue Navier 75017 Paris.

50 C.F patients aged 1 month to 36 years old were investigated from March 1981 to January 1984 for possible Aspergillosis Fumigatus (A.f.) infection. Routine examinations were :
clinical findings (dyspnea, wheezing), biological tests :
A.f. search in direct sputum and bronchial aspirate (10 cases),
hemoagglutination test by indirect technique (Fumouze
laboratory), precipitin and IgE levels, blood eosinophilia.
Chest radiography was made in every suspicious case.
Results : 5 had symptomatic Aspergillosis and were treated,
14 patients had high levels of A.f. Haemagglutinin, over
1/1280. Therapy was : Ketoconazole 10 mg/24 h in a case of
Aspergilloma ; Ketoconazole 10 mg/24 h + 5 Flucytosin
140 mg/Kg/24 h in a case of allergic bronchopulmonary
aspergillosis ; Intravenous amphotericin B : 1 mg/Kg/every
48 h for a total dose of 2 g + 5 Fucytosin 140 mg/Kg/24 h
in a case of invasive Aspergillosis ; Ketoconazole 10 mg/24 h
+ 15 days of Steroïd·therapy (prednisone) 2 mg/Kg/24 h in
2 cases of invasive Aspergillosis.

CONCLUSIONS :

(1) A.f. is a common feature in Cystic fibrosis
(2) A.f. found into sputum is not always invasive and has
    to be compared with precipitin levels and IGE levels
(3) Treatment is not univocal.

**POSTER GROUP SEVEN No. 7.24**

A SURVEY OF IgG AND IgA SERUM ANTIBODIES TO PURIFIED
ASPERGILLUS FUMIGATUS ANTIGENS IN 157 CF-PATIENTS.

Henrik Schønheyder[1], Tim Jensen[2], Niels Høiby[3], and
Christian Koch[2].
[1] Institute of Medical Microbiology, University of
Aarhus, [2] Department of Pediatrics, Rigshospitalet,
and [3] Department of Clinical Microbiology, Rigshospitalet, Copenhagen, Denmark.

Pulmonary aspergillosis may add to morbidity in patients with CF. Aspergillus fumigatus may cause infection or hypersensitivity reactions. The immunological
response to A. fumigatus antigens may play a role in the
pathogenesis of aspergillosis and is also of diagnostic
importance. New insights in the humoral immune response
to A. fumigatus antigens in CF-patients are therefore
needed.
We have studied IgG and IgA serum antibodies to purified A. fumigatus antigens by enzyme-linked immunosor-
bent assay (ELISA) in 157 patients from the Danish national center for CF at Rigshospitalet, Copenhagen. Antigens were prepared by hydrophobic interaction chromatography and gel filtration and comprised fractions of
molecular weight (MW) 470,000, 250,000 and 25,-50,000.
Antibody levels in a single serum sample from each patient were related to age, presence and duration of
chronic pseudomonas infection, number of Ps. aeruginosa
precipitin lines, and the frequency of A. fumigatus in
sputum cultures within a period of approximately one
year. The most distinctive correlations observed were
between the frequency of A. fumigatus isolates and 1.
IgG antibodies to the low MW antigen fraction which
exhibites protease activity, and 2. IgA antibodies to
the high MW antigen fraction which is of glycoprotein
nature. For levels of IgG antibodies to the low MW
fraction the correlation was positive, suggesting that
this ELISA test may be useful for monitoring A. fumigatus colonization in CF-patients. For levels of IgA
antibodies to the high MW fraction the correlation was
negative which is in accordance with a conception of
locally produced antibodies being protective against
fungal colonization within the respiratory tract.

AN INVESTIGATION OF ASPERGILLUS FUMIGATUS ANTIGENICITY IN CYSTIC
FIBROSIS PATIENTS.

D.J. Reen, J. McDonnell and M.X. FitzGerald

Children's Research Centre, Our Lady's Hospital for Sick Children,
Crumlin, Dublin 12, Ireland & Dept. of Medicine, UCD, St. Vincent's
Hospital, Dublin 4.

Aspergillus fumigatus is a common opportunistic pathogen which gives
rise to a number of pulmonary disorders in humans depending on the
immunological response of the host to the organism.  Allergic
aspergillosis is a common occurrence particularly in older CF
patients and both precipitating antibodies and specific IgE
antibodies to A. fumigatus have been demonstrated in these patients.
In order to understand the variable immunological response to
Aspergillus in CF patients, methods are required which can identify
clinically relevant antigens of A. fumigatus which give rise to the
variable immune response seen in infected patients.  In this study
crude A. fumigatus extracts were separated by polyacrylamide gel
electrophoresis and the antigenicity of individual polypeptide
bands was investigated following electroblotting of the separated
components onto nitrocellulose membranes.  The specificity of
patient antibodies which reacted with individual polypeptide bands
was identified using peroxidase labelled anti-human immunoglobulin
antibodies.  At least 50 protein bands were seen following
separation of A. fumigatus extract on polyacrylamide gel electrophoresis using a silver stain.  Following blotting, identification
of anti-human IgG, IgA and IgM antibodies to A. fumigatus, revealed
discrete antigenic regions of the A. fumigatus electrophoretogram.
A major antigenic band (molecular weight = 55,000 daltons approx.)
was identified which reacted with serum from patients with
Aspergilloma.  In CF patients antibodies of all immunoglobulin
classes reacted with polypeptides greater than 70,000 daltons.
This study demonstrates the complexity of A. fumigatus antigenicity
in patients with Aspergillus related disease.

380

**POSTER GROUP SEVEN No. 7.26**

MYCOBACTERIAL ISOLATIONS IN YOUNG ADULTS WITH CYSTIC FIBROSIS

M.J. Smith, J. Efthimiou, M.E. Hodson and J.C. Batten
Cardiothoracic Institute, Fulham Road, London SW3 6HP.

Mycobacterial infections in cystic fibrosis (CF) are apparently rare. Wood et al[1] found only two cases of active pulmonary tuberculosis from over 700 patients with CF over an 18year period. Non-tuberculous mycobacteria have also been isolated from the sputa of CF patients, particularly rapidly growing organisms (Runyon group IV)[1,2], however their clinical significance in this context is not clear.

In a series of 223 patients with CF we have isolated mycobacteria from the sputa of seven of them. All of these cases were identified over a six year period following the introduction of routine examination and culture of sputum from CF patients for acid fast bacilli. The organisms isolated were M. tuberculosis in three patients, M. chelonei in one, M. fortuitum in one, and unidentified mycobacteria in two. The diagnosis was not suspected on clinical grounds in any of the cases, however in one patient night sweats were a prominent feature prior to diagnosis. In four of the patients direct sputum smear examination was negative, the organism being subsequently grown in culture. An unusual phenomenon of liquifaction of the Lowenstein-Jensen culture medium was encountered in five of the seven patients described, which in one case made identification and sensitivity testing of the organism impossible. This phenomenon has been observed in sputum cultures from other patients with CF but not in other pulmonary diseases. Immunological studies performed in three of the patients showed normal peripheral blood T and B lymphocyte numbers in all three, however in vitro lymphocyte transformation to tuberculin PPD was reduced in the patient with extensive M. fortuitum infection which proved fatal. The treatment regimens used and the difficulties associated with the management of mycobacterial isolations in CF patients are discussed.

Mycobacteria may be present in the sputa of CF patients more often than previously recognised and therefore sputum examination and culture for mycobacteria should be performed periodically and improved methods of culture for these organisms must be sought.

References
1. Wood RE, Boat RF, Doershuk CF. State of the Art: Cystic Fibrosis. Am Rev Respir Dis 1976; 113: 833–878.
2. Boxerbaum B. Isolation of rapidly growing mycobacteria in patients with cystic fibrosis.J.Paediatric.1980;96:689-91.

VIRAL (V) AND MYCOPLASMA (M) INFECTIONS IN CYSTIC FIBROSIS (CF):  DO
THEY PLAY A SIGNIFICANT ROLE IN PULMONARY EXACERBATIONS?
Bonnie W. Ramsey, M.D., Marion K. Cooney, PhD., Arnold L. Smith, M.D.
Children's Orthopedic Hospital and Medical Center, University of
Washington, Seattle, Washington 98105

We are continuing to prospectively study the effect of V and M
infections on acute lower respiratory symptoms, airway disease, and
bacterial colonization in CF patients.  Thirty-four patients [17 CF
and 17 normal siblings (NS)] have been followed on a two monthly basis
since July, 1982.  Two patients have died leaving 15 sibling pairs.  At
each visit V cultures and serology, M serology, pulmonary function
tests, anthropomorphic measurements, vital signs, white blood counts
and sputum samples are obtained.  Clinic symptomatology is given a
numerical exacerbation score;[1] a sick visit is defined as a score
greater than 10.
   The following results represent the first 15 months of the study
including 83 CF well, 49 CF sick, 106 NS well and 13 NS sick visits.
There have been sixty agents identified by either culture or serology;
an isolation rate of 23%.  Twenty positive V cultures (2 Influenza A,
1 Influenza B, 2 Coxsackie, 4 ECHO, 11 Rhinovirus) and 40 greater than
four-fold serologic titer rises (17 RSV, 4 Parainfluenza type 1, 2
Parainfluenza type 2, 4 Parainfluenza type 3, 4 Influenza A, 2 Influenza B, 7 M. pneumoniae).  There was no significant difference in the
number of positive cultures or serologic titer rises between CF (N=28)
and NS (N=32).  In 9/60 CF patients with positive isolates, their
siblings yielded the same organism within 6 weeks.
   In 13/28 (46%) of the V infections, CF patients had increased pulmonary symptoms compared with 3/32 (9%) of NS (p< .05).  We serially
measured changes in FVC, $FEV_{1.0}$, sputum density of Pseudomonas aeruginosa (Pa), and Staphylococcus aureus, and antibody to Pa exotoxin A
to determine changes in airway resistance or bacterial infection which
explain  the increased clinical symptoms.  CF patients increased their
$FEV_{1.0}$ by 10% (p< .05) at the time of viral infection.  There appears
to be an increase in the density of the Pa and a decrease in exotoxin A
antibody titer.  We attempted to analyze individual agents, particularly RSV, but the number of cases is currently insufficient.
   In summary, there appears to be no increased susceptibility to V and
M infections in CF patients.  They have more lower respiratory symptoms
at the time of infection than siblings.  These respiratory symptoms do
not appear to be associated with increased airway resistance but, may
be secondary to changes in bacterial colonization.

Reference:  Ramsey, BW, et al.  CF Club Abstracts  1983  24:43

Supported by Grant G049-3 from the Cystic Fibrosis Foundation

382

WHY ARE SOME CYSTIC FIBROSIS PATIENTS FREE OF PSEUDOMONAS COLONIZATION
L.L.Kulczycki,M.D.; R.L.Wientzen,M.D.; J.A.Bellanti,M.D.;T.Heller,M.D.
Dept. of Pediatrics, Georgetown University Medical Center,Washington,
D.C. 20007

In over 95% of C.F. patients respiratory tract pathology determines morbidity and mortality. Several investigators have confirmed
that the respiratory tract in C.F. patients has a selective propensity
for pseudomonas colonization. In an effort to identify factors which
may contribute to prevention of colonization of the respiratory tract
(R.T.) of cystic fibrosis (C.F.) patients with pseudomonas, we compared during a 3-year period, 1981-1983, clinical, laboratory and
microbiological features of two groups of C.F. patients: Group A, 24
patients, pseudomonas-free and Group B, 28 patients, pseudomonas
infected. Bacterial flora of each patient was analyzed on the basis of
cultures from sputum, bronchial washings or throat and nasopharyngeal
secretions. It appears that the pseudomonas positive group does far
worse in terms of clinical course and laboratory findings. Five
patients who expired during the 3-year study were all colonized by
pseudomonas and had advanced respiratory tract pathology. DiSant'Agnese
and Andersen in the pre-antibiotic era (1946) failed to demonstrate
evidence of pseudomonas infection in the respiratory tracts of C.F.
patients. Subsequent studies have reported a lower incidence of
pseudomonas colonization in C.F. patients not receiving antibiotics.
Twenty-four patients in this study remaining free of pseudomonas,
received antibiotics, for short time-periods, amounting to less than
30 days per year. These patients had a significantly higher incidence
of Staph. aureus colonization. On the other hand, the pseudomonas
positive group received frequent oral and intravenous antibiotics,
including aminoglycosides, but still remained colonized by pseudomonas
and mucoid pseudomonas, once Staph aureus had been eradicated. It
appears that the prolonged use of antibiotics combined with the eradication of Staph. aureus from the respiratory tract of C.F. patients,
heralds the onset of persistent pseudomonas colonization. An equally
plausible but less likely possibility is that the colonization with
pseudomonas seen in Group B may be related to a biological susceptibility of this group to bacterial colonization. Clearly additional
studies are required to verify the spectrum of host factors contributing to pseudomonas colonization as well as protective factors which
prevent colonization.

1) Kulczycki,L.L.,Murphy,T.M.,Bellanti,J.A.: Pseudomonas colonization
   in Cystic Fibrosis. JAMA, 240:30-34, 1978.

2) Hoiby,N. and Schiotz, P.O.: Pulmonary infections in Cystic Fibrosis
   Acta Paediatrica Scandinavica. Suppl. 301, 1982.

3) Smalhout, B.; Hill-Vaugham,A.D.: The Suffocating Child. Broncho-
   scopy. A guide to Diagnosis and Treatment. Boehringer Sohn, 1980.

**POSTER GROUP SEVEN No. 7.29**

SPHEROPLASTS OF HAEMOPHILUS INFLUENZAE ARE A POTENTIAL RESERVOIR FOR
RE-INFECTION IN CHRONIC BRONCHIAL SEPSIS BUT CAN THEORETICALLY BE
ERADICATED.

David Roberts, Andrew Rutman, Elizabeth Higgs and Peter Cole.
Host Defence Unit, Department of Medicine, Cardiothoracic Institute,
Brompton Hospital, Fulham Road, London SW3 6HP, England.

The use of selective medium (Roberts DE, Cole PJ. Lancet, 1980;
1: 796) has increased the isolation rate of Haemophilus influenzae
from the sputum of patients with chronic bronchial sepsis despite the
presence of many vigorously growing organisms, including Pseudomonas,
which would overgrow cultures employing conventional media. In spite
of this, some purulent sputum specimens still fail to yield pathogens.
This prompted us to supplement the selective medium with cell wall
constituents in case the organisms had been rendered unable to form a
cell wall by previous chemotherapy. The addition of N-acetyl-D-
glucosamine (NAG) was found to promote growth of colonies of
H.influenzae from some specimens of sputum which yielded no growth on
medium lacking this additive. By light microscopy the organisms were
found to be large spheroplasts similar to those which can be induced
intentionally with amoxycillin in vitro (Roberts DE et al, J Clin Path
1974; 27: 560). They reverted to normal on subculture. We suggest
that spheroplasts of H.influenzae may represent a reservoir from which
recurrence of respiratory infection could occur.

During in vitro titrations to determine minimal inhibitory and
minimal bactericidal concentrations (MIC and MBC, respectively) of
amoxycillin for H.influenzae, we noted that such spheroplasts were
commonly induced at concentrations ($< 1$ $\mu$g/ml) of antibiotic usually
achieved in sputum by conventional oral dosage. These abnormal forms
should be susceptible to cell wall-attacking antibiotics because
electron microscopy showed the spheroplasts to possess intact cell
walls, but the concentration of antibiotic required in the bronchial
lumen for this to occur would need to approximate to, or exceed, the
MBC for H.influenzae (3-3.5 $\mu$g/ml). To achieve this requires an appropriately higher dose of oral drug. The more so, because these concentrations derived from in vitro titrations of MIC and MBC are obtained under ideal laboratory conditions whereas access of antibiotic
to the lumen is reduced in patients with chronic bronchial sepsis and
a scarred bronchial tree. Furthermore, secretions within the bronchial
lumen of such patients often contain antibiotic-destroying enzymes.

We have in vivo evidence that this reservoir of H.influenzae
spheroplasts, which may be induced by treatment of such patients with
sub-optimal antimicrobial therapy, can be eradicated by treatment
with appropriage dose of oral drug.

**POSTER GROUP EIGHT No. 8.01**

NUTRITIONAL REHABILITATION OF MALNOURISHED CYSTIC FIBROSIS PATIENTS BY SUPPLEMENTAL NOCTURNAL GASTROSTOMY FEEDING.

P.Pencharz, L.Levy, P.Durie: Departments of Paediatrics & Nutritional Sciences, The University of Toronto and The Research Institute, The Hospital for Sick Children, 555 University Avenue, Toronto, Ontario Canada    M5G 1X8

Progressive malnutrition associated with deteriorating lung function in CF patients is a major clinical problem. Our initial approach is intensive dietary counselling and oral supplementation.  This approach not infrequently fails, particularly in adolescents due to a combination of early satiety, anorexia and nausea. We attempted nasogastric (NG) nocturnal supplemental feeding but found it to be of limited usefulness as it provoked coughing and on occasion, facilitated regurgitation and vomiting. The longest period any of our CF patients were able to tolerate NG feedings was 2 months. Nonetheless, the NG feeding did improve the patients' nutritional status. We therefore sought and found a more suitable access to the stomach by use of an incisionless gastrostomy (G-tube) placed (usually) under local anaesthesia and not requiring a laparotomy. Fourteen patients (5 male, mean age 15.6 yr; 9 female, mean age 11.4 yr) with moderately severe lung disease (mean $FEF_{25-75}$, $30\pm18.0\%$ predicted; $PaO_2$, $64.0\pm7.0$mmHg; $PaCO_2$, $39\pm2.0$mmHg) were studied prospectively with nocturnal supplementation (1200 kcal) of an elemental diet delivered via a G-tube. Daytime meals with exogenous pancreatic enzymes were as usual. Changes in growth, body composition and habitual physical activity were measured. Growth rates in all subjects were initially reduced ($\bar{X}$ height velocity = 69% predicted $\bar{X}$ weight velocity = 25% predicted). In response to G-tube supplementation, height and weight growth, body fat, fat free mass and total body potassium (TBK) were significantly increased. Catch-up growth in weight and height (where growth potential existed), was evident in the initial stages of refeeding. Total body nitrogen (TBN) also increased but not significantly ($\Delta$TBN (kg) +0.10 NS). There was a significant rise in haemoglobin for the group although only 2 of the 14 received therapeutic iron ($\Delta$group $\bar{X}$ Hb(g/L) 10.2, $p<0.005$). The table shows changes seen after a mean period of 0.8 yr (range 0.3-2.5 yr) of supplementation.

|   | Δ% Body Fat | ΔFFM(kg) | Δ% Ht V | Δ% Wt V | ΔTBK(g) |
|---|---|---|---|---|---|
| M | +4.9($p<0.05$) | +2.28 | +163.0 | +596.0 | +8.5 |
| F | +3.1($p<0.005$) | $p<0.005$ | $p<0.25$ | $p<0.005$ | $p<0.025$ |

Two subjects with the worst lung disease died which points to the need for careful patient selection criteria for G-tube placement. In the remaining 12 subjects with restoration of a positive energy balance, there has been marked improvement of habitual physical activity. We conclude that in CF patients unable to meet energy needs orally, supplemental nocturnal G-tube feeds offer a reasonable and important alternative.

**POSTER GROUP EIGHT No. 8.02**

EFFECT OF HIGH ENERGY SUPPLEMENTATION ON GROWTH
IN CHILDREN WITH CYSTIC FIBROSIS

By:   B. Armitage
      P. Brennan
      Sheffield Children's Hospital,
      Western Bank,
      SHEFFIELD 1

Aims

This trial was to determine the effect of a 20% energy increase to the diets of children with cystic fibrosis using a synthetic high energy supplement including linoleic acid, monoglyceride and MCT, and also to determine the palatability of this product.

Method

Fifteen prepubertal children with cystic fibrosis with poor weight gain were asked to use the energy supplement (RD 157) to increase their previously assessed dietary intake by at least 20% to a minimum of 120% recommended intake for their age.  They could take the supplement

       (1)   mixed with food
       (2)   as a milk shake
       (3)   as a medicine or a combination of these.

Height, weight, and skinfold thickness were taken every 6/52 for 3/12 before and during supplementation.  Linoleic acid levels were measured at the beginning and end of the trial.  Bone age was also taken.

Stool frequency, abdominal pain, distension, and amount and type of pancreatic supplements were recorded for 1/12 prior to - through supplementation;  and comments on palatability were requested from patients and parents.

After this trial, a smaller group will be asked to continue the energy supplement to enable us to monitor their growth over a longer period.

The results of the first 6 patients recruited will be available by May 1984.

**POSTER GROUP EIGHT No. 8.03**

MAINTAINING WEIGHT GAIN IN WASTED CHILDREN WITH
CF USING ENTERAL FEEDING

Margaret P. Boland, M.D., F.R.C.P. (C), John Patrick, M.B.(Lond), D.
Med., Deanna S. Stoski, R.N., Noni E. MacDonald, M.D., F.R.C.P. (C),
Pierre H. Beaudry, M.D., F.R.C.P. (C). Departments of Pediatrics and
Biochemistry, University of Ottawa, 401 Smyth Road, Ottawa, Ontario,
Canada K1H 8L1.

Thirteen wasted children with CF who had failed to gain weight
appropriately in the previous year, despite dietary counselling, were
treated by enteral feeding (5 by nasogastric tube and 8 by jejunostomy). Eleven had severe pulmonary disease (FEF 25-75 ≤28%
predicted), two were too young to obtain measurements.

Weight gain was achieved in all cases ranging from 7.7 to 18% of
initial weight. The rate of gain during catch-up growth varied from
1 to 9.6 g/kg/day. Of the initial 5 patients who were treated with
nasogastric feeding, only 2 (aged 16 mos and 17 yrs) maintained the
weight gain. The next 8 children were therefore fed via long-term
jejunostomy tubes. These children have now been followed during a
mean of 8 months jejunostomy feeding. No major problems have been
encountered: two tubes blocked and were replaced, minor infection
around the exit site occurred in one. On several occasions, 24-48
hours before the onset of a severe exacerbation of pulmonary
infection, the children's tolerance of enteral feeding decreased
dramatically and it was not possible to re-establish adequate
nutrition until the infection was controlled. Weight lost during
infections was rapidly replaced by increased feeding afterwards.
Nocturnal feeding was usually sufficient to maintain the improved
nutritional status. In addition to weight gain, we also noted a small
increase in height velocity and encouraging preliminary evidence of
stablized clinical state. In the 12 months preceeding feeding, FVC
decreased by a mean of 6.8% predicted and in the 12 months following,
by 2.9%. There was also a reduction in family anxiety and conflict
over eating and improved mood and energy in the patients while weight
was maintained. We conclude that this chronic jejunostomy treatment
may be of considerable benefit, but at least two more years will be
required to substantiate this initial impression.

**POSTER GROUP EIGHT No. 8.04**

USE OF AN INDWELLING JEJUNOSTOMY FEEDING TUBE AS A MEANS OF CALORIC SUPPORT FOR CYSTIC FIBROSIS PATIENTS.

Paula Partch, David Hicks, Donald Bendig, Barbara Towne, Carrie Worcester and Ralph Rucker, Childrens Hospital of Orange County. Orange, California.

Cystic Fibrosis (CF) is often associated with severe pulmonary disease, growth failure and malnutrition.  A large percentage of CF patients have been shown to have dietary intakes which are inadequate for their needs( 1).   Patients and family compliance with voluntary caloric supplementation is poor.  Nocturnal nasogastric feeding has almost a zero patient compliance and is frequently accompanied with post-tussive vomiting.  Parental alimentation is very expensive and has significant potential complications.  R.H. Mathisen et. al reported 4 patients receiving nocturnal feeds utilizing a fine needle jejun-ostomy(2).  We have chosen to use an indwelling t-tube jejunostomy(j-tube) because there is less fear of dislodgement and for its ease of replacement.  Over a period of 2 1/2 years (March 1981 to October 1983) 9 CF patients were selected for placement of the J-tube.  4 of the patients were female, 5 were male.  Ages varied from 16 months to 13 1/2 years.  All patients had demonstrated a plateau in weight gain for 6 to 12 months, in spite of maximum dietary and pulmonary support. Caloric supplementation with Vital (Ross Labs), one calorie/cc, varied from 400 to 1500 cc per night, depending on age, size and tolerance. The feedings were delivered at a constant rate for 8-12 hours.  Sig-nificant weight gain was apparent in all cases.  Complications in-cluded: gastric stasis with early AM vomiting of the evening meal (4 cases), nocturnal enuresis (1 case), prolapse and rectal passage of the tube (1 case) and lact of parental and patient acceptance(1 case). Several teenagers reported improved self image associated with the weight gain.  Persistant dumping syndrome was not observed.  It is our feeling that an indwelling t-tube feeding jejunostomy is a prac-tical, safe and effective means to deliver caloric supplementation to CF patients.  Questions to be answered include the optimal time for placement of the tube, patient selection and appropriate enzyme supp-lementation.

(2) Mathisen,R.H. et al: Evaluation of a New Method of Nutritional Intervention in Cystic Fibrosis Via Feeding Jejunostomy, CF Club Abstracts 1982.

(1) Hubbard, J.S. and Mongrum, P.J.: Energy Intake and Nutrition Counseling in Cystic Fibrosis JADA 127-131,February 1982.

388

OUTCOME OF PERIPHERAL HYPERALIMENTATION (PH) IN PATIENTS WITH CYSTIC
FIBROSIS (CF): RELATIONSHIP TO BASELINE NUTRITIONAL STATUS

Lucille A. Lester, M.D., Angelita Lopez, R.D., Zenaida Corpuz, R.N.,
Richard M. Rothberg, M.D.    Department of Pediatrics, The University
of Chicago School of Medicine, Box 133, 5841 So. Maryland Ave.,
Chicago, Illinois 60637.

   The efficacy of supplemental (PH) has been evaluated in selected
CF pts in ongoing studies at our CF center over the past 5 years. It
was the purpose of this analysis to determine whether assessment of
nutritional status would allow prediction of a sub-group of pts more·
likely to benefit from nutritional intervention. Over a 3 yr period,
15 pts (age 4-26 yrs, NIH clinical scores 45-75) who were hospitalized
for treatment of pulmonary symptoms received PH in form of Freamine
(amino acid solution) (up to 2.5 gms/kg/day), 10% Intralipid (up to
2.5 gms/kg/day) and dextrose (up to 10%). Pts received PH as a constant infusion for 9 to 18 days (mean = 13 days) in addition to their
usual diet ad lib. All pts had a history of poor weight gain or a
2 to 5 kg weight loss in the 6 months prior to admission. Clinical
scores and anthropometric measurements (triceps skinfold thickness
(TSF) and arm circumference (AC) expressed as % predicted normal for
age) were performed on admission. The recommended daily allowances
(RDA) for calories and protein were also calculated for each pt.
Response to PH was defined as a minimum of 2.0 kg wgt gain together
with maintenance or increase in wgt in the 6 months following hospitalization. Pertinent data is summarized below: (Non-responders = NR,
Responders = R).

| | age | NIH score | TSF | AC | wgt gain (kg) | mean calories/day %RDA(IV) | %RDA(total) |
|---|---|---|---|---|---|---|---|
| NR's (n=4) | 6.7±2 | 61±13 | 77±33% | 87±18% | 1.4±0.8 | 31±13% | 68±20% |
| R's (n=11) | 15.6±4 | 62±9 | 56±20% | 79±9% | 3.4±1.3 | 45±12% | 141±40% |
| t-test p= | <.002 | ns | ns | ns | <.005 | ns | <.001 |

Conclusions:(1) Analysis of nutritional assessment parameters did not
allow a prediction of which CF pts would benefit optimally from supplemental PH. The group responding favorably to PH included pts with
a wide range of nutritional impairment and pulmonary disease severity.
         (2) Supplying >100% of the (RDA) for calories and protein
for the full period of PH resulted in a good response (% RDA calories
vs wgt gain (kg) r=0.76). Poor wgt gain and lack of improvement in
subsequent clinical course occurred in 4 younger pts and appeared to
be related to inability to maintain a high level of oral and intravenous calories.

**POSTER GROUP EIGHT No. 8.06**

AN EVALUATION OF SUPPLEMENTAL OVERNIGHT NASOGASTRIC FEEDING IN CHILDREN WITH CYSTIC FIBROSIS (C.F.).

L.A. Daniels, G.P. Davidson, A.J. Martin.
Departments of Nutrition and Dietetics, Gastroenterology and Pulmonary Medicine, The Adelaide Children's Hospital Inc., North Adelaide, South Australia.   5006.

Fourteen pre-pubertal C.F. children were evaluated to determine the effect of overnight nasogastric nutrition during courses of standard intravenous antibiotics for chronic chest disease. Only children with discrepancies between height and weight of one standard deviation or greater, were selected.  Each child was admitted on two occasions, in random order, approximately six months apart.  During one admission the diet was supplemented by continuous nasogastric vivonex, overnight, to provide an additional 50% to the usual calorie intake.  Eleven children, mean age 7.75 years (range 1.9 - 13.5 years), completed the study.

Supplementary feeding significantly increased energy intake (P<.01) by a mean of 52 ± 14% despite a spontaneous fall in oral intake.  No significant differences in energy intake, after admission, short term (3 to 16 weeks) or long term (13 to 49 weeks), were noted.  The mean percentage increase in weight during the supplemented admission was 9.4 ± 4% and was significantly greater (P<.001) than that during the unsupplemented admission 2.6 ± 2.1%. Following the supplemented admission, subjects lost a mean of 0.6 kilograms in weight, in the short term, compared to a mean weight gain of 0.15 kilograms (P<.05) following the unsupplemented admission.

This study showed that overnight nasogastric supplementation significantly improved both energy intake and weight gain during admission and consideration should be given to trials of longer term energy supplementation.

390

CORRECTION OF GROWTH FAILURE BY NUTRITIONAL SUPPLE-
MENTATION VIA NOCTURNAL JEJUNOSTOMY FEEDINGS

Harris, R. O., III, M. D. and Miller, S. C., M. D.
University of South Alabama College of Medicine
2451 Fillingim Street, Mobile, AL   USA 36617

Growth failure occurs in a high percentage of patients
with Cystic Fibrosis.  We previously reported that every
one of our severely growth-retarded patients had markedly
reduced total caloric intakes in relation to their calculated needs.  If this, as well as pulmonary disease, might
be the cause of growth failure, then dietary correction
should cause a reversal of growth failure in many cases.
Improved nutrition might also have a favorable effect in
reducing the frequency and severity of pulmonary infections, as it is well known that undernourished children are
more susceptible to infection.  Finally, correction of
undernutrition in early life could have a salutary effect
in later life and result in an increased life expectancy.
This study investigates the effect of supplemental nocturnal jejunostomy feedings on growth failure.  Silastic
feeding tubes are surgically implanted in the jejunum. C.F.
patients are selected on the basis of 1) request of parents
for nutritional intervention, 2) age 6 to 11 years, 3)
height and weight below the 5th percentile for age, 4) mild
to moderate pulmonary disease, 5) ability of family members
to properly care for and administer feedings.  Total daily
caloric requirements are calculated at 175 K cal/kg., the
supplemental jejunostomy feedings to provide approximately
30% of this requirement. The formulas chosen contain 1 K
cal/ml with the appropriate carbohydrate, protein and fat
content for CF patients.  A protein allowance of 3 to 4
gms/kg is used. Jejunostomy feedings are administered during the hours of sleep, generally 8 P.M. to 4 A.M. via a
calibrated pump, and are planned to continue for one year.
Five patients have completed this program.  All but one
child achieved a significant weight gain which continued
throughout the period of the study.  Two gained over 10 kg.
in less than one year. Several also experienced significant
increases in height. All children who have completed the
program thus far have maintained the increased growth a-
chieved by supplemental jejunostomy feedings and have continued to gain weight and grow in height.  Also, all have
experienced remarkable subjective feelings of well-being
and gratifying personality changes.

**POSTER GROUP EIGHT No. 8.08**

PREVENTION OF GROWTH RETARDATION IN INFANTS WITH CYSTIC FIBROSIS. Philip Farrell, Sherie Sondel, Mari Palta, Elaine Mischler. University of Wisconsin, Madison, WI 53792, U.S.A.

Because neonatal screening for CF has made it possible to initiate treatment before malnutrition occurs and growth is impaired, an approach to infant feeding needs to be established that will routinely insure normal growth rates. Predigested formula has been shown in a limited number of CF infants to enhance absorption of macronutrients that supply energy; however, a clinical trial has not yet been reported on groups of CF infants fed predigested formula. The goal of this project, therefore, was to compare the growth rates of CF babies fed various diets and test the hypothesis that the weight of infants could be normalized by one year of age if they were placed on predigested formula before age 6 months. A group of 19 consecutively diagnosed CF patients who were referred to our Center on standard (nondigested) formula or breast milk were placed on Pregestimil (Mead Johnson Nutritional Division, Evansville, IND, USA) without pancreatic enzyme supplements. They were compared to a group of 19 previously diagnosed infants with CF who were fed standard formula, with each feeding being preceded by the administration of pancreatin powder in applesauce. The recommended caloric intake for each infant was 120 kcal/kg/day. Both groups were given vitamin supplements.

Birth weights were not significantly different between the two groups, nor was the weight at diagnosis (mean ± SD = 4.66 ± 0.99 kg in the Pregestimil group compared to 5.07 ± 1.97 kg in the controls) or the weight percentile (19 ± 24 vs. 20 ± 29). The sex distribution was 10 female and 9 male in each group. At one year of age, the Pregestimil group showed significantly greater length (p<.05) and weight (9.43 ± 0.67 kg compared to 8.39 ± 1.27 kg in the patients fed standard formula; p<.01). Average weight percentile, based on U.S. National Center for Health Statistics standards at 12 months of age, was twofold higher (40 vs. 20, p<.01) in the group fed Pregestimil; weight/length ratio was also markedly better (p<.001). Growth velocity was determined for the period between diagnosis and 12 months of age, revealing a better rate of growth (p<.001) for babies raised on Pregestimil (556 compared to 423 g/month); the same was true when calculations were made with birthweight as the starting point. Using weight percentile as the major growth index and values less than the fifth percentile as abnormal at 12 months of age, we found that all 19 babies were normal in the group fed Pregestimil, whereas nine were below the fifth percentile in the group fed regular formula (p=.0006). We conclude that the routine use of predigested formula in babies with CF promotes significantly better growth than standard formula and that normalization of weight and length can be readily achieved in infants with cystic fibrosis.

**POSTER GROUP EIGHT No. 8.09**

HYPOVITAMINOSIS D, OSTEOPENIA AND RESPONSE TO VITAMIN D
SUPPLEMENTATION IN OLDER PATIENTS WITH CYSTIC FIBROSIS.

J. Hanly, M.J. McKenna, C. Quigley, R. Freaney,
F.P. Muldowney and M.X. FitzGerald.
Departments of Metabolic Medicine and Respiratory Medicine,
St. Vincent's Hospital and University College Dublin.

Limited studies of vitamin D status and bone mineral
content in older patients with cystic fibrosis (C.F.) have
yielded conflicting results.  This study reports serum
25-hydroxy vitamin D (25-OHD) levels, bone mineral content,
and bony maturation in 20 adolescent and adult C.F. patients,
and their response to the internationally recommended dose
of supplementary vitamin D (800 i.u./day).

Serum 25-OHD values were below normal in 75% of patients,
the levels being undetectable ( < 5 nmol/l) in 65% of cases.
Serum alkaline phosphatase values, corrected for age, were
increased in 60% of patients.  Bone mineral content, measured
by photon beam absorptiometry, was below the normal range in
45% of patients, and bone age retarded in 45%.  Following
short-term supplementation with vitamin D (800 iu/day), 43%
of patients failed to achieve normal serum 25-OHD levels, and
repeat measurements after twelve months of therapy showed
similar results.

We conclude that profound hypovitaminosis D occurs
frequently in older C.F. patients, and is accompanied by
osteopenia and retarded bony maturation.  The recommended
dose of vitamin D (800 i.u./day) failed to correct this
deficiency in almost half of the patients studied.  Higher
supplementary doses of vitamin D with regular monitoring of
serum levels is necessary if prolonged exposure to low
circulating levels of 25-OHD is to be avoided in older C.F.
patients.

**POSTER GROUP EIGHT No. 8.10**

SONICATED EMULSION OF SAFFLOWER OIL (SESO) IN TREATMENT OF ESSENTIAL FATTY ACID (EFA) DEFICIENCY IN CYSTIC FIBROSIS

Melanie M. Hunt, R.D., Assistant Professor of Clinical Pediatrics, and Helen K. Berry, M.S., Professor of Research Pediatrics. The Children's Hospital Research Foundation and the Department of Pediatrics, University of Cincinnati College of Medicine, Cincinnati, Ohio 45229 U.S.A.

The purpose of this study was 1) to determine the extent of EFA deficiency in CF patients by comparing EFA levels in CF children and non-CF children matched for age, 2) to determine if the oral administration of a stable aqueous emulsion of safflower oil would alter the EFA levels of children with CF and 3) to compare the effect of linoleic acid supplementation on sweat sodium and chloride concentrations and on saliva sodium and calcium concentrations.

Sixteen CF subjects between 1 and 30 years of age were divided into two groups and were matched as nearly as possible on the basis of initial linoleic acid levels, severity of disease, diet, etc. One subject of each pair received supplemental linoleic acid in the form of SESO. The emulsion (30cc-60cc) was prescribed in an amount which supplied approximately 4% of the recommended daily calories in the form of linoleic acid. There was no other change in treatment for either group. Non-CF control subjects (N=16) were matched by age with CF subjects. EFA were measured before and every three months during a period of twelve months.

The fatty acid pattern of CF individuals was different from non-CF subjects. Significant differences were seen between CF and non-CF subjects for palmitoleic ($p < .05$), oleic ($p < .001$), linoleic ($p < .001$) and the abnormal fatty acid 5,8,11-eicosatrienoic acid ($p < .01$). CF subjects who took SESO showed a significant increase in linoleic acid ($p < .01$) after a 12 month period when compared to CF subjects who did not take the emulsion. Oleic acid declined in the experimental group but was not statistically different from the control group of CF subjects. Saliva and sweat electrolytes were not altered by the use of SESO.

Growth phases which occur during childhood are associated with increased requirements for EFA. Increased amounts of EFA are necessary to prevent biochemical deficiencies, clinical symptoms of deficiencies and histological abnormalities. Intravenous fat emulsions have been shown to raise EFA levels but they are expensive and difficult to administer to the patient. The use of an oral sonicated emulsion is an effective and inexpensive way to increase the serum linoleic acid levels of individuals who have CF.

394

ESSENTIAL FATTY ACIDS INFUSION TO THIRTY CF INFANTS

I. Garcia*, E. Bannier*, D. Michelon*, A. Revol* and
R. Gilly**

* Laboratoire de Biochimie, Secteur Ste-Eugenie et
** Clinique Pediatrique, Centre Hospitalier Lyon-Sud,
69310 Pierre-Benite, France.

Analysis of serum lipids of children with CF has
indicated a deficiency in essential fatty acids (EFA).
Since brain maturation is not complete at birth, we think
that it is very important to prevent or correct EFA
deficiency during the first two years of life. Soybean
oil emulsion has been administered intravenously to 30
babies with CF, diagnosed at birth by systematic
screening or during the first three months of life by
clinical symptoms. 5 ml/kg of 20% Intralipid was
perfused once every three weeks for a period of two
years. Clinical evaluation is based on the following
parameters: weight, height, Shwachman score and pulmonary
X-rays. Biochemical tests included determination of the
phosphoglyceride fatty acid patterns in serum and
erythrocyte membranes by gas-liquid chromatography, and
quantitative determination of total cholesterol,
triglycerides and total phospholipids in serum.

Patients can be divided into two groups according to the
extent of EFA deficiency. When correction of deficiency
is possible, it occurs after one or two infusions and
continues throughout the treatment. The improvement is
seen both for serum and erythrocyte membranes. On the
other hand, some patients with poor clinical evolution of
the disease never correct their essential fatty acid
deficiency despite repeated Intralipid infusions. The
results will be discussed taking into account concomitant
oral food intake and eventual occurence of neonatal
meconium ileus.

Clinically, it seems that there is a little improvement
at the age of 2 years, but it is not known whether this
is due to our intensive attention and care or to EFA
treatment.

**POSTER GROUP EIGHT No. 8.12**

HIGH, MODERATE OR LOW FAT DIETS FOR CYSTIC FIBROSIS?

MacDonald, Anita.   Regional Cystic Fibrosis Unit, St James's
                    University Hospital, Leeds 9.

What is the best diet for cystic fibrosis (CF) patients – a high,
moderate or low fat diet? The total fat intake, determined by seven
day diet histories, of 64 CF patients (aged from 3–24 years) was
related to total energy intake, anthropometric measurements, fat
absorption and abdominal symptoms.

Patients were divided into 4 groups. Group 1 (14 patients) consumed
>120%, Group 2 (22 patients) 100–119%, Group 3 (19 patients) 80–99%
and Group 4 (9 patients) <80% of the Department of Health and Social
Security (DHSS) (1979) recommended energy intakes. The results are
tabulated below.

| Group | % DHSS RDI for energy | Mean fat (g) daily intake | Fat g/kg/day | Mean % fat absorption | Mean standard deviation scores | |
|---|---|---|---|---|---|---|
| | | | | | Ht | Wt |
| 1 | >120 | 108 | 3.9 | 65 | −0.09 | −0.4 |
| 2 | 100–119 | 77 | 3.2 | 68 | −0.46 | −0.94 |
| 3 | 80–99 | 71 | 3.0 | 68 | −1.66 | −1.57 |
| 4 | <80 | 44 | 2.0 | 78 | −1.348 | −1.287 |

Data on mean subscapular and triceps skinfold thicknesses will also be
presented.

Mean standard deviation scores for height and weight were better for
patients in Groups 1 and 2 with higher energy and fat intakes than
for patients in Groups 3 and 4. Only 5 patients suffered from severe
abdominal symptoms when eating fatty foods and none of these were in
Group 1. Symptoms were not related to the degree of malabsorption.
Although many patients felt they should moderately restrict fat in
their diet, in practice the majority could tolerate fatty foods.

From the results it can be seen that CF children who consumed energy
intakes in excess of the DHSS (1979) recommended amounts achieved
better growth. As fat restriction makes it difficult to achieve an
adequate energy intake and fat is generally well tolerated, more
emphasis should be placed on encouraging generous fat intakes and an
appropriate dose of pancreatic enzyme supplements. The traditional
low fat diet is unnecessary for the majority of CF patients.

**POSTER GROUP EIGHT No. 8.13**

A DOUBLE DUMMY CROSS-OVER STUDY COMPARING THE EFFECT OF PANCREATIC ENZYME AS ACID-RESISTANT MICROSPHERES (PANCREASE[R] CILAG CHEMIE) TO GRANULES (PANCREATIN[R] ROSCO) IN CYSTIC FIBROSIS.

W. Petersen, C. Heilmann, S. Garne. Cystic Fibrosis Center, Department G University of Copenhagen, Rigshospitalet Blegdamsvej 9, DK-2loo Copenhagen Ø, Denmark.

11 patients apparently well controlled on Pancreatin were randomly allocated to treatment with either Pancreatin or Pancrease in approximately equipotent doses according to manufactures recommandations. Patients previously receiving less than 15 ml Pancreatin were given 1 capsule Pancrease per meal, and patients previously receiving above 15 ml received 2 capsules. Treatment was given for one month, whereafter the alternative treatment was given for one month. During both periods placebo preparation was given in form of capsules or granules.

1 ml of Pancreatin contains 525 U trypsine, 12ooo U lipase and 1275o U amylase. Each Pancrease capsule 4ooo U lipase, 2oooo U amylase and 25ooo U protease.

Clinical effect was judged by a 3 days fat absorption test done at the end of each treatment period, with the children being hospitalized. Symptom score card was filled in daily giving stoll frequency, consistency, colour and odor and abdominal cramps. The parents and/or children were asked for preference before breaking the code.

Results showed Pancrease was slightly superior to Pancreatin in reducing dyspeptic symptoms. Fat absorption was slightly better on Pancrease. Results of statistical analysis are at the moment pending. The results of a similar, but open study involving more patients and a longer treatment period, but not yet completed, will be presented and discussed.

**POSTER GROUP EIGHT No. 8.14**

PULMONARY INFECTION AND PROTEIN TURNOVER IN CYSTIC FIBROSIS.
Holt, T.L.[1], Ward, L.C.[2], Thomas, B.J.[3], Cooksley, W.G.E.[2],
Shepherd, R.W.[1].
Departments of Child Health[1] and Biochemistry[2], University of
Queensland and Department of Medical Physics[3], Queensland Institute
of Technology, and Royal Children's Hospital, Brisbane, Australia.

Despite improved treatment, underweight in cystic fibrosis (CF)
patients remains a major problem. Relative underweight has been shown
to be a major factor adversely affecting survival. We have previously
documented abnormalities of body composition and myofibrillar protein
catabolism in CF, and that adequate nutritional support can favourably
affect growth and clinical status in some patients suggesting a role
for reversible nutritional factors in the pathogenisis of the disease.
To further investigate determinants of protein-energy balance in CF,
studies of the effects of acute-active pulmonary infection, a common
and recurring feature of the disease, on whole body protein turnover
were conducted. Total body protein synthesis and catabolism were
determined in 5 CF children with acute exacerbations of pulmonary
infection at the time of study (CF I), a group (n=5) of healthy
children, and a group of CF children with chronic but stable
pulmonary disease (CF II). Protein synthesis was determined via the
method of Waterlow using a single oral dose of $^{15}$N glycine and
protein catabolism derived from nitrogen balance.

Protein Turnover (g Kg$^{-1}$ 24hr$^{-1}$)

|          | Synthesis | Catabolism | Deposition |
|----------|-----------|------------|------------|
| Controls | 4.5±0.8   | 3.3±2.1    | 1.5±0.6    |
| CF I     | 2.8±0.5   | 1.2±0.2    | 1.5±0.4    |

Protein synthesis was decreased ($p<0.01$) in the CF (I) group compared
with controls and with CF children with chronic but stable pulmonary
disease (CF II). Protein catabolism was also decreased ($p<0.05$) such
that there was no significant difference in net deposition. These
findings contrast strongly to studies in normal children and those
with mild protein-energy malnutrition (PEM) and infection, where
infection increased protein synthesis, but are consistent with the
observed decrease in protein turnover where severe PEM is accompanied
by infection. We conclude that repeated pulmonary infection can
adversely affect protein-energy balance and that adequate nutritional
support should be considered in management during and after each
episode.

**POSTER GROUP EIGHT No. 8.15**

NITROGEN LOSS FROM SPUTUM IN CYSTIC FIBROSIS:  AN UNEXPECTED FACTOR
IN ASSESSING PROTEIN-ENERGY BALANCE.

Ward, L.C.[1], Holt, T.L.[2], Thomas, B.J.[3], Cooksley W.G.E.[1] and
Shepherd, R.W.[2].
Departments of Biochemistry[1], Child Health[2], University of
Queensland and Institute of Technology[3] and Royal Children's
    Hospital, Brisbane, Australia.

Nitrogen balance studies form the basis for assessment of protein-
energy requirements, and studies of protein-turnover in man.  In
diseases such as cystic fibrosis (CF) all factors affecting protein-
energy balance need to be taken into account.  Previous studies in
CF have emphasised the necessity to account for faecal losses but
sputum losses have hitherto been largely ignored.  As part of an
investigation to assess factors contributing to an unfavourable
protein-energy balance in CF we measured 72 hour nitrogen loss from
sputum in ten randomly selected CF patients.  The sputum losses ranged
up to 2g N 24 hr$^{-1}$ (Table 1).

TABLE 1

| Subject Ages Yrs | Sputum Production g 24 hr$^{-1}$ | Sputum N concentration mg g$^{-1}$ | Nitrogen loss g 24 hr$^{-1}$ |
|---|---|---|---|
| 3-5→19.5 | <10→233 | 2.3→10.3 | <0.1→1.98 |

Sputum nitrogen did not correlate with sputum volume, pulmonary
function or clinical score.  We have previously determined total
urinary and faecal N loss in children with CF to vary between
7.4 gN 24 hr$^{-1}$ and 15.1 gN 24 hr$^{-1}$.  This indicates that sputum N loss
may represent up to 13% of total nitrogen loss and correspond to a
maximum protein loss of up to 12 g 24 hr$^{-1}$.  The contribution of
sputum N losses to protein-energy deficit varies with the severity
of lung disease, presence of ongoing active infection and other
factors but not withstanding the variability that was observed
between subjects, this study highlights the extent of sputum N
losses in some patients and suggests that these losses may be a
significant protein-energy drain in these patients.  The preliminary
findings documented here require further study, but raise several
important issues regarding the relationship between lung disease and
malnutrition in CF, and may have an influence on the assessment of
protein-energy requirements.  In addition the present findings
further elucidate the aetiology of the protein-energy deficit and
altered protein metabolism observed in CF patients, and suggest that
undernutrition does not result from an energy deficit alone.

**POSTER GROUP EIGHT No. 8.16**

## OVARIAN ULTRASONOGRAPHY, SERUM GONADOTROPHIN CONCENTRATIONS AND MENSTRUAL FUNCTION IN WOMEN WITH CYSTIC FIBROSIS

R.J.Stead, M.E.Hodson, J.C.Batten, Cardiothoracic Institute, Brompton Hospital, London SW3 6HP.
H.D.Mason, S.Franks, St Mary's Hospital Medical School, London W2 1PG.
J. Adams, Middlesex Hospital, Mortimer Street, London W1N 8AA.

Disturbances of menstruation are common in women with cystic fibrosis (CF). The aim of the present study was to investigate the relationship between ultrasound appearances of the ovaries and serum gonadotrophin concentrations in a group of CF women with various menstrual patterns.

Eight female patients (mean age 23·2 years, range 15·7-35·5) attending an adult CF clinic were studied. Five patients had secondary amenorrhoea, one patient was pre-menarchal (age <16), one patient was peri-menarchal and one patient had regular menstrual cycles. Six of the eight patients were below acceptable body weight for height. Mean body mass index (weight/height$^2$) was 16·0 (acceptable range 18·7 - 23·8). Pelvic ultrasonography was performed and ovarian volumes calculated from ovarian diameters. The sizes of intra-ovarian cystic structures were also determined. Serum LH and FSH concentrations were measured by a standard double antibody radioimmunoassay. In three patients sequential samples of serum were taken at 15 minute intervals over an eight hour period for determination of gonadotrophins.

Four patients (Group 1) had amenorrhoea with normal sized or small ovaries (mean volume 3·1cm$^3$) containing a few follicles mainly 2-4mm in diameter. There were no follicles >12 mm in diameter. Four patients (Group 2) had normal sized or large ovaries (mean volume 5·5 cm$^3$) with a 'megalocystic' appearance containing around 8-10 cystic structures measuring 6-10mm in diameter. Basal LH was lower in Group 1 patients, mean 1·9 iu/l ± 1·5 (SD) than in Group 2 patients, mean 6·6 ± 1·9 (p<0·02). Similarly mean basal FSH in Group 1 was 2·05 iu/l ± 1·3 compared with 5·5 ± 3·9 in Group 2. All three patients sampled sequentially had secondary amenorrhoea. Two of them had 'megalocystic' ovaries and had gonadotrophin pulses. The third patient had normal sized ovaries with a few small follicles and showed very low gonadotrophin concentrations with no pulses.

'Megalocystic' ovaries are associated with normal puberty and with an intermediate stage of 'recovery' from weight loss related amenorrhoea in otherwise healthy women. Women with 'megalocystic' ovaries have evidence of pulsatile gonadotrophin secretion whereas patients with amenorrhoea and normal sized or small ovaries do not. Our findings in CF are consistent with this. Our patients with amenorrhoea and 'megalocystic' appearances have all subsequently had menstrual cycles whereas none of the patients in Group 1 have done so.

**POSTER GROUP EIGHT No. 8.17**

AMENORRHOEA IN CYSTIC FIBROSIS
R.J.Stead., M.E.Hodson, J.C.Batten, Cardiothoracic Institute,
Brompton Hospital, London SW3 6HP.
J.Adams, H.S.Jacobs, Middlesex Hospital, Mortimer Street, London
WIN 8AA.

Delayed puberty is a common complication of cystic fibrosis (CF) including delay in menarche in girls. We report a prospective study of the relationship between amenorrhoea, body composition and respiratory status in CF. Forty-two female patients (age range 15·5 - 40·0 years) attending an adult CF clinic were assessed. Primary amenorrhoea was defined as absence of menstruation by age 16 and secondary amenorrhoea as absence of menstruation for four months at any time after menarche. The height and weight of the subjects were used to derive body mass index (weight/height$^2$) and percentage body fat. Percentage body fat was also derived from measurements of skinfold thickness at four sites. Forced vital capacity (FVC) was recorded as percentage predicted for age and height. Pelvic ultrasonography was performed on 22 patients. Ovarian diameters were measured to estimate ovarian volume. Uterine cross-sectional area was calculated from length and anteroposterior diameter as a biological assay of oestrogenic activity.

Twenty-seven patients had regular menstrual cycles, ten patients had primary or secondary amenorrhoea, two patients were pre-menarchal (age <16 years) and two patients were assessed at the time of menarche. Lastly, five patients had irregular menstrual cycles. Four patients were therefore assessed twice. The median age of menarche was 14·5 years. All three measures of body fat were greater in patients with regular menstrual cycles than those with primary or secondary amenorrhoea (p<0·001). Respiratory function was also better in those with regular cycles than those with amenorrhoea (0·01>p>0·001). Patients with regular cycles had a greater mean uterine cross-sectional area than those with primary or secondary amenorrhoea (0·01 > p >0·001) and in patients with amenorrhoea there was a positive correlation between uterine cross-sectional area and $\log_{10}$ sum of the skinfold thicknesses ($\tau = 0·611$, $p < 0·05$). There was no correlation between uterine cross-sectional area and percentage predicted FVC. The ovaries in seven patients (32%) had a 'megalocystic' appearance containing cystic structures between 6 and 10 mm in diameter, usually with ovarian enlargement.

This study demonstrates a relationship between poor nutritional status and amenorrhoea in women with CF. The correlation between 'fatness' and uterine size in women with amenorrhoea suggests a critical effect of body fat on oestrogen production. 'Megalocystic' ovaries have been associated with amenorrhoea in women without CF, but the full significance of this appearance is not yet clear.

**POSTER GROUP EIGHT No. 8.18**

## THE PHARMACOKINETICS OF CONTRACEPTIVE STEROIDS IN CYSTIC FIBROSIS

R.J. Stead, M.E. Hodson, J.C. Batten, Cardiothoracic Institute, Brompton Hospital, London SW3 6HP.
S.F.M. Grimmer, W.L.Allen, M.L'E. Orme, Department of Pharmacology and Therapeutics, University of Liverpool, Liverpool L69 3BX.

Increasing numbers of girls with cystic fibrosis (CF) are reaching maturity and those with regular menstrual cycles probably have near normal fertility, hence creating a need for effective contraception. Combined oral contraceptives containing an oestrogen and progestogen are the most effective method in healthy women. However, information on the bioavailability of these steroids in CF is needed in view of the possible effects of gastrointestinal disease and use of antibiotics. The aim of this study was to examine the pharmacokinetics of two such steroids.

Five girls with proven CF (mean age 22·8 years, range 17·4-26·5) were studied. All had exocrine pancreatic insufficiency and were clinically stable. All had been taking a combined oral contraceptive for at least two months and none received systemic antibiotics within 10 days of the study. Patients were randomised to receive either an oral or intravenous (iv) dose of ethinyloestradiol 50 mcg and levonorgestrel 250 mcg after an overnight fast having not taken any contraceptive steroids within the previous 36 hours. Samples of plasma were taken for ethinyloestradiol and levonorgestrel concentrations at 0, ½, 1, 1½, 2, 3, 4, 6, 8, 10, 11, 12, 13, 14, and 24 hours after dosing. The study was repeated after a minimum of four days using the alternative route of administration. Plasma steroids were measured by radioimmunoassay. The areas under the plasma concentration time curves (AUC's) were calculated and hence systemic bioavailability. Plasma clearance and elimination half-life were also calculated. The results were compared with data obtained on healthy female volunteers.

The mean AUC after oral levonorgestrel was similar to the controls. However, the mean AUC after iv dosing was greater in CF patients, and mean bioavailability of levonorgestrel was 76% compared with 99% in controls. The mean clearance in CF was 121 ml/hr/kg as against 113 ml/hr/kg in controls. However, one patient had a markedly elevated clearance of 347 ml/hr/kg whereas in the other four patients it was below 75 ml/hr/kg. The mean elimination half-life was 12 hours compared with 8·8 hours in controls. None of these differences were statistically significant. However, the results suggest reduced bioavailability of levonorgestrel in CF compared with normal women and further studies will be reported together with the results for ethinyloestradiol.

**POSTER GROUP NINE No. 9.01**

CYTOSOLIC FREE $Ca^{2+}$ CONCENTRATION AND INTRACELLULAR $Ca^{2+}$ DISTRIBUTION IN CF LYMPHOCYTES

Dorr G. Dearborn, Robert L. Waller & William J. Brattin, Case Western Reserve Univ., Cleveland, Ohio 44106, U.S.A.

Cytosolic free $Ca^{2+}$ concentration is important in the regulation of many cellular processes, including stimulus-secretion coupling. Cytosolic free $Ca^{2+}$ levels are determined by a balance between transport and diffusion across the plasma membrane and intracellular organelles such as mitochondria and the endoplasmic reticulum. To investigate whether altered intracellular $Ca^{2+}$ homeostatsis is important in the cellular dysfunctions observed in cystic fibrosis (CF), we measured the cytosolic free $Ca^{2+}$ and the distribution of total intracellular $Ca^{2+}$ in CF and control lymphocytes. Cytosolic free $Ca^{2+}$ was monitored in intact lymphocytes using the $Ca^{2+}$ sensitive indicator, quin-2, first described by R.Y. Tsein (Biochemistry 19, 2396-2404, 1980). In 10 experiments, the mean concentration of free $Ca^{2+}$ in control lymphocytes was $98\pm5$ nM, and in CF lymphocytes was $102\pm7$ nM. Measurement of total intracellular $Ca^{2+}$ revealed that CF lymphocytes contained about 25% more total $Ca^{2+}$ than control ($54\pm5$ vs $43\pm4$ nmol/mg cell protein). Two lines of evidence suggest that this extra $Ca^{2+}$ is stored primarily in the mitochondria: when 10 uM carbonyl cyanide p-trifluoromethoxyphenyl-hydrazone (FCCP) is added to lymphocytes, there is a much larger increase in cytosolic free $Ca^{2+}$ in CF lymphocytes than in controls ($28\pm9$ vs $12\pm5$ nM). (FCCP is believed to cause specific release of intramitochondrial $Ca^{2+}$ stores). The FCCP-releasable intracellular $Ca^{2+}$ pool (measured as the difference between total intracellular $Ca^{2+}$ and FCCP non-releasable $Ca^{2+}$ ) is larger in CF lymphocytes than in controls ($7.1\pm2.8$ vs $1.1\pm3.5$ nmol/mg cell protein)(cf. Feigal & Shapiro, Pediat Res 13, 764-8, 1979, who found increased mitochondrial $Ca^{2+}$ content in CF fibroblasts). To determine if CF lymphocytes have a diminished capacity to restore cytosolic $Ca^{2+}$ levels to normal after perturbation, we incubated control and CF lymphocytes at $0^{\circ}C$ (this results in an increase in both cytosolic and total $Ca^{2+}$ content). The cells were then warmed and the rate of removal of $Ca^{2+}$ from the cytosol was measured using quin-2. The data fit a single exponential function ($Ca^{2+} = Ae^{-kt} + B$); no significant differences between control and CF lymphocytes were found in any of the kinetic parameters. In summary, comparison of CF and control lymphocytes revealed no change in cytosolic free $Ca^{2+}$ concentration and no significant difference in the kinetic parameters of $Ca^{2+}$ disappearance from cold-loaded cells. However, an increase in total intracellular $Ca^{2+}$ was found in CF cells, and this appears to be located primarily in the mitochondria. (Supported by NIH Grant AM27651).

**POSTER GROUP NINE No. 9.02**

CALCIUM EFFLUX AND CELL MORPHOLOGY CHANGES IN RED BLOOD CELLS FROM
NORMAL SUBJECTS AND PATIENTS WITH CYSTIC FIBROSIS.

Vivian Siegal and C.T. Settlemire, Biology Department, Biochemistry
Committee, Bowdoin College, Brunswick, Maine, USA and Zoology Department, University College of Wales, Aberystwyth, Dyfed, Wales.

Several workers have reported that red blood cells from cystic
fibrosis patients have an abnormal calcium translocation process.
Much of this work has been done with rbc ghosts or energy depleted
cells. These experiments were designed to ask whether intact rbc
from normal and CF sources loaded with calcium by the use of an
ionophore would efflux calcium at different rates.

The cells were loaded with $^{45}Ca^{++}$ using the ionophore A23187,
based on the procedure of Sardeki et al (J. Memb. Biol., 26:357,
1976). After removal of the ionophore the cells were suspended in
an isotonic KCl solution.

Red blood cells from both normal and CF sources effluxed $^{45}Ca^{++}$
at approximately linear rates for 30 minutes but the rbc from CF
sources had a decreased efflux rate which was 29.4% $\pm$ 4.8% (n=10)
lower than that of aged-matched cells from normal sources. At
approximately 40 minutes, cells from normal sources had returned
to normal intracellular $Ca^{++}$ concentrations. RBC from CF sources
required 120 minutes to return to normal concentrations.

Examination by SEM techniques indicated that calcium loaded cells
have a echinocyte morphology. As the calcium was effluxed, the
cells returned to the characteristic biconcave disc. The difference
in percent cells returning to a biconcave morphology was correlated
with the difference in $^{45}Ca^{++}$ efflux. During the initial 40 minute
phase, 30.4% $\pm$ 4.0% fewer CF cells were returned to a biconcave
morphology.

**POSTER GROUP NINE No. 9.03**

LYSOSOMAL ENZYMES EXOCYTOSIS IN CF NEUTROPHILS: EFFECT OF
CALCIUM MODULATION.
Cabrini G., *De Togni P., Mastella G.
Centro Fibrosi Cistica,Ospedale B. Trento,37126 Verona, Italy
*Istituto Patologia Generale,Strada Le Grazie, 37134 Verona,Italy

Among the alterations at the cellular level which accompany CF disease, an increase in cytosolic calcium concentration and an enhanced
release of lysosomal enzymes have been described. Since redistribu-
tion of cytosolic calcium is known to play an important role in
stimulus-secretion coupling, we studied lysosomal enzyme secretion
by neutrophils of CF patients in condition which alter the levels of
free calcium inside the cell.Neutrophils were obtained after dextran
sedimentation, Ficoll gradient and, after lysis of contaminating
erythrocytes,resuspended in Hepes 20mM, NaCl 154 mM, KCl 2.7 mM,
glucose 5.6 mM (pH 7.40) and Cytocalasin B (5 μg/ml). Exocytosis was
studied by assaying the release of β-glucuronidase and α-glucosidase
in the supernatant of cells incubated at 37°C for 20 minutes. LDH
release served as a marker of cell lysis and was always < 2%.
Enzyme release was studied in unstimulated cells (spontaneous exocytosis) either in the presence of calcium (0.5 mM) or of the $Ca^{2+}$
chelator EGTA (0.1 mM). Spontaneous exocytosis was compared with
that induced by the $Ca^{2+}$ ionophore A23187 (1.0 μM), which induces
passive $Ca^{2+}$ intake, and by the peptide N-formyl-L-methionyl-L-leu
cyl-L-phenilalanine (FMLP)(100 nM), which promotes the release of
$Ca^{2+}$ from intracellular stores.

| % EXOCYTOSIS OF CF PATIENTS REFERRED TO CONTROLS = 100% | | |
|---|---|---|
| | β-GLUCURONIDASE | α-GLUCOSIDASE |
| Spontaneous (EGTA) | 211.7+ 68.3 (4) | 261.3+71.2 (3) |
| Spontaneous (calcium) | 98.9+ 29.8 (4) | 155.7+14.8 (3) |
| A23187 stimulated | 126.8+ 29.5 (4) | 104.2+ 5.9 (3) |
| FMLP stimulated | 102.4+ 15.7 (4) | 82.3+11.3 (3) |

mean + S.E. (number of experiments)

The significantly higher exocytosis in CF neutrophils in the absence
of calcium (EGTA) suggests cytosolic calcium could be increased in
these cells and that calcium homeostasis could play an important
role in the derangment of CF secretory processes.

**POSTER GROUP NINE No. 9.04**

CHLORIDE PERMEABILITY PROPERTIES OF CYSTIC FIBROSIS SWEAT DUCTS

J. Bijman and P. Quinton, Biomedical Sciences, University of California, Riverside, CA 92521, USA

Microperfused sweat ducts from control and cystic fibrosis (CF) subjects were compared with respect to changes in the transepithelial potential as a function of Cl concentration at the luminal and contraluminal surfaces in an attempt to gain insight as to the nature of the Cl permeability defect in CF (1). Segments of sweat ducts were prepared for microperfusion as described previously (2). The Cl concentration was varied independent of other components in the bathing and perfusion solutions by substitution with gluconate (taken as impermeant). When Cl was present in the perfusion medium, the spontaneous luminal potential relative to the bath in normal ducts was $-11.9 \pm 3.6$ mV* (n=14) and $-102.4 \pm 7.2$ mV (n=12) in CF ducts. Removal of Cl from the luminal medium caused no change in the potential in CF ducts ($-101.2 \pm 5.4$ mV; n=12), but in control ducts, the potential increased to about the same level ($-94.8 \pm 4.4$ mV; n=20) as in CF ducts with or without Cl. The electrical response of the luminal surface of the control duct was 3.3 times greater than that of the contraluminal surface to a 15 fold change in the Cl concentration, but the response of each surface of the control duct was at least 3 times greater than either surface of the CF duct which responded only slightly to the changes in Cl. After the application of ouabain to block active Na reabsorption in normal Cl containing solutions, the luminal potential in both groups of ducts was essentially abolished. But while the electrical response of the luminal surface of the control duct was only 1.1 times larger than the contraluminal surface, the response at both surfaces was at least 3 times greater than that of either surface of the CF duct to the same changes in Cl concentration. However, the response of the contraluminal surface of the CF duct after ouabain, was more than 6 times larger than the response of the luminal surface to changes in Cl. In the presence of normal Cl, amiloride at the luminal surface reduced the spontaneous potential of the control duct to $+0.1 \pm 1.7$ mV (n=5) but raised the luminal potential of the CF duct to $+22.0 \pm 5.7$ mV (n=8). When luminal Cl was removed in the presence of amiloride, the potential in both groups of ducts was hyperpolarized by about $-25$ mV. These results are consistent with an electrodiffusive pathway for Cl which is defective in the CF duct. Results will be discussed in terms of abnormal transcellular or paracellular anion shunts.

\* mean $\pm$ S.E.M.

1. Quinton, P.M. and Bijman J., N. Engl. J. Med. 308: 1185 (1983).
2. Quinton, P.M., Pflugers Arch 391: 309 (1981).
We deeply appreciate the assistance of Dr. Chun-I Wang, Children's Hospital, L.A. and Dr. R.C. Dooley, Dept. Pediatrics, SBCMC. Supported by grants from the Getty Oil Co., Gillette Co., and the USPHS-NIH No. 26547.

**POSTER GROUP NINE No. 9.05**

A MEMBRANE ABNORMALITY IN RED CELLS OF PATIENTS CARRYING THE
CYSTIC FIBROSIS GENE

Carol A. Seymour and J. A. Davis - Physiological Laboratory,
Downing Street, Cambridge, CB2 3EG and Department Paediatrics,
Addenbrooke's Hospital, Cambridge, CB2 2QQ

We have demonstrated a consistent defect in calcium transport
in the red blood cells of patients with cystic fibrosis which
appears to be also a marker for the heterozygote.

We have used red cells, from cystic fibrosis and control
patients, to study the calcium pump (Ca/Mg ATPase) in relation
to total membrane protein, to haemoglobin and to other membrane
markers (Na/K ATPase).  The number of active calcium pumps per
red cell has been measured using lanthanum to trap Ca/Mg ATPase
in the partly phosphorylated form.

A significant reduction in Ca/Mg ATPase activity and in
calcium-dependent phosphoenzyme occurred in cystic fibrosis
cells compared with controls, which was independent of calmodulin,
indicating an absolute reduction in the number of active pumps
per cell.

Free intracellular calcium concentration has been measured
using a non-disruptive method for chelator loading of red cell
ghosts, which depends on hydrolysis of the chelator ester by
cytoplasmic esterases.  Surprisingly, the levels were unchanged
from controls suggesting a similar reduction in passive calcium
permeability to the reduction in number of calcium pumps.  These
changes were independent of any circulating inhibitory factor.

**POSTER GROUP NINE No. 9.06**

IMBALANCE BETWEEN ALPHA- AND BETA-ADRENOCEPTOR BINDING SITES IN MARKER CELLS IN CYSTIC FIBROSIS

Kazuji Tawara, Gunnar Alván, Birgitta Strandvik
Departments of Clinical Pharmacology and Pediatrics, Karolinska Institutet, Huddinge University Hospital, S-141 86 Huddinge, Sweden.

There have been suggestions that altered alpha- and beta-adrenoceptor response could be related to the basic defect in cystic fibrosis (CF) (J Lab Clin Med 1980; 96: 75; N Engl J Med 1980; 302: 1453; J Clin Invest 1981; 68: 253).
Six CF patients with clinical score ranging between 32 and 95 and 20 age-matched controls were investigated when free from acute infection. They did not take beta-adrenergic agonists, methylxanthines and aspirin for at least two weeks prior to the study. Platelets were recovered from a 45 ml fresh blood sample and stored at $-70^{\circ}$. Polymorphonuclear leukocytes (PMNs) were isolated from the same sample, homogenized, washed and stored. The binding to alpha2-receptors was assessed by a $^3$H-yohimbine assay after thawing and homogenizing the platelets. Non-specific binding was determined by incubating platelet homogenates with $^3$H-yohimbine in the presence of 10 umol of phentolamine. The binding to beta-2-receptors was assessed by use of ($^{125}$I)-hydroxybenzylpindolol (IHYP). Unspecific binding was determined by incubating the PMN fragments in the presence of 0.5 umol (-)-propranolol.
There was a tendency ($p = 0.08$) in this small material towards a difference in Kd values of IHYP binding in PMNs from CF patients (113.0 pM $\pm$ 32.8, SD) and controls (84.3 pM $\pm$ 30.4, SD). The Kd values for ($^3$H)-yohimbine were not significantly different between the two groups. We found no consistent differences in Bmax values for neiter ($^3$H)-yohimbine nor IHYP bindings between the two groups. However, the ratio of ($^3$H)-yohimbine versus IHYP binding sites was significantly greater in CF patients (1.51 $\pm$ 0.48) than in controls (1.07 $\pm$ 0.34, $p < 0.05$).
Inverse trends of a higher Bmax of ($^3$H)-yohimbine and lower Bmax of IHYP binding can be interpreted as an altered balance between alpha-2- and beta-2-receptors. This provides a possible explanation for the increased vasoconstriction and decreased heart rate response to adrenergic stimulation in CF. We did not find significant changes in density or affinity of alpha-2- and beta-2-receptors in CF compared to controls. The reason for this difference to other studies could be that our patients were in good condition and had not in relation to the study used drugs known to interfere with these receptors.

Further Investigation of Biological Membranes in
Children with Cystofibrosis.

B.Ja.Reznik. I.L.Babiy.
Odessa Pirogov Medical Institute,Odessa,USSR.

Observations of 32 patients with pulmonary and pulmono-
enteric forms of cystofibrosis have shown that due to
primary defect secondary lipodistrophia may take place.
Hipodistrophia is connected with changes in absorption,
transport and metabolism of lipids, phospholipids, in particular, and fatty acid spectrum, composing membrane
structures.
The studies of phospholipid spectrum of cellular membranes in patients with cystofibrosis using two-way chromatography method revealed considerable changes in composition of minor fractions, the increase of phosphatidili-
nozite to 1.06%,while in healthy children only traces of
this phospholipid-0.03% were revealed. And the second point to be mentioned is the increase of lipophospatidil-
choline up to 0.81%, which is the product of membrane
disintergation.
While investigating the fatty acid spectrum of erythrocyte membranes the increase of quantitative content of
saturated pulmitic and begenic fatty acids,in particular,
was established.
The general content of unsaturated fatty acids in patients with mucoviscidosis decreased. In unsaturated acid
spectrum the considerable decrease of oleic and linoleic
acids was observed.
Simultaneously a disorder of transmembraneous distribution of potassium ions was noted.
While determining $Na^+ K^+-ATF$ activity its evident increase in patients with cytofibrosis was revealed. It compo-
sed 1.67 micromoles of inorganic phosphorus per 1mg of
protein (in healthy child group, this index was equal to
1.04.).
Thus the determined by us changes of $Na^+K^+ATF$ are coor-
dinated with previously revealed changes of potassium
membrane porosity. Alteration of ATF enzyme activity
leads to disturbances of cell energetic and metabolic
breakages.
The determined changes in membrane structure and its
function is the foundation for conducting the basic therapy with purposeful influence on metabolic defects.

**POSTER GROUP NINE No. 9.08**

ESSENTIAL FATTY ACID SUPPLEMENTATION: ABSORPTION AND METABOLISM

M.C. Goodchild, S. Laing, J. Custance, M. Vaughan and J.A. Dodge,
Department of Child Health, Welsh National School of Medicine,
Cardiff, U.K.

Deficiency of 'essential' fatty acids (EFA) derived from dietary linoleic acid has been widely reported in CF. Biochemical evidence of EFA deficiency may exist at birth, and increased turnover of EFA in red blood cell (RBC) membranes has been reported. Prostaglandins (PG) are important EFA derivatives and EFA deficiency leads to reduced $PGE_2$ synthesis. This study examined the effect of dietary EFA supplements (oil of evening primrose 1g/kg/day to maximum 25g) on plasma and RBC membranes, and on PG metabolism in 20 patients aged 3-23 years. The study is still in progress and numerous biochemical parameters are being monitored. Significant observations at the start of treatment (a), after 6 weeks (b) and 6 months (c) include the following;
1. Before supplementation, linoleic acid (18:2) levels in whole plasma (19.96±3.97%, normal 26.86±5.18%) and RBC (10.02±1.41%, normal 13.10±1.23%) were low.
2. Linoleic acid levels in plasma and RBC rose at 6 weeks but reverted almost to pretreatment levels at 6 months (plasma b 25.64± 6.24, c 22.84±5.10, a:b p=0.0005, b:c p=0.10, a:c p=0.025).
3. Eicosatrienoic acid (20:3) increased significantly in both plasma (p=0.0005) and RBC (p=0.0005) at 6 weeks and remained elevated at 6 months (b:c not significant).
4. Arachidonic acid (20:4) levels in plasma and RBCs were in the normal range throughout.
5. Plasma PGFα levels increased at 6 weeks and fell at 6 months (a:b p=0.15, b:c p=0.025, a:c p=0.05).
    Sweat PGFα fell significantly by 6 months (a:c p=0.05).
    24 hour urine PGFα metabolites fell slightly but not significantly at 6 weeks and 6 months.
6. Plasma $PGE_2$ levels did not change significantly.
    Sweat $PGE_2$ levels fell by 6 weeks (p=0.0125) then stabilised.
    24 hour urine $PGE_2$ metabolites were unchanged at 6 weeks but increased significantly after 6 months (p=0.005).
7. There was a negative correlation between the levels of urinary metabolites of PGFα and $PGE_2$ (p=0.001).
8. Sweat electrolytes showed no significant change.

From these observations, we conclude that linoleic acid is absorbed from evening primrose oil, but that increased absorption is followed by increased metabolism. The rise in urinary $PGE_2$ metabolite excretion suggests that inhibition of $PGE_2$ synthesis and enhanced $PGF_2α$ synthesis caused by EFA deficiency is being corrected.

410

INTRINSIC ABNORMAL FATTY ACID TURNOVER IN THE RED CELL MEMBRANES OF CYSTIC FIBROSIS.

V. Rogiers[*], I. Dab[°], A. Vercruysse[*], R. Crokaert[¨] and H.L. Vis[°].
[*]Department of Pharmacognosy, Phytochemistry and Toxicology,
[°]Department of Pediatrics, [¨]Department of Biochemistry.
Free University Brussels, Laarbeeklaan, 103, 1090 Brussels, Belgium.

A study has been carried out in order to investigate whether the abnormal "in vitro" turnover of fatty acids of cystic fibrosis (CF) patients (1) is intrinsic to the membrane, whether it is induced by extrinsic serum factors. Red blood cells of CF patients and healthy subjects were labeled "in vitro" with [$^{14}$C]-linoleic acid, bound to albumin. The labeled cells were reincubated in autologous and homologous serum. The radioactivity present in the serum lipids and in the major phospholipid fractions of red cell membranes was measured. Conclusions of this study are :

- not all of the CF patients examined individually show an abnormal "in vitro" turnover of the red cell fatty acids, although they all presented abnormal fatty acid patterns for the red blood cell phospholipids, the platelet phospholipids and the plasma lipids.
- the "in vitro" abnormal fatty acid turnover occurs only in the incubations, where red cells of CF patients are involved and not where red cells of healthy subjects are incubated in serum of CF patients. Consequently, the abnormal turnover is intrinsic to the red cells and is not induced by extrinsic serum factors.

(1) V. Rogiers et al. Pediatr. Res. 16; 761-768 (1982).

**POSTER GROUP NINE No. 9.10**

CORRECTION OF ESSENTIAL FATTY ACID DEFICIENCY AND EFFECT ON PROSTAGLANDINS IN CYSTIC FIBROSIS. Elaine H. Mischler, Philip M. Farrell, Sara W. Parrell, William J. Raynor, Richard J. Lemen. Department of Pediatrics, Department of Statistics, University of Wisconsin, Madison, WI 53792 and Arizona Medical Center, Pediatric Pulmonary Division, Tucson, AZ 85716.

Controversy exists regarding the significance of linoleic acid(18:2) deficiency, an essential fatty acid abnormality described in cystic fibrosis (CF) patients. Although 18:2 deficiency is not the primary metabolic defect in CF, the deficiency could have several important secondary effects such as growth retardation, membrane dysfunction, and derangement of prostaglandin (PG) metabolism as 18:2 is a potential precursor for PG synthesis. We studied the feasibility and effectiveness of 18:2 supplementation in patients with CF as well as the influence of supplementation on clinical status and biochemical parameters.

Sixty-four patients with CF had plasma fatty acids analyzed by gas chromatography and 67% were found deficient in plasma linoleate. This abnormality was also uniformly present in tissues taken at autopsy from 7 CF adolescents. Fifteen patients aged 10 to 24 years agreed to take 7% of their total daily calories as Microlipid (safflower oil emulsion with 72% linoleate) along with pancreatic enzymes for one year. Thirteen completed the study, 2 patients dying at 7 and 9 months. Five patients aged 10 to 37 years served as controls. Plasma and red blood cell (RBC) fatty acid composition and prostaglandin metabolites were monitored. Sweat Na and Cl, arterial oxygen saturation, NIH scores, and growth were followed.

Results proved that biochemical correction of plasma and erythrocyte 18:2 levels can be achieved with oral supplementation. Plasma % 18:2 levels described as mean±S.D. increased from 22.8 ± 3.8 prior to supplementation to 28.7 ± 4.2 after supplementation (normal=26), at $p<0.0001$. Erythrocyte % 18:2 levels also increased significantly only in supplemented patients ($p<0.0005$). Prostaglandins were evaluated for time trends over 1 year using a pooled Kendall's tau statistic. Focusing on the last 6 months of the study, the controls show only a significant increase in 6-keto-$F_{1\alpha}$ and decrease in $PGF_{2\alpha}$ (which causes bronchial conconstricton) whereas all of the metabolites including $PGE_2$ (which causes bronchial relaxation) show a significant increase in the supplemented group except $PGF_{2\alpha}$ which showed a significant decrease at $p<0.02$. At autopsy, one of the study patients showed normal linoleate tissue levels whereas tissues from 7 non-supplemented CF patients were abnormal. Nine of 13 supplemented patients gained more weight while taking the supplement than in the previous year and 2 controls gained more weight during the study year. NIH clinical severity scores, sweat Na and Cl, and arterial oxygen saturation did not change significantly for either group. In conclusion, oral supplementation can effectively correct 18:2 deficiency in plasma, erythrocytes and other tissues of CF patients.

**POSTER GROUP NINE No. 9.11**

GLYCOPROTEINS AND GLYCOSAMINOGLYCANS OF THE CELL SURFACE OF CULTURED SKIN FIBROBLASTS FROM CONTROL AND CYSTIC FIBROSIS PATIENTS.

Brigitte HERMELIN, France BERTRAND and Jacques PICARD.

Faculté de Médecine Saint-Antoine, Laboratoire de Biochimie INSERM U. 181, 27 rue Chaligny, 75571 Paris Cédex 12, France.

The glycoproteins and glycosaminoglycans of the cell surface of cultured skin fibroblasts were studied after incubation in the presence of $\{^{14}C\}$-glucosamine or $\{^{35}S\}$-sodium sulphate. Pericellular macromolecules were obtained after trypsinization of the cultured cells and were fractionated by gel filtration, ion exchange chromatography and affinity chromatography on concanavalin A-Sepharose and characterized by enzymatic degradation (chondroitin AC and ABC lyase) and nitrous acid treatment. Three groups of glycoconjugates were obtained : glycosaminoglycans, O-glycosyl proteins and N-glycosyl proteins.

1. No difference in the $\{^{14}C\}$-glucosamine labelling of glycosaminoglycans and glycoproteins from control and cystic fibrosis cells was observed.

   a. The relative proportions of radioactivity in O-glycosyl proteins and N-glycosyl proteins were similar for control and cystic fibrosis cells.

   b. The profile on concanavalin A-Sepharose of the N-glycosyl proteins did not reveal changes in the relative proportions of N-glycosyl proteins of the oligomannosidic and N-acetyllactosaminidic types.

   c. The relative proportions of the different glycosaminoglycans (chondroitin sulphate, dermatan sulphate and heparan sulphate) and of the O-glycoproteins from control and cystic fibrosis cells was not modified.

2. After incubation with $\{^{35}S\}$-sodium sulphate, changes appeared in the relative proportions of the different glycosaminoglycans and in particular a decrease in the incorporation into heparan sulphate from cystic fibrosis cells.

3. The quantitative analysis of the O-glycosyl proteins from cystic fibrosis cells revealed a fucose content twice that of the control cells.

Thus the examination of pericellular glycoproteins and glycosaminoglycans of cells from cystic fibrosis patients revealed the presence of an O-glycosyl protein belonging to the mucin-type particularly rich in fucose. This anomaly may be the result of either a modification in the biosynthesis or a decrease in the catabolism of this glycoprotein in agreement with low levels of $\alpha$-fucosidase in cystic fibrosis cells. The abnormally high level of fucose observed in cystic fibrosis cells may be related to the modifications in the physico-chemical properties of bronchial mucins particularly rich in O-glycosyl proteins.

**POSTER GROUP NINE No. 9.12**

ACTIVITIES OF SOME GLYCOLYTIC ENZYMES IN CULTURED FIBROBLASTS FROM CF
HOMOZYGOTES, HETEROZYGOTES AND NORMAL CONTROLS
A. Bardoń[1,2], O. Ceder[1], H. Kollberg[1,3]

[1]Department of Pediatrics, University Hospital, S-901 85 Umeå, Sweden;
[2]Department of Biochemistry, Institute of Sport, Warsaw, Poland;
[3]Department of Pediatrics, University of Kuwait, Safat, Kuwait.

In previous work we have shown that CF homozygotes and heterozygotes
at rest have a higher concentration of lactate and pyruvate in their
saliva than healthy controls (Bardoń et al., Ceder et al.).
   The purpose of the present work was to investigate the regulatory
enzymes of the glycolytic pathway in cultured skin fibroblasts, a
frequently used system for basic research in cystic fibrosis.
   Hexokinase (HK), phosphofructokinase (PFK), pyruvate kinase (PK)
and lactate dehydrogenase (LDH) were estimated in homogenates of fibroblasts from the three genotypes. The mean levels of activity of all
four enzymes expressed per g of protein were found to be higher in
fibroblasts from CF homozygotes than in fibroblasts from matched controls. Fibroblasts from heterozygotes had intermediate activities.
   The above results, as well as those in earlier publications (Bardoń
et al., Ceder et al.), indicate that in CF the activity of the glycolytic pathway is increased. This increase leads to lactic acidosis of
the exocrine glands. The disturbance in glucose metabolism also can
be responsible for some of the clinical finding;  e.g. release of
enzymes and mucus and increased concentrations of electrolytes (Kollberg et al.).

Bardoń et al. Clin Chim Acta 1983; 113: 311-316.
Ceder et al. Acta Paediatr Scand 1983; Suppl 309: 25-39.
Kollberg et al. Acta Paediatr Scand 1983; Suppl 309: 41-47.

This study was financially supported by the Torsten and Ragnar Söder-
berg Foundation and the Swedish National Association of Heart and
Chest Diseases.

**POSTER GROUP NINE No. 9.13**

Regulation of hyaluronic acid synthesis by reversible phosphorylation of hyaluronate synthase in isolated plasma membranes from normal and CF skin fibroblasts

N. MIAN. Department of Physiology, St. George's Hospital Medical School, Cranmer Terrace, Tooting, London SW17 ORE.

Hyaluronic acid is synthesized by hyaluronate synthase complex which is tightly bound to plasma membranes in human skin fibroblasts. Recent experiments suggest that initiation and chain growth of hyaluronic acid, both $Mg^{2+}$ dependent reactions, are carried out by this enzyme without the involvement of a signal sequence or a primer. Autophosphorylation of tyrosyl residues in the inactive native enzyme by ATP in the presence of UDP-GlcNAc and UDP-GlcA is essential for the activation of the enzyme activity. These phosphotyrosyl residues act as 'anchors' during the formation of GlcNAc ($\beta 1 \rightarrow 4$) GlcA and GlcA ($\beta 1 \rightarrow 3$) GlcNAc linkages. The hyaluronic acid chain grows on its non-reducing end and the rate of chain growth is about 1 dissacharide per second. Removal of UDP-GlcNAc and UDP-GlcA even in the presence of ATP results in auto-dephosphorylation of phosphotyrosyl residues and causes enzyme inactivation. The activity of hyaluronate synthase phosphoprotein is further regulated by a soluble protein kinase – phosphatase enzyme system by reversible phosphorylation of serine residues in the hyaluronate synthase protein. Phosphorylation of serine residues by this soluble protein kinase in the presence of calmodulin and n mole concentrations of $Ca^{2+}$ considerably reduces hyaluronate synthase activity. On the other hand dephosphorylation of phosphorserine residues by this soluble phosphatase in the presence of $\mu$mole concentrations of $Ca^{2+}$ restores the hyaluronate synthase activity to its normal base line level. Plasma membranes prepared from CF skin fibroblasts (2 cell lines investigated in the present study) exhibit higher hyaluronate synthase activity compared with normal skin fibroblast membranes. The soluble protein kinase – phosphatase enzyme system from CF cells also shows quantitative differences in phosphorylation/dephosphory-lation activities compared with the enzyme system from normal fibroblasts.

**POSTER GROUP NINE No. 9.14**

ELECTROPHYSIOLOGICAL STUDIES ON ISOLATED HUMAN ECCRINE
SWEAT GLANDS*

By Christopher J. Jones, David Hyde, Catherine M. Lee[#]
and Terence Kealey[#]
Department of Zoology, University of Durham and [#]Depart-
ment of Clinical Biochemistry, University of Newcastle-
upon-Tyne, U.K.

As part of an investigation into human exocrine
mechanisms with special reference to cystic fibrosis,
eccrine sweat glands isolated from human abdominal and
thoracic skin were studied electrophysiologically, either
directly, or following maintenance for 24-48 hours in
supplemented RPMI-1640 tissue culture medium.  Glands were
superfused with bicarbonate/$CO_2$ buffered Krebs Ringer,
pH 7.4 and cells penetrated with bevelled glass microelectrodes of tip resistance 80-120 megohms.  An assessment of membrane potentials in secretory coil cells of
cultured glands gave a mean membrane potential of 50.26
mV ± 1.36 S.E.M. (n = 91).  Acetylcholine ($10^{-5}$-$10^{-6}$M)
produced hyperpolarizing responses in secretory coil cells
of both fresh and cultured glands and increased input
impedance, an unexpected finding.  These responses were
reversibly inhibited by atropine (1.4 x $10^{-5}$M) and either
completely or partially abolished by ouabain (5 x $10^{-4}$M).
Occasionally, acetylcholine would produce electrode
dislodgement, possibly by an action on contractile
elements.

Presently, the responses of cells to changes in
external $Na^+$, $K^+$ and $Cl^-$ are being studied and these
together with the superimposed effects of acetylcholine
will be discussed.

*Supported by the Cystic Fibrosis Research Trust (U.K.)

416

MONOLAYER CULTURE OF HUMAN SWEAT
GLAND EPITHELIAL CELLS.

Peter Steen Pedersen
Section of Clinical Genetics, dept. of Paediatrics ( G )
Rigshospitalet    Copenhagen    Denmark

Investigation of the abnormal electrolyte transport in the
reabsorbtive part of sweat glands from CF patients has
been accelerated after P.M.Quinton's discovery of abnormal
anion transport in CF. The need for a more stable material
is obvious and the new techniques in cell culture should be
used in attempts to produce a epithelium monolayer culture
from this organ suited for morphological, biochemical and
endochrinological study.
Our experiences in developing such a culture is presented.

**POSTER GROUP NINE No. 9.16**

INCREASED PLASMA LACTOFERRIN LEVELS IN CYSTIC FIBROSIS
PATIENTS.

C.Figarella*,J.P.Estèvenon*,J.R.Harlé*, and C.Galabert°,
*INSERM U31, 46 Bd. de la Gaye, 13009, Marseille, and
°Hopital R.Sabran, Giens.

A series of reports on the possible identification of
cystic fibrosis (CF) as beeing a lysosomal disorder has
appeared during the past years. Among others, an increase in the number and size of lysosomes, the presence of
metachromatic granules, and an increased content of total acid mucopolysaccharids in fibroblasts cell cultures
of CF patients have afforded indirect evidence of an impaired lysosomal activity. More recently, increased
"leakage" of lysosomal enzymes from CF fibroblasts into
the medium has been reported and an increase of total
activity of several hydrolases in serum from CF patients
compared to normal controls have been described. These
findings led us to study the behaviour of plasma lactoferrin in CF patients. Lactoferrin is not a lysosomal
enzyme, since it is an iron binding glycoprotein devoi-
ded of enzyme activity, but it is present in a large
amount in specific granules of polymorphic granulocytes
and collaborate with lysosomal hydrolases to phagocytosis.   Two series of experiments were performed: in the
first one, 73 plasma were studied (controls:28, obligate
heterozygotes:25, CF:20). Plasma were collected on crus-
hed ice and immediatly centrifugated. Lactoferrin was
assayed by a specific and sensitive immunoassay.
The results showed a statistically significant increase
($2p < 0.05$) between the level of plama lactoferrin in CF
patients ($255.20 \pm 39.06 \mu g/l$) compared to controls ($171.17
\pm 20 \mu g/l$) and heterozygotes ($151.70 \pm 16.03 \mu g/l$). Since it
is well established that plasma lactoferrin level was
not influenced by external gland production, but by neutrophils , a second set of experiments was performed on
17 CF patients with a concomitant numeration of leucocytes counts. 3 of these patients with a neutrophil level
over than 9 giga/l were discarded. The other 14 had a
level of neutrophils between 2 and 6 giga/l, and their
mean plasma lactoferrin level was $321.53 \pm 32.77 ug/l$, far
above the normal value. In conclusion, lactoferrin level
is significantly increased in plasma of CF patients compared to controls and obligate heterozygotes. The possibilities of an over-production and/or an impaired removal of neutrophilic lactoferrin are currently under investigation.

418

THE EFFECT OF ACETYLCHOLINE ON NON-ELECTROLYTE TRANSPORT ACROSS RABBIT MANDIBULAR GLAND EPITHELIUM

A.J. Potter, M.C. Steward and R.M. Case, Department of Physiology, University of Manchester, Manchester M13 9PT, UK.

The permeability properties of the epithelium comprising the rabbit mandibular salivary gland have been studied by observing the effect of acetylcholine on non-electrolyte transport in an isolated, perfused preparation of the gland.

A trace amount of a radio-labelled non-electrolyte was added to the perfusate and the concentration of the tracer in the saliva measured. From the ratio of the concentrations of tracer in the perfusate ($Cp$) and secretion ($Cs$) and the secretory rate ($Jv$) it is possible to determine the filtration coefficient ($1-\sigma$), where $\sigma$ is the reflection coefficient, using the following version of the Kedem/Katchalsky solute flux equation:

$$\frac{Cs}{Cp} = \frac{1-\sigma}{1-\sigma \exp\left[-\frac{(1-\sigma)Jv}{P}\right]}$$

The effect of acetylcholine on the filtration coefficient has been determined for three non-electrolytes (sucrose, erythritol and ethanediol) as indicated below:

| | Hydrated molecular radius ($\overset{o}{A}$) | Filtration coefficient ($1-\sigma$) at different acetylcholine concentration (M) | | |
|---|---|---|---|---|
| | | $8\times10^{-7}$ | $8\times10^{-6}$ | $8\times10^{-5}$ |
| $^{14}$C-sucrose | 5.05 | $0.0033\pm0.0013$ | $0.014\pm0.0045$ | $0.028\pm0.0067$ |
| $^{14}$C-erythritol | 3.21 | $0.036\pm0.010$ | $0.040\pm0.005$ | $0.113\pm0.011$ |
| $^{14}$C-ethanediol | 2.43 | $0.47\pm0.01$ | $0.63\pm0.02$ | $0.66\pm0.01$ |

The data represent the mean $\pm$ s.e.m. of 3 - 5 experiments.

The dependence of $1-\sigma$ on molecular size may indicate that the tracer crosses the epithelium via channels. The dependence of $1-\sigma$ on acetylcholine concentration further suggests that acetylcholine may have an effect on the size of these channels.

**POSTER GROUP NINE No. 9.18**

NASAL TRANSEPITHELIAL POTENTIAL DIFFERENCE AND CHLORIDE PERMEABILITY IN NORMAL, CYSTIC FIBROSIS, AND DISEASE CONTROL SUBJECTS. Michael R. Knowles, John T. Gatzy, and Richard C. Boucher, University of North Carolina School of Medicine, Chapel Hill, NC 27514

The transepithelial potential difference (PD) is raised across cystic fibrosis (CF) respiratory epithelia. This abnormality may reflect both an increased rate of active $Na^+$ absorption and a reduced $Cl^-$ permeability. To assess the specificity of the reduced $Cl^-$ permeability for CF, the nasal epithelial $Cl^-$ permeability of non-CF patients with chronic suppurative respiratory diseases (disease controls) was compared to CF and normal subjects. The figure below displays the basal PD (abscissa) and the voltage response to nasal superfusion with a $Cl^-$-free solution (ordinate; $\Delta$ PD = hyperpolarization) for these three groups of subjects.

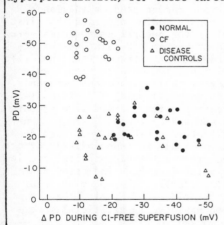

Δ PD DURING Cl-FREE SUPERFUSION (mV)

As previously reported, 1) the mean nasal PD for the CF patients ($48.6 \pm 1.3$ mV; n=24) is approximately twofold greater than that noted for normal ($23.7 \pm 1.0$ mV; n=22) or disease control ($19.4 \pm 1.4$; n=25) subjects and 2) the mean nasal $Cl^-$ permeability (as reflected by the voltage response to $Cl^-$ free solution superfusion) is lower for CF ($\Delta$PD = $12.0 \pm 1.4$ mV) as compared to normal ($\Delta$PD = $33.1 \pm 1.9$ mV) subjects and there is little overlap between these two groups. In contrast, the mean $Cl^-$ diffusion PD of the disease control subjects is intermediate ($\Delta$PD = $24.0 \pm 3.0$ mV) and overlaps with both CF and normal subjects. Because the voltage response to $Cl^-$ free superfusion can be increased by isoproterenol (Iso) superfusion onto normal ($\Delta$PD = $11.7 \pm 2.0$ mV; n =10) but not CF ($\Delta$PD = $-0.9 \pm 2.3$ mV; n=7) nasal epithelia, we tested the response to Iso superfusion in 5 disease control subjects whose $Cl^-$ diffusion PD before Iso ranged from 19-37 mV. The $Cl^-$ diffusion PD was increased by Iso in each disease control subject (mean $Cl^-$ diffusion PD = $27.2\pm3.8$ mV pre, $39.1\pm3.0$ mV post Iso). The mean Iso-induced augmentation of the $Cl^-$ diffusion PD in disease control subjects ($\Delta$PD = $11.9 \pm 1.1$ mV) was similar to that seen in normal subjects. We conclude that 1) reduced nasal epithelial $Cl^-$ permeability is not specific for CF, 2) the nasal PD is not raised in non-CF disease control subjects who have reduced $Cl^-$ permeability, and 3) $Cl^-$ permeability can be increased by Iso superfusion in normal and disease control but not in CF subjects.

**POSTER GROUP NINE No. 9.19**

METABOLITE TRANSPORT AT THE BLOOD-TISSUE INTERFACE OF EXOCRINE ORGANS
EVALUATED USING A RAPID PAIRED TRACER DILUTION TECHNIQUE

By D.L. Yudilevich, S.M. Wilson, P. Banks and G.E. Mann. Department of
Physiology, Queen Elizabeth College, Univ. London, London W8 7AH.

Until recently very little was known about the transport processes
mediating amino acid and sugar uptake at the blood-side (basolateral)
of exocrine epithelia.  The introduction of a rapid paired-tracer dilution technique (1) has enabled us to characterize the specificity
and kinetics of different membrane carriers in the cat submandibular
salivary gland.  The uptake (U) of a labelled substrate is determined
relative to an extracellular reference tracer such as D-mannitol:
U = 1 - test/D-mannitol.

Competitive inhibition assessed in non-secreting glands in vivo
suggested the presence of separate transport systems for short- and
long-chain neutral amino acids (2).  More recent studies in glands
perfused with a Krebs-Henseleit bicarbonate medium provided the first
kinetic evidence that these two carriers for neutral amino acids were
distinct : a high affinity, Na-dependent System ASC (alanine-serine-
cysteine) and a lower affinity, Na-independent System L (leucine) (3).
The metabolic inhibitor dinitrophenol inhibited unidirectional amino
acid uptake.  A detailed kinetic study of the interactions between
neutral and basic amino acids revealed no overlapping affinities (4).
Thus, the identified Na-independent cationic transport system appears
to be operating in parallel with the neutral Systems ASC and L.  Unlike other epithelia these transport systems exhibit a very high degree of specificity, and it should be possible to independently detect
changes in each of the systems.  Concurrent autoradiographical studies
of amino acid uptake by the salivary epithelium have indicated that
the acinar, striated ductal and demilunar cells take up amino acids
differentially (5).  In this context the effect of Cystic Fibrosis
serum on amino acid transport has been explored in artificially perfused glands and serine uptake was unaffected.

(1)*Yudilevich, D.L. & Mann, G.E. (1982). Fedn. Proc. 41, 3045-3053.
(2) Bustamante, J.C., Mann, G.E. & Yudilevich, D.L. (1981).
        J. Physiol. 313, 65-79.
(3)*Mann, G.E. & Yudilevich, D.L. (1984). J. Physiol. 347, 111-127.
(4)*Mann, G.E., Wilson, S.M. & Yudilevich, D.L. (1984).  J. Physiol.
        (paper in press).
(5)*Mann, G.E., Moller, M. & Poulsen, J.H. (1982). J. Physiol. 332,75P.

*These publications have been supported by a research grant from the
Cystic Fibrosis Research Trust, U.K.

**POSTER GROUP NINE No. 9.20**

INSULIN RECEPTOR BINDING IN ERYTHROCYTES (IB) IN PATIENTS WITH
CYSTIC FIBROSIS (CF)

O. Andersen, S. Garne, K. E. Petersen, W. Petersen & C. Heilmann

Diabetes Centre, dept. of Obstetrics and Gynaecology, Cystic
Fibrosis Centre, dept. of Paediatrics G, Rigshospitalet, University
of Copenhagen, DK-2100 Copenhagen Ø, and Steno Memorial Hospital,
Gentofte, Denmark.

The AIM of the study was to investigate whether IB differs in
patients with CF from that in controls.

MATERIALS AND METHODS: Nine patients with CF entered the study (six
males and three females before menarche). Age: 12 - 32 years. Bodyweight as percentage of mean for height (BW): 86.8 $\pm$ 10.5 (SD). All
had normal fasting blood glucose concentrations (BG) and were without glucosuria. Nine healthy normal subjects served as controls
( five males and four females before menarche). Age: 10 - 17 years.
BW: 88.6 $\pm$ 9.7 (SD). Oral glucose tolerance test (OGTT) was performed with 1.75 g/kg bodyweight to a maximum of 100 g. $IB$ was measured by conventional competition binding technique: $6 \times 10^8$ cells
were incubated in 250 µl samples for 3 1/2 hours at $15°C$. Mono-$^{125}I$-
(Tyr A14)-insulin (NOVO) was used as tracer at a concentration of 34
pmol/l, monocomponent insulin being added in increasing concentrations. Cells were separated from incubation-medium by centrifugation
through oil. IB was expressed as insulin bound to cells as fraction
of free insulin and was corrected for non-specific binding by sub-
traction of binding at a concentration of insulin at 11.7 µmol/l. BG
was measured by a glucose oxidase method. Plasma insulin will be
measured by radioimmunoassay.

RESULTS: All controls had normal glucose tolerances (GT). Four CF-
patients had pathological GT: Three had impaired GT (BG at two hours
> 6.7 mmol/l) and one was diabetic (BG at two hours > 10.0 mmol/l).
The integrated areas under the OGTT-curves were significantly greater
in CF-patients both with normal and with pathological GT compared to
controls ($\underline{p}$ < 0.05). IB was similar in CF-patients and controls and
no difference was found in IB between CF-patients with normal and in
CF-patients with pathological GT. The non-specific binding was also
similar.

CONCLUSION: IB is similar in CF-patients and in controls of comparable BW despite significant differences in GT.

422

VIP RECEPTORS ON LYMPHOCYTES

F.A. McEvoy, Liverpool Polytechnic
J.M. Walker

Vasoactive Intestinal Peptide (VIP) is present in the central and peripheral nervous system. VIP is reported to stimulate adenyl cyclase of intestinal, brain and lung tissues. We have shown that receptors for this substance are present in human circulating lymphocytes. Several papers published in 1983 have confirmed the existence of these receptors.

We have tested for the presence of VIP receptors in circulating lymphocytes from Cystic Fibrosis patients. Four adults and five age-matched controls were tested. All cells tested showed the presence of receptors for VIP.

The binding capacity of the CF samples was similar to that of the control cells, suggesting there was a similar number of receptors. The affinity constant of the CF cells was slightly higher than the control cells and further experiments are being carried out to determine the significance of this observation. The cells had an affinity for secretin which was three orders of magnitude less than the affinity for VIP.

A recent publication of Davis *et al* [J.C.I. 71 p.1787 1983] showed that lymphocyte receptors for beta-adrenergic agonists had less response in CF samples than control samples, as measured by the cAMP contents of the cells after stimulation with isoproterenol.

We are now measuring the cAMP response of CF and control lymphocytes to VIP and adrenergic agents.

**POSTER GROUP NINE No. 9.22**

GLUCOCORTICOID RECEPTORS IN CYSTIC FIBROSIS

M. Brönnegård*, B. Strandvik*, O. Broberger*, J. Carlstedt-Duke**.
*Dep. of Paeditrics and **Dep. of Medical Nutrition, Karolinska Institutet, Huddinge University Hospital, Stockholm, Sweden.

Patients with Cystic Fibrosis (CF) have a deficiency of essential fatty acids i.e. linoleic acid and arachidonic acid, in serum and in membranes of erytrocytes. Substitution with these essential fatty acids under a long period will improve but not normalize the concentrations in serum. In vitro, there are evidences that these essential fatty acids are consumed or metabolized to a higher extent than normal ( Rogiers 1981), suggesting that the turnover of arachidonic acid is increased. Arachidonic acid is released from cell-membranes by phospholipase $A_2$. Phospholipase $A_2$ shows an increased activity in patients with CF (Roscher 1981). Phospholipase $A_2$ can be inhibited by glucocorticoids if these steroid hormones are added to cell systems. A non-responsive cell would therefore show an increased phospholipase $A_2$ activity due to a defect in the biological action of glucocorticoids. Glucocorticoids bind to an intracellullar cytoplasmic receptor and after an activation step the receptor-steroid complex translocates to the nucleus, binds to DNA and initiates transcription. Hirata et al (1980) reported a phospholipase $A_2$ inhibitory protein induced by glucocorticoids and Geoffray et al (1980) proposed a similar theory calling this induced protein "macrocortin". A defect of the glucocorticoid receptor or a defect of the biological action of receptor-hormone complex could affect steroid binding, activation of the complex, DNA-binding of the complex or transcription of DNA. A defect in any of these steps concerning the biological action of glucocorticoids would lead to an increased activity of phospholipase $A_2$. We have studied 5 patients with CF concerning steroid-receptor affinity and number of binding sites per cell using lymphocytes from whole blood. Only one of the patients hitherto studied had normal receptor levels compared to the controls (1700 sites/cell). Control values according to our material are 1000-5500 sites/cell and this is in agreement with the litterature. Three patients had very high receptor levels 6800-48000 sites/cell and one patient only 270 sites/cell. The affinity constant was normal in all cases. It is interesting to note the variation in receptor levels. Breslow et al (1978) found no difference in receptor activity but he could not role out other receptor abnormalities responsible for steroid resistance. Further studies of glucocorticoid receptors in patients with CF will elucidate if the receptor is defect concerning size, DNA-binding or other biochemical parameters.

424

**POSTER GROUP NINE No. 9.23**

CHARACTERISTICS OF STIMULATION OF MUCIN SECRETION FROM RAT SUB-
MANDIBULAR ACINI BY AUTONOMIC NEUROTRANSMITTERS AND CF SERUM.
M.A. McPherson, Department of Medical Biochemistry, Welsh National
School of Medicine, Heath Park, Cardiff, U.K.

Autonomic neurotransmitters released from sympathetic nerves are
physiological stimulators of mucin secretion from mammalian submandibular acinar cells.   Abnormal factor(s) in the serum of CF patients
may also cause pathological stimulation of mucin secretion, since we
have shown (McPherson, Dodge and Goodchild, Clin. Chim. Acta 135, 181;
1983) that CF serum stimulates mucin secretion from rat submandibular
acini to a significantly greater degree than control serum.

My aim was to define the type of receptors controlling mucin
secretion under physiological conditions and to investigate the characteristics of the mucin-secreting activity of CF serum, which may
contribute to the pathophysiology of the disease.   Mucin release from
isolated acini or tissue fragments was measured by incorporation of
$^{14}$C-glucosamine into mucins and measuring release of $^{14}$C-labelled
mucins into the medium.   Secretory responses of isolated acini were
similar to those of intact tissue.   Isoproterenol, a β-adrenergic
agonist and noradrenaline, a mixed α- and β-agonist, stimulated mucin
release in a dose-dependent manner, 10 μM giving maximum effect.
Increased secretion in response to either neutrotransmitter was inhibited by the β-blocker propranolol, but not by the α-blocker, phentolamine, indicating that stimulation of β- but not α-adrenergic
receptors increases mucin secretion from rat submandibular acini.

The action of CF serum in stimulating mucin release was not
blocked by propranolol, but was destroyed by heating (60°C for 30 min)
or during storage for 16 - 18 weeks at -70°C, suggesting a labile
protein or peptide factor.   A possible candidate might be the mucociliary inhibiting peptide, purified from CF serum, which increases
mucus secretion from rabbit trachea (Blitzer & Shapira, Ped. Res. 16,
203; 1982).   However I have found no difference in activity of this
CF peptide and a corresponding peptide from control serum in stimulating mucin release from rat submandibular acini.   It is possible that
our assays may have different sensitivities or that activity of the
CF peptide was lost in transit.   However, the results suggest that
the mucin-secreting activity of CF serum which we have demonstrated
is unlikely to be due to the mucociliary inhibiting peptide.

In conclusion, I have defined the type of adrenergic receptor
controlling rat submandibular mucin secretion and have further characterized the properties of the mucin-secreting activity of CF serum.

I am very grateful to Dr. J.A. Dodge and Dr. M.C. Goodchild for
providing serum samples and to Dr. M. Blitzer and Dr. E. Shapira for
supplying purified control and CF (mucociliary inhibiting) peptides,
isolated from serum.   I thank the CF Trust for financial support.

**POSTER GROUP NINE No. 9.24**

FIBRONECTIN AND CYSTIC FIBROSIS

M. FILLIAT - C. GALABERT - J. P. CHAZALETTE - C. HEINEMANN
Hopital Renée SABRAN - Giens - 83400 HYERES - FRANCE

Introduction

The fibronectins are high molecular weight adhesive glycoproteins present on the cell surface and circulating in the blood.
Several authors have described a significant decrease of this blood protein in adult respiratory distress syndrome and in acute pneumonia as well as in acute circulatory failure.
This profile in cystic fibrosis was studied.

Material and Methods

21 cystic fibrosis from 4 to 18 year olds were studied during hospitalisation.
Plasma fibronectin was evaluated by the Mancini Method

Results

$1^o$ ) The pulmonary condition of the patients was compared with their blood fibronectin values :
- good............................ 302 mg$^o$/oo ;
- quite good....................... 222 mg$^o$/oo ;
- fair............................ 167 mg$^o$/oo ;
- poor............................ 137 mg$^o$/oo.
$2^o$ ) The blood fibronectin rate of 9 patients was evaluated during a therapeutical period with more or less clinical improvement :
- 6 children showed a fibronectin increase (from 150 to 250 mg$^o$/oo) with a significant improvement ;
- 3 children had a stable fibronectin rate (150 - 170 mg$^o$/oo) with no amelioration.

Comments

This work has no statistical value and, no definitive conclusion can be reached. However, even though the exact meaning of these results is not known, the plasma fibronectin concentration is a good parameter to appreciate the pulmonary condition and prognostic value in cystic fibrosis.

**POSTER GROUP NINE No. 9.25**

ALTERATION OF DOPA, DOPAMINE AND 5-HYDROXYINDOLEACETIC ACID IN
PLASMA AND URINE OF PATIENTS WITH CYSTIC FIBROSIS.

M.H. Schoeni*, K. Türler*, H. Käser* and R. Kraemer**.

*Institute for Clinical & Experimental Cancer Research and ** Dept.
of Paediatrics, University of Berne, Switzerland.

In 43 patients ( age 8-23 years, 26 boys and 17 girls ) with cystic
fibrosis (CF), attending a summer holiday camp, as well as in 25
parents ( heterozygotes, HZ ), plasma and urinary DOPA, catecholamines, their main catabolites and the metabolic breakdown product
of serotonin, 5-hydroxyindoleacetic acid ( 5-HIAA ), were measured.
   The 24 hour excretion of the free urinary amines epinephrine (E),
norepinephrine (NE), dopamine (DA), of their O-methylated products
metanephrine (MN), normetanephrine (NM), 3-methoxytyramine (MT) and
the phenolic acids vanilmandelic acid (VMA) and homovanillic acid
(HVA) was normal compared to age matched controls (C). For CF
patients a significantly elevated DOPA concentration ( $0.076 \pm$
$0.025$ nmol/umol creatinine vs $0.021 \pm 0.014$ for C ) in the 24 hour
urine was found. Furthermore, an age dependent increase of 5-HIAA
excretion, correlated to lung involvement, was present in CF.
   Normal concentrations of phenylalanine, tyrosine, E and a normal
enzymatic activity of dopamine-beta-hydroxylase (DBH) were observed
in CF plasma. Plasma DOPA and NE were slightly elevated whereas
3-O-methyl-DOPA, as well as DA, were significantly increased ( 3-O-
methyl DOPA: $130.2 \pm 45.4$ nmol/L for CF vs $62.5 \pm 11.3$ for C;
DA: $2.4 \pm 0.6$ nmol/L for CF vs $0.42 \pm 0.34$ for C ). The percentage
of sulfated E, NE, DA in plasma and of DA in urine of CF patients
was normal. The increased levels of catecholamines did not correlate
to the disease state, to electrolytes in plasma and sweat, to drug
intake, to blood pressure and to pulse rate.
   No abnormalities at all were observed in plasma of HZ.
Therefore, it is concluded, that an autonomic dysfunction is present
in CF, which is due to a disturbed metabolism of DOPA. The stereo-
chemical and electrochemical properties of this amino acid might
affect the physico-chemical behaviour of glycoproteins and peptides,
when erroneously integrated into these substances. A single gene
defect could selectively affect the integration of DOPA into proteins
and might therefore be responsible for the basic defect of cystic
fibrosis.

The determinations of 3-O-methyl-DOPA and of sulfated catecholamines
were kindly performed by M. Da Prada and G. Zürcher ( Research Dept.
Hoffmann-LaRoche, Basle,Switzerland).

**POSTER GROUP NINE No. 9.26**

ALTERATION OF FMLP-INDUCED DEGRANULATION AND CHEMILUMINESCENCE IN CYSTIC FIBROSIS POLYMORPHONUCLEAR LEUCOCYTES.

T.Kemp, A. Schram-Doumont, R. Kram[†], R. Van Geffel[x] & C. Szpirer, Laboratoire de Biologie du Développement, Université libre de Bruxelles, Rue des Chevaux, 67,1640 Rhode-St-Genèse & [x] Service de Pédiatrie, Hôpital de Braine-l'Alleud (Belgium).

Polymorphonuclear neutrophils (PMN) are easily accessible cells which, under adequate circumstances, can behave as secretory cells. These features make them particularly attractive for the study of cystic fibrosis, a disease characterized by a generalized exocrinopathy. Exocytosis from PMN is induced by a great variety of stimuli (both soluble and particulate). We have used three of them to investigate the possible alterations of lysosomal enzymes secretion from cystic fibrosis neutrophils: the synthetic chemotactic peptide N-formyl-methionyl-leucyl-phenylalanine (FMLP), opsonized zymosan and the calcium ionophore A23187. When purified neutrophils from normal and cystic fibrosis children were compared using FMLP as a stimulus, cells from the affected children exhibited a reproducible and significantly impaired response. On the contrary, when stimulated by A23187 or opsonized zymosan, CF neutrophils did not differ from normal cells. Another aspect of neutrophil response to stimulation has been studied,namely chemiluminescence, dependent on the stimulation of the membrane enzyme NADPH-oxidase. Chemiluminescence of FMLP-stimulated neutrophils, monitored without ("native chemiluminescence") or with amplifiers like luminol and lucigenin, confirmed the results obtained for exocytosis, although amplifiers gave sometimes equivocal data. In order to localize the source of this alteration in neutrophil response, we have characterized FMLP receptors from normal and CF neutrophils. The number of receptors was greater in CF neutrophils but the dissociation constant $K_D$ was identical in the two populations. Thus, the origin of the observed deficiency of CF cells has to be searched in the stimulus-secretion coupling sequence following the formation of the receptor-ligand complexes, and probably in the plasma membrane itself since both exocytosis and chemiluminescence are membrane-dependent phenomena.

[†] Deceased.

428

FRACTIONATION AND PARTIAL CHARACTERIZATION OF CF SERUM
ULTRAFILTRATES. Bruce I.Bogart, Thomas Taylor, Puerza F. Gaerlan*
and Carolyn R. Denning*. Departments of Cell Biology and
Pediatrics, New York University Medical Center and St. Vincent's
Hospital and Medical Center, New York, NY 10016.

Low molecular weight serum ultrafiltrates from Cystic
Fibrosis patients possess several biological activities. Using
liquid chromatography and isoelectric focusing techniques, several
investigators have identified CF serum factor(s) as low molecular
weight substances. This report briefly describes our experiences
with fractionation of CF and control serum ultrafiltrates utilizing
high performance liquid chromatography (HPLC) and subsequent partial
characterization of subfractions that correspond to OD peaks.

Serum samples were obtained after informed consent and were
subjected to ultrafiltration using Amicon PM10 membranes.
Fractionation by HPLC of the control serum ultrafiltrates produced a
characteristic profile of 7-8 OD peaks with specific retention times
and magnitudes in OD units. The characteristic control profile was
readily reproducible in the 10 control serum samples tested to
date. Fractionation of the ultrafiltrates from CF patients produced
profiles with many similarities to the control population. However,
fractionation of CF ultrafiltrates did produce a consistent increase
in magnitude (OD units) of the peak with a retention time of 10-12
minutes and a distinctive new peak with a retention time of 18.5-21
minutes. This latter new OD peak was also observed upon
fractionation of serum from heterozygotes, but in diminished amounts
(OD units). Subfractions collected by HPLC of CF ultrafiltrates
corresponding to OD peaks with retention times of 10-12 and 18.5-21
minutes produced $K^+$ efflux above basal levels from rat
submandibular gland fragments.

Constituents of the complement cascade have been implicated
in the ciliary dyskinesia response to CF serum. Radioimmune assay
(RIA) demonstrated the presence of significant levels of C3a des
Arg. and C4a des Arg. in CF ultrafiltrates even though these serum
samples were not collected in a manner to maximize the presence of
these proteins. RIA of collected subfractions corresponding to OD
peaks from concentrated ultrafiltrates indicated the presence of C3a
des Arg. and C4a des Arg. in subfractions with retention times of
10-14 minutes. OD peaks with retention times of 10-14 minutes are
reduced upon incubation with Concanavalin A and subsequent removal
of the lectin-ligand complexes. However, the OD peak with a
retention time of 18.5-21 minutes is not reduced in magnitude (OD
units) after Concanavalin A treatment. C3a has previously been
identified as one of the components in CF and asthmatic serum that
produced ciliary dyskinesia, while C4a has many of the physical
properties of the CF protein described by Wilson and co-workers.

**POSTER GROUP NINE No. 9.28**

GLYCATED HEMOGLOBIN IN CF PATIENTS WITH AND WITHOUT
SYMPTOMATIC HYPERGLYCEMIA AND THE TREATMENT WITH
SULPHONYLUREA.

H.K.HARMS, R.M.BERTELE, J.ROSENEGGER, W.ENDRES, Y.SHIN
Universitätskinderklinik München

Out of 196 CF patients 10 ( 5.1 % ) developed symptomatic
hyperglycemia ( SHG ) at 10-17 years of age (mean 14.3
years). In 8 of these 10 patients we determined the
glycated hemoglobin by the chemical method ( 1 ) at time
of SHG diagnosis and before starting any treatment. Hb $A_1$
was significantly elevated in all patients ( 4.85-6.03
nmol HMF/mg Hb vs. normal range of 2.0-3.3 ).

We have further analysed Hb $A_1$ in 49 CF patients older
than 10 years of age but without SHG. In 11 patients
(22.4 %) Hb $A_1$ was above the normal range and beyond the
values of the group with SHG, reaching 3.74 nmol HMF/mg Hb.
One patient with a Hb $A_1$ level of 3.6 has developed SHG
three months after the measurement. Since Hb $A_1$ reflects
the glycemic state of 1-3 months, it seems to be a better
index for an imminent SHG than oral or i. v. glucose
tolerance tests.

In contrast to the  widespread opinion of ineffectiveness
of sulfonylurea ( SU ) in the treatment of SHG in CF
(2,3), we found SU to be the treatment of first choice,
even in the younger patients ( 4 ). In 7 patients treated
exclusively with 2.5-7.5 mg glibenclamid ( Euglucon[R] ) in
addition to dietary restricitons, the mean urinary
glucose excretion fell to 1 g/day from 93.5 g/day within
6 weeks. All patients remained well controlled during
the following two years.

We now consider the early use of SU in CF patients without
SHG but elevated Hb $A_1$.

1) Shin Y.et al.Clin.Biochem. in press 1984
2) Barbero G.J. et al in: Cystic Fibrosis, Projections
   into the Future, Stratton Intercontinental Medical
   Book Corporation 1976
3) Doershuk C.F. and T.F.Boat in Nelson: Textbook of
   Pediatrics 1983
4) Stead, R.J. et al. abstr. 12th annual meeting of
   EWGCF  Athen 1983

## POSTER GROUP NINE No. 9.29

RENAL ELIMINATION OF CEPHALOSPORIN ANTIBIOTICS IN PATIENTS WITH CYSTIC FIBROSIS AND NORMAL SUBJECTS AS MARKERS FOR POSSIBLE DIFFERENCES IN TUBULAR TRANSPORT

G. Alván, A. Arvidsson, A. Hedman, Y. Adan-Abdi and B. Strandvik Departments of Clinical Pharmacology and Pediatrics, Karolinska Institutet, Huddinge University Hospital, S-141 86 Huddinge, Sweden.

In a comparison of the renal excretion of cefsulodin in patients with cystic fibrosis (CF) and a control group, we found that differences in renal handling of the drug occurred (Acta Paed 1983; 72: 293).

Cefsulodin is normally excreted by net secretion adding to glomerular filtration, which can be seen in the table by a cefsulodin/inulin renal clearance ratio larger than one. The CF-patients, however, received a ratio equal to unity. The interpretation of this finding is that either a reduced secretion or an increased tubular reabsorption is present in CF. To further elucidate this differential renal elimination pattern, we studied the excretion of ceftazidime, which in healthy subjects is considered only to be filtered. Ceftazidime was given in exactly the same way as was cefsulodin, i.e. an intravenous single dose of 2g to healthy controls and 50 mg/kg to CF-patients, followed by constant infusion of inulin. Blood samples were frequently drawn and urine collected hourly during six hours. The results this far are shown below

|  | Subjects with CF | Normal subject |
|---|---|---|
| Cefsulodin | n = 7 | n = 5 |
| Plasma clearance ml/minx1.73m$^2$ | 178+81 S.D. | 189+43 |
| Renal clearance ($Cl_{cefs}$)  " | 140+34 · | 141+36 |
| (T 1/2)  (h)  " | 1.33+0.22 | 1.50+0.31 |
| Inulinclearance ($Cl_{inul}$)  " | 142+38 (n=5) | 102+15 |
| Clcefs/Clinul | 1.01+0.14 | 1.37+0.21 |
| Ceftazidime | n = 3 | n = 6 |
| Plasma clearance  " | 125+2 | 112+22 |
| Renal clearance ($Cl_{ceft}$)  " | 111+11 | 101+9 |
| (T 1/2)  (h)  " | 1.54+0.13 | 1.73+0.16 |
| Inulinclearance ($Cl_{inul}$)  " | 122+10 | 104+13 |
| Clceft/Clinul | 0.92+0.16 | 0.98+0.10 |

These preliminary data reveal that, in contrast to the cefsulodin finding, no difference is to be seen in renal excretion of ceftazidime between the groups. This supports the assumption that the changed renal handling of cefsulodin in CF-subjects is due to a deficient tubular transport.

**POSTER GROUP NINE No. 9.30**

ARACHIDONIC ACID METABOLISM IN HUMAN SKIN FIBROBLAST CULTURES OF
PATIENTS WITH CYSTIC FIBROSIS AND OF CONTROLS.

R.Moser,H.J.Leis,E.Zenzmaier,A.Roscher,B.Hadorn and H.Gleispach
University of Graz,Department of Pediatrics,Graz,Austria.

Alterations in the metabolism of arachidonic acid (AA) and of prostaglandins (PG) have been postulated to be involved in the pathogenesis
of cystic fibrosis (CF).Since enzymes responsible for AA metabolism
are present in human skin fibroblasts (HSF) it seems likely that a genetic disturbance in AA metabolism would be expressed in HSF cultures.
The present study was carried out with HSF derived from 5 CF patients
and 5 healthy,age matched donors.Confluenced monolayers ($75 cm^2$ flasks),
matched for passage number and protein content,were investigated for
basal,as well as for bradykinin and ionophore A 23187 stimulated AA
metabolism.The growth medium was decanted,the cultures were washed
and equilibrated for 3o min.in serum free Dulbecco's minimal essential medium containing o.o2% albumin(fatty acid free).This medium was
replaced by a fresh 1o ml portion and the incubations were carried
out in duplicate,for 15 min.at $37^\circ C$ in the presence or absence of the
stimulators.The medium was then decanted and extracted with ether,the
extracts were preseparated by thin-layer-chromatography into fractions
containing PG-E1 and PG-E2,PG-F2$\alpha$ and 6-oxo-PG-F1$\alpha$,and unsaturated
fatty acids (HETEs and HHT).The different fractions were scraped off,
eluted and derivatised for gaschromatography-mass spectrometry.In unstimulated HSF a higher mean level of PG-E1 and PG-E2 was detected in
the CF group than in the controls.Under stimulation mainly PG-E2 was
formed in both groups.Under basal conditions the mean PG-E2 production
was 6.4 ng/mg protein in CF cultures and 2.5 ng/mg protein in contols.
Bradykinin stimulated PG-E2 formation to 75o ng/mg protein in CF and
to 54o ng/mg protein in controls.Ionophore stimulation resulted in
61o ng PG-E2/mg protein in CF and in 45o ng PG-E2/mg protein in the
control cultures.

INTERNATIONAL CYSTIC FIBROSIS (MUCOVISCIDOSIS) ASSOCIATION

The initiative for the formation of the International Cystic Fibrosis (Mucoviscidosis) Association was taken by the US and Canadian CF Foundations. Invitations were issued to individuals in various countries known to be interested, and a steering meeting was held at the Grand Hotel, Paris, in July 1964, chaired by Mr. George Barrie of the US Foundation.

It was agreed that the purposes of the Association would best be served by a corporate membership, consisting exclusively of one national association for each country. As one of the purposes was to foster the development of such associations in countries where they did not yet exist, provision was also made for the election of individuals, as associate members, who would provisionally represent their countries until such time as a national association had been formed, and had been accepted by the ICF(M)A as properly constituted to represent the country concerned.

Further discussions took place in the course of a CF Research Conference arranged by the United States Foundation, in Bethesda, Maryland, in September 1964; and the first formal meeting of the ICF(M)A, registered as a charity in the State of Delaware, USA, was held in Paris in March 1965. Mr. George Barrie was elected president, and representatives from 14 countries attended. It was also a scientific meeting on a small scale, and a number of papers were presented and discussed.

A Scientific/Medical Advisory Council was constituted. This full council, consisting of one nominated member from each national association, meets at 4 year intervals at major international conferences, and elects an Executive to carry out its functions between such conferences. This Executive consists of a chairman, vice-chairman, secretary and nine other members. Members normally serve about two terms. The president of the ICF(M)A, and the presidents of the CF Club of America, and the European Working Group for Cystic Fibrosis, are ex officio members. Past chairmen enjoy permanent non-voting membership.

International Conferences are held under the auspices of the ICF(M)A at about 4-yearly intervals, and are hosted by the national association of the country in which the conference is being held.

There was some initial confusion about the numbering of these conferences. Numbers 1 - 3 seem to have included the Paris steering meeting in 1964, the Bethesda Conference of 1964 (which was arranged by the American CF Foundation), and the first formal meeting of the ICF(M)A in Paris in 1965. Thus the first major international conference arranged by the ICF(M)A itself was number 4, after which the record is clear.

        Fourth   -  Berne, Grindelwald,
                    Switzerland 1966
        Fifth    -  Churchill College,
                    Cambridge, England 1969
        Sixth    -  Washington, USA 1973
        Seventh  -  Paris, France 1976
        Eighth   -  Toronto, Canada 1980
        Ninth    -  Brighton, England 1984

Annual business meetings of the ICF(M)A have been held each year, in parallel either with an international conference, or with a scientific meeting of the European Working Group for Cystic Fibrosis - a body which was formed at Cambridge in 1969 to provide for Europeans an annual continuity similar to that provided for North Americans by the meetings of the CF Club of America.

The combination of ICF(M)A lay meetings were scientific/medical conferences, has provided a valuable and very pleasant international forum in which personal, organisational, social, and technical problems of cystic fibrosis can be discussed.

The United States have from the very beginning provided much of the impetus for the creation and development of the Association, which has benefitted enormously from the expertise acquired by some of their officers and advisers in prior service with the long-established US CF Foundation.

Our current president, Mr. Bob McCreery, has over the past eight years proved a highly efficient and extremely stimulating president and chief executive. He has been tireless in his efforts to maintain and increase the momentum and effectiveness of the Association's work.

It is difficult to define exactly the achievements of a loose federation of people from all over the world, all dedicated in their varying ways, and in their widely differing communities, to the pursuit of the goals of the Association.

Perhaps the most tangible result has been the formation of new national associations, reflected by the list of accession dates of associations given earlier.

Through the ICF(M)A the experience of well-established associations
has been offered to newer members, but the ICF(M)A has always borne
firmly in mind that different countries vary widely in a number of
respects and that the problems of developing associations can only
be resolved in the context of their own cultures. Some of the more
important differences are in the following fields:

1.  Traditions relating to the development of and participation
    in voluntary charitable work, including the collection and
    management of funds.

2.  The extent to which medical and social services and research
    facilities are state-provided or state-aided.

3.  The attitude of governments and communities to independent
    charitable activities.

4.  Variations in national wealth and economic priorities in the
    fields of health and sickness.

5.  National cultural patterns in the techniques of fund-raising,
    and their relationship to national taxation policies.

While each country needs therefore to develop its own appropriate
structure, and its own descriptive and advisory literature, there
is much to be gained by national associations from the experience
of other members.

The United States in particular has throughout been extremely
generous in making their well-developed resources of literature
available to other members.

In particular, the US Quarterly Annotated reference system was so
well-developed by the time the ICF(M)A was formed, that there has
been no need for the ICF(M)A to consider any further action in
this field other than gratefully to accept the American output.

It is a matter of regret that the annotated references have now
ceased publication.

World-wide distribution of literature both to national associations
and to a rapidly increasing number of individuals with changing
addresses soon became an unmanageable problem; and the ICF(M)A
have established a firm modus operandi which is as follows:

> The ICF(M)A and any association which makes its own
> literature available to other associations will send
> one or two copies only, to national associations only.
> National associations are solely and fully responsible
> both for duplication, and for appropriate circulation
> within their own countries.

This arrangement is fully in line with the agreed structure of the ICF(M)A as having a corporate membership only. It is also felt that these arrangements will assist in building up close relationships between national associations and interested people in their own countries.

The ICF(M)A is affiliated to the World Health Organisation and to the International Paediatric Association.

As a result of a personal initiative by the President, Mr. Robert McCreery, who had for several years been conscious of the need to broaden the knowledge of CF throughout the world, contacts were established with the World Health Organization. Dr. A. Kuliev from the Division of Non-Communicable Diseases, WHO, Geneva, attended the ICF(M)A Meeting in Brussels in 1982, and from discussions held there the proposal emerged to hold a joint workshop of the two organizations. This workshop took place in Vienna in October 1983. The Working Party identified major objectives requiring multi-national support and co-operation as follows:

1.  To increase the awareness of Cystic Fibrosis among the general population and health professionals worldwide.

2.  To define standards for screening and diagnosis.

3.  To provide guidelines for health care in developed and developing countries relevant to cystic fibrosis and other similar chronic disorders, and

4.  To identify key research areas, including fundamental research in molecular genetics and pathophysiology as well as treatment.

Participants at the Workshop were: E. Abdel-Salam, T. Boat, C. Coutelle, J. Dodge, E. Ginter, A. Kuliev   J. Mangos, P. Roussel, J. Sturgess, M. Wagner, R. Williamson

The Working Party produced a detailed report which was submitted to WHO for final approval and distribution.

PURPOSES OF ICF(M)A

At their 1979 meeting in Holland, the ICF(M)A redefined their goals as follows:

"The International Cystic Fibrosis (Mucoviscidosis) Association, is a non-profit making organisation, whose membership consists of affiliated national associations devoted to the problems of the disease of cystic fibrosis (mucoviscidosis).

"Its purposes, in common with those of its affiliated national associations, are as follows:

A.    The furtherance of the interests of children and adults who have cystic fibrosis: and the improvement of the medical care available to them, and of the psychological and social care available to them and their families.

B.    The stimulation, support and advancement of research into the nature, cause, prevention, treatment, alleviation and cure of cystic fibrosis.

C.    The co-ordination of information services and the interchange of information on all phases of cystic fibrosis.

D.    To assist in the formation of national associations devoted to cystic fibrosis, where they are required, but do not yet exist.

E.    The holding of, arrangements for, and promotion of meetings of representatives of government agencies, organisations, and individuals interested in the prevention, treatment and cure of cystic fibrosis."

## Past Presidents of ICF(M)A

George Barrie (USA)        1965-70
Lyle Blackwell (Canada)    1970-76

## Past Chairmen of Executive of Scientific/Medical Advisory Council

Elected 1965    Dr. Paul di Sant Agnese (USA)
        1969    Professor Ettore Rossi (Switzerland)
        1973    Dr. Harry Shwachmann (USA)
        1976    Dr. David Lawson  (UK)

For current chairmen and members see page (iii).

Author   Index

438

Author Index

Author Index

Author Index

Author Index

Author Index

Author Index

# Author Index

Author Index

# Author Index